Translationality

This book defines "translationality" by weaving a number of sub- and interdisciplinary interests through the medical humanities: medicine in literature, the translational history of medical literature, a medical (neuroscience) approach to literary translation and translational hermeneutics, and a humanities (phenomenological/performative) approach to translational medicine. It consists of three long essays: the first on the traditional medicine-in-literature side of the medical humanities, with a close look at a recent novel built around the Capgras delusion and other neurological misidentification disorders; the second beginning with the traditional history-of-medicine side of the medical humanities, but segueing into literary history, translation history, and translation theory; the third on the social neuroscience of translational hermeneutics. The conclusion links the discussion up with a humanistic (performative/phenomenological) take on translational medicine.

Douglas Robinson is Chair Professor of English at Hong Kong Baptist University, and most recently authored *Critical Translation Studies* (Routledge).

Routledge Advances in Translation and Interpreting Studies

For a full list of titles in this series, please visit www.routledge.com

17 **Consecutive Notetaking and Interpreter Training**
Edited by Yasumasa Someya

18 **Queer in Translation**
Edited by B.J. Epstein and Robert Gillett

19 **Critical Translation Studies**
Douglas Robinson

20 **Feminist Translation Studies**
Local and Transnational Perspectives
Edited by Olga Castro and Emek Ergun

21 **Studying Scientific Metaphor in Translation**
An Inquiry into Cross-Lingual Translation Practices
Mark Shuttleworth

22 **Translating Frantz Fanon Across Continents and Languages**
Edited by Kathryn Batchelor and Sue-Ann Harding

23 **Translation and Public Policy**
Interdisciplinary Perspectives and Case Studies
Edited by Gabriel González Núñez and Reine Meylaerts

24 **Translationality**
Essays in the Translational-Medical Humanities
Douglas Robinson

25 **The Changing Role of the Interpreter**
Contextualising Norms, Ethics and Quality Standards
Edited by Marta Biagini, Michael S. Boyd and Claudia Monacelli

Translationality

Essays in the Translational-Medical Humanities

Douglas Robinson

Routledge
Taylor & Francis Group
LONDON AND NEW YORK

First published 2017 by Routledge

2 Park Square, Milton Park, Abingdon, Oxfordshire OX14 4RN
52 Vanderbilt Avenue, New York, NY 10017

Routledge is an imprint of the Taylor & Francis Group, an informa business

First issued in paperback 2019

British Library Cataloguing-in-Publication Data
A catalogue record for this book is available from the British Library

Library of Congress Cataloging-in-Publication Data
A catalog record for this book has been requested

ISBN: 978-1-138-72704-5 (hbk)
ISBN: 978-1-315-19103-4 (ebk)

Typeset in Galliard
by Apex CoVantage, LLC

Contents

Figures and Table

Figures

Table

Preface

My title, I suspect, is a bit difficult to parse. What is "translationality"? What are the "translational-medical humanities"?

Let us unpack all that slowly.

0.1 Translationality

Things/events change; things/events keep emerging; things/events remain in process. As we respond to change, we keep "translating" the old regimes into new patterns. For translation scholars "translation" is a transfer of textual features from one language to another; but in the world at large the term is used for a wide variety of transformations. Translation can mean the conversion of a thing from one form to another (transformation), or various kinds of transfer or conveyance from place to place: of a human body to heaven without dying (Elijah was "translated" to heaven in a chariot of fire), of a bishop from one diocese to another, of a holy relic from one shrine to another, or of a disease from one part of a body to another. The medieval historiographical theory of the *translatio imperii,* derived from the biblical Book of Daniel (the four-kingdom scheme in Dan. 2 and 7), posited the "translation of empire" from Greece to Rome to whatever local kingdom was doing the imagining. Closely connected with that theory was the metaphor of the *translatio studii,* the "translation of learning" from Eden to Jerusalem to Babylon to Athens to Rome to Paris, and perhaps from there on to London, and perhaps even – according to George Herbert (1593–1633) – on to America.

We translate thoughts or ideas or principles into action – and that is considered a necessary and beneficial transformation. Woody Allen used subtitles in *Annie Hall* to translate what the leading couple actually said into what they actually meant; and at the 2015 White House Correspondents' Dinner President Obama brought in "Luther, Anger Translator" to provide a similar kind of translation from what he says in politically constructive/conciliatory terms to the deeper frustrations he actually feels (www.youtube.com/watch?v=G6NfRMv-4OY).

The terminological shift made by the French sociologists Michel Callon and Bruno Latour (1981/2006, 12–13) in their "sociology of translation" *(sosiologie du traduction)* is arguably the inverse of Obama's:

> By "translation" we mean the set of negotiations, intrigues, acts of persuasion, calculations, acts of violence by which an actor or a force accords or allows itself

> to be accorded the authority to speak or to act in the name of another actor or force: "your interests are our interests," "do what I want," "you cannot succeed without me." As soon as an actor says "we," he or she translates other actors into a single aspiration of which she or he becomes the master or spokesperson.
> (quoted in Pym 2010, 155)

Gayatri Spivak (2007, 261) uses the word "translation" to characterize the infant's transition into social interaction and socialized subjectivity by grabbing things: "This grabbing *(begreifen)* of an outside indistinguishable from an inside constitutes an inside, going back and forth and coding everything into a sign system by the thing(s) grasped. One can call this crude coding a 'translation.'"

More directly relevant to this book, around the turn of the millennium medical professionals too began to speak of translationality, first in the term translational medicine, later as translational psychiatry and other forms of translational research seeking to cross the gap between science and medical care. Other disciplines too have jumped on the translational bandwagon, from biology ("translational termination," "translational misincorporation") and physics ("translational momentum of the molecule") to computing ("translational freedoms" and "translational motion") to aviation ("translational lift"). Translationality as change, force, impact, motion, energy.[1]

My title, "Translationality," is itself a translation: the Slovak translation theorist Anton Popovič's (1975, 22) own English translation of his Slovak term *prekladovosť*. For Popovič *prekladovosť*/translationality is "a communicative relation in the communicative chain between the author of the original communicate and the receiver of the translation who may or may not be aware that the literary communicate has been translated from the original." For him, that communicative relation simply has "a semiotic or modeling character" (22) of some unspecified kind; I am pushing his coinage in a specific, perhaps tendentious direction, namely into the realm of the inevitability of *change*. To paraphrase the second sentence of his definition, with my addendum in italics: "From the textual standpoint, the translationality is a relation holding between the proto-[source] and meta-[target] text and having a *transformative* semiotic or modeling character." I would argue, however, that my addendum is already implicit in Popovič's Peircean term "semiotic": for Peirce iconic modeling is an abstract First that can only keep believing in the possibility of exact reproduction until it crashes into the resistant turbulence of Seconds, for example a target language, or a target audience, or the interpretive predilections of a reader who becomes the target author (translator). Semiosis is rife with transformation. To fuse Popovič's coinage with Dinda L. Gorlée's (1994, 231; see Robinson 2016c for discussion), what we are concerned with here is *semiotranslationality*.

Since I am a humanist, oriented intellectually to phenomenology and hermeneutics, I tend to direct my explorations of translationality through felt experience. But an attentive engagement with felt experience will reveal that we not only *feel* the processuality I'm calling translationality: we *perform* it with our bodies, interactively. We co-perform it. Performed translationality would be shorthand for *felt-becoming-mobilized-becoming-performed translationality*. We first feel the change, feel the need to respond actively to the change, to participate in translationality. As we also feel the others around us feeling the same processual or translational impulses, we collectively *mobilize* those impulses for action. The performance of the mobilized action that ensues is collective as well, but continues to be felt and mobilized in each individual member of the group.

Translationality as transformationality: the constant emergingness of everything, through embodied, situated, performative interactions.

I also want to complicate the performativity of translationality through the notion of *peri*performativity, first theorized by Eve Kosofsky Sedgwick in *Touching Feeling* (2003) as the communal interactivity that makes performativity possible: if "I" do something to "you" with words, my performative is *witnessed*, and so ratified and guided, by "them," the people around us. Periperformativity as *alongside* performativity, guiding and shaping the performative construction of the social world. What is interesting and useful about Sedgwick's intervention into performative theory is that performativity is big, visible action on the social stage – people *doing things to each other with words* – and so relatively easy to notice (not that philosophers of language, historically, found noticing it all that easy). Periperformativity is much less visible: still action on the social stage, but support action, facilitative action, auxiliary action. If performativity is the action onstage, periperformativity is the work done by directors, stage managers, technicians, and the audience in the house on any given night. If literary translationality is "performed" by writers, translators, and adapters, it is "periperformed" by audiences, including editors and critics – and who ever notices them? Translationality as performed by brilliant artists is about cultural change brought about by creative innovators (studied by literary scholars, especially those working on literary history, literary translation, and adaptation); translationality as periperformed by audiences is about cultural change as an almost imperceptible "groundswell," as a "watershed" without inciting events, indeed as "reality," as "human nature," as "the way things are."

I have no desire to choose between the two, however. I assume that periperformativity encompasses performativity, and want to study the interdisciplinary interactions between "performed translationality" as creative rewriting and "periperformed translationality" as the emerging social construction of "reality" – between, to put that in disciplinary terms, transnational literary history and cognitive/medical (neuro)science.

A rather cumbersome (Hegelian or Deleuzean) -becoming- construction that I use for this (peri)performance of translationality is "affective-becoming-conative-becoming-(peri)performative." We participate in it affectively. And because we tend to have an interest in the outcome of such processes, we also tend to convert affect into conation, which is to say, feeling into pressure. We exert pressure on ourselves and others to bring our shared feelings into some kind of "neurocultural" organization, which, we hope, will increase predictability and so homeostatic control over our environments and ourselves. And then we periperform that organization, not only on the world's stage, in situated/distributed social interactions staged as full-body movement in space and time, but on the body's stage as well, in social interactions staged as expressive/receptive/mimetic body language. We periperform social organization by organizing social performance, and in so doing periperform social organization. This is the continual reciprocal/reticulatory through-put of periperformative social regulation.

Of course by "we" I mean normals: there are many neural disorders that make it impossible to feel those things, and I will be exploring one of those disorders at some length here, especially in Essay 1 – the Capgras delusion. We tend to believe, commonsensically, that reality *just is* real, and we feel its reality because it *is* real. As we will see, cognitive neuroscientists, building on Immanuel Kant's so-called "Copernican Hypothesis,"[2] have shown that commonsensical view to be simply untrue. Studies of the Capgras delusion and other so-called misidentification brain disorders have shown conclusively that normal people *construct* reality, and that a deficit or defect in the neural systems that manage that construction causes disruption to the sufferer's sense of reality:

- Alice in Wonderland syndrome causes space and time to shrink or expand disturbingly. I once experienced this during a migraine, and panicked, because my legs stretched all the way across the room.
- Cotard syndrome causes the person to believe seriously that s/he is dead.
- In alien hand syndrome, one hand seems to be possessed by a demon: it refuses to obey your wishes, fights you, undoes things your other hand does.
- Akinetopsia deprives you of the ability to experience motion: life comes at you in isolated snapshots at five-second intervals. Without the ability to watch the liquid level rising gradually in a cup, it becomes very difficult to pour a cup of tea.
- So-called category deficits disrupt our ability to tell things apart, say, dogs from cats, or animals from furniture, or, in a case Oliver Sacks (1998) made famous, a wife from a hat.
- Mirror touch synesthesia intensifies the normal empathic mirroring we do of others' body states (tactile, kinesthetic, emotional, etc.) so radically that we are constantly acutely conscious of fusing with other people's body states, precariously eroding the boundary between self and other. Their felt reality becomes our felt reality – but serially. We experience other people's felt realities one at a time, depending on where our visual focus is trained.
- There is a disorder called aprosodia that deprives the person of the ability to feel the somatics of language – the affective (prosodic) charge of speech, the tonalizations, the rhythms, everything that not only makes language feel alive but helps us detect subtle nuances like irony, wistfulness, and secret delight. The aprosodiac experiences speech the way twentieth-century linguists used to study it: as an abstract sign system. I have been studying the somatics of language for three decades, and can't begin to tell you how many times reviewers and skeptics in the audience have scornfully dismissed the very idea of a somatics of language, insisting that I had made the whole thing up out of some misguided sixties touchy-feely mysticism. As we will see below, one called it "mystical biologism." *It's not real.* I just think it's real because I am somehow psychologically warped, perhaps overemotional.

> What is ironic about this reaction to my talk of the somatics of language is that for aprosodiacs the somatics of language is *not* real – but for my critics it is. They just don't know that it is, because their understanding of language and other humanistic phenomena has been shaped by bad theory.

And by "bad theory," of course, I mean hegemonic Western rationalism, as informed by Platonism, Christianity, and Enlightenment science. The fact that over the past century or two brain science has increasingly overturned that bad theory is just another historical irony.

0.2 Medical humanities

Now let us move into the subtitle, "Essays in the Translational-Medical Humanities," where you are intended to hear echoes of both translational medicine (TM) and the medical humanities (MH). Take the latter first.

The interdiscipline of MH is variously defined: "history of medicine, bioethics, narrative medicine, medicine in literature, creative writing, disability studies, and various social sciences (for example, medical anthropology and sociology) can all be part of medical humanities programs or curricula," as Brian Dolan (2015, 1) writes in the introduction to his hundred-year reader. Dolan also adds in his preface that the question of "why the medical humanities [are] important to medical education" is "one that almost everyone teaching medical humanities in medical schools needs to answer, repeatedly" (x). In other words, the medical humanities are primarily a part of medical education in medical schools. Future medical professionals need to be "humanized" – taught to engage humanistically not only with patients but with themselves, their colleagues, and the public. These various MH interventions are a necessary corrective to the tendency to focus on the scientific side of medicine, at the expense of the human.

I have no desire to impose a single narrow (re)definition on the field; rather, I would simply (initially) like to propose a slight expansion, to include people like me who are not medical professionals and do not teach in medical schools, but who have not only been patients (who hasn't?) but may even have engaged intellectually with some of the scientific subfields that contribute to medical science. I first began exploring the pathways in the autonomic nervous system that control somatic response back in the mid-1980s, because it seemed to me – a student of language and literature – that any explanatory model of human communication that ignored the neurological substrate of human behavior was woefully deficient.

An example of that deficiency to which I keep recurring through this book is the theory Jean Baudrillard offered in the 1970s and 1980s of "simulacra" – especially his claim that in the postmodern age signs refer only to other signs, no longer to "reality," which as a consequence has lately become "impossible" – without the slightest interest in whether his theory made sense physiologically:

> Simulating is not pretending: "Whoever fakes an illness can simply stay in bed and make everyone believe he is ill. Whoever simulates an illness produces

> in himself some of the symptoms" (Littré). Therefore, pretending, or dissimulating, leaves the principle of reality intact: the difference is always clear, it is simply masked, whereas simulation threatens the difference between the "true" and the "false," the "real" and the "imaginary." Is the simulator sick or not, given that he produces "true" symptoms? Objectively one cannot treat him as being either ill or not ill. Psychology and medicine stop at this point, forestalled by the illness's henceforth undiscoverable truth. For if any symptoms can be "produced," and can no longer be taken as a fact of nature, then every illness can be considered as simulatable and simulated, and medicine loses its meaning since it only knows how to treat "real" illnesses according to their objective causes. Psychosomatics evolves in a dubious manner at the borders of the principle of illness. As to psychoanalysis, it transfers the symptom of the organic order to the unconscious order: the latter is new and taken for "real" more real than the other [*sic*] – but why would simulation be [stopped?] at the gates of the unconscious? Why couldn't the "work" of the unconscious be "produced" in the same way as any old symptom of classical medicine? Dreams already are.
>
> (1981/1994, 3)

The stereotype of "medicine" on which this riff is based is a familiar one, of course; MH scholars invoke it repeatedly as a call to arms. It is precisely because "illness" and "symptomatology" and the conscious and unconscious human motivations behind both are far more complex than mechanical etiological models will allow that medical professionals have been stressing the importance of the humanities in medical education for roughly the past century. But Baudrillard's binaries are painfully simpleminded: because "simulation threatens the difference between the 'true' and the 'false,' the 'real' and the 'imaginary,'" and it becomes "objectively" impossible to "treat him as being either ill or not ill," "psychology and medicine stop at this point" and "medicine loses its meaning." The key word there is "objectively": this is an Enlightenment stereotype of science as either perfectly objective or perfectly worthless. If the human phenomenology of illness is more complicated than a mythically objectivized diagnosis would allow, medicine is impossible. There is no middle ground. Medicine is only possible if it operates on a simple Newtonian mechanics of causation: X causes Y. Cue ball to eight ball to corner pocket. If human beings turn out to be more complicated than that, everything falls apart. Not only is medicine impossible, reality itself is impossible. All human endeavor becomes a frantic effort to "escape the interrogation posed by simulation – the knowledge that truth, reference, objective cause have ceased to exist" (3). As a result, "reality" or "the real" too has ceased to exist. "In fact, it is no longer really the real, because no imaginary envelops it anymore. It is a hyperreal, produced from a radiating synthesis of combinatory models in a hyperspace without atmosphere" (2).

In that kind of postmodern world, obviously, it also becomes possible to theorize anything we like in any way we like. Since we can never test our theories against an impossible "objective reality," we can confabulate the most glorious fictions, and no one can challenge us. Deprived of reference to a shared sense of the real, we are freed from the heavy burden of communal engagement and responsibility.

I personally find it disturbing that I have never seen a humanistic study of Baudrillard's theory that showed the slightest interest in explaining – let alone testing – this notion of simulacra through neuroscience. And let me hasten to add that by "explaining" and "testing" I don't mean *reducing* the theory to the biochemistry of neurotransmitters; I mean creating a dialogue, an intellectual engagement, in which the humanistic theory might even drive the inquiry, but interactively, in a spirit of give-and-take and mutual learning.

I mean, for example, the interesting convergence between the "humanistic" philosophies of Kantian Idealists who insist that we have no direct access to "reality" (Kant's *Ding an sich* or Thing in Itself), but construct cognitive images that we take for reality, and the "medical" thinking of neo-Jamesian cognitive neuroscientists who insist that all reality-construction is a production of the human nervous system, which builds what it takes to be reality out of interpreted sense-data. In that confluence, *all* "reality" is what Baudrillard calls simulacra. We have *never* had a stable objective reality with which to compare our images of reality. Viewed through that lens, Baudrillard's theory of simulacra is nostalgic (as Jean-François Lyotard charged) not so much in the sense of longing for a lost time when we had access to reality but rather in the meta-sense of longing for a lost time when we *believed* we had access to reality – when naïve objectivism had not yet been neurophilosophically discredited.

And there are two layers to my critique of ostrich humanists here. On the first and most obvious layer, post-Kantian thought – often called social constructivism – is the basis of what is typically called "critical theory," the best thinking in the humanities. Humanities scholars should be aware of this stuff, and should be disinclined to take a literal reading of Baudrillard seriously. On the face of it there would seem to be no excuse, other than sheer ignorance of *humanities* thinking, for humanities scholars to buy into the absurdity of claims like "never again will the real have the chance to produce itself" (Baudrillard 1981/1994, 2).

On the second layer, however, it would appear that a century and a half of brain science has tended to confirm Kant's philosophical insight – and, as humanists and scientists find common ground, as cognitive and social neuroscientists are inspired by post-Kantian philosopher-psychologists like William James, the narrow territorial tensions of C. P. Snow's Two Cultures theory begin to dissipate. Scientists and humanists don't have to fear and despise each other.

It is of course an intriguing puzzle that neurologists have used objective, empirical science to prove that *everything* we know – including the findings of objective, empirical science – is what I will be calling a "neurocultural" construct. Don't those two impulses cancel each other out? They would, certainly, for a nostalgic binarist like Jean Baudrillard; but it turns out that life is more complicated than that old bad theorizing would have it. It also turns out, I suggest, that the places where the "new" – which is to say, newly recognized – complexity of life tends to be recognized and appreciated are interdisciplinary intersections between the Two Cultures: places like cognitive and affective science, chaos theory, complexity theory, dynamic systems theory, emergentism, performance studies, and the medical humanities. It begins to seem likely that "reality" is not only a collective performative construct but an *emerging ecological* construct. It also begins to seem very likely, as I argue in Essay 3 (section 3.4.2), that ancient Chinese thinkers from Laozi to Mengzi understood this ecological constructivism far better than the reductive-rationalist tradition that began to dominate Western thinking around the same time; but it seems equally likely, as I show in *The Deep Ecology of Rhetoric in Mencius and Aristotle* (Robinson 2016a), that very much the same ecological model of emergent reality-construction is right there in the *Rhetoric* of the quintessential Western reductive rationalist, Aristotle.

Understood as a form of practical reason (Aristotle's *phronesis*) guided by narrativized and value-laden social interaction – a core MH competence – the medical study of human neurological disorders and deficits over the last several centuries looks very different from the old stereotype invoked by Baudrillard, which leads him to the dogmatic conclusion that "psychology and medicine stop at this point" and "medicine loses its meaning." No: that's where psychology and medicine *start;* that's where medicine *develops* its meaning. The clinician presented with a baffling symptomatology is the *beginning* of medicine, and of medical knowledge. And if the clinical work leads through diagnosis, or a series of exploratory diagnoses and treatments, to a cure, or an amelioration of pain and dysfunction – or, barring that amelioration, to an enhanced understanding of the problem – it doesn't really matter whether the *metaphysics* of "objective science" works according to the idealized old models or cancels itself out. The interpersonal phenomenology of medical treatment is a klugey trial-and-error work-around driven primarily by human care for fellow humans, secondarily by the need for scientific understanding, and only tertiarily, if at all, by some disciplinary need for metaphysical consistency.

What I find exciting about MH and other interdisciplinary crossovers is that integrating humanistic and scientific thinking helps us push harder on the established views that we still feel as intuitively right but have begun inchoately to suspect may not be the final word. If I lean strongly but conflictedly toward a "counterintuitive" conclusion, but that conclusion is seconded in another discipline, that helps me overcome the conflicts that might otherwise hold me back from embracing a deviant or disruptive discovery.

But of course as the history of medicine shows clearly – I track one such history in Essay 2 (section 2.3.1): Renaissance physicians like Andreas Vesalius struggling to free medical science from calcified Galenic errors and traditionalists like Jacobus Sylvius continuing to cling to Galen as if to Scripture – hegemonic thinking can so powerfully command intellectual allegiance from even very intelligent people as to shut down critical receptivity to anomalies and resulting proposed reframings of the established models (what Thomas Kuhn calls revolutionary science). I have, for example, been accused of "biologizing" the humanities – even, once, of perpetrating what one (poststructuralist/Marxist) reviewer called "mystical biologism." Since my "biologism," if that's even an accurate descriptor of my somatic theory of human communication, came out of an engagement with brain science without the tiniest shred of mysticism, I assume that at base the "mystical" part of that accusation meant something like "I have no idea what this guy is talking about." This reviewer's accusation was almost certainly also conditioned by the discursivist orthodoxy in the poststructuralist critical theory of the early 1990s, according to which, as Brian Massumi (2002, 2) put it, the body "could only be a 'discursive' body: one with its signifying gestures. Signifying gestures make sense. If properly 'performed,' they may also unmake sense by scrambling significations already in place. Make and unmake sense as they might, they don't *sense*." From within the dogmas of that orthodoxy, *any* focus on the somatic body became "mystical biologism."

In other words, I come to MH from the humanistic side, with no axe to grind regarding the training of medical professionals. My unground axes mostly hang in the hall of the non-medical humanities: those humanistic scholars who remain content to compartmentalize knowing into the Two Cultures, "humanistic understanding" (our team) and "science" (the enemy), and to dismiss integrative approaches blithely as "not my field." If those "scientists" over there in the enemy camp (goes the thinking in our camp) look on in amazement as humanistic theorists like Baudrillard make extremist claims that have no apparent basis in what they know to be true about the situated human brain, so be it: let them think what they want. Their derision has no impact on us, over here. After all, they don't sit on our promotion-and-tenure committees. We do things differently in the humanities.

While my hope for the medical humanities is primarily directed at these colleagues in the traditional humanities, however, it is more broadly aimed at building bridges between the Two Cultures – and bringing researchers, teachers, and practitioners from both sides into an expanded middle.

What I embrace enthusiastically in MH is the focus on *phenomenology,* how it feels to be alive in the body, to experience life in specific embodied situations (see e.g. Morrissey 2014); and especially *hermeneutics,* the phenomenology of interpretation that forms the core professional experience of all medical clinicians in every moment of their working lives. (Essay 3 is concerned with the social neuroscience of empathic hermeneutics.) As specialists in "narrative medicine" have long insisted, "physicians need the ability to listen to the narratives of the patient, grasp and honor their meanings, and be moved to act on the patient's behalf. This is narrative competence, that is, the competence that human beings use[ ] to absorb, interpret, and respond[ ] to stories" (Charon 2015, 210).

0.3 Translational-medical humanities

Now add "translational-" to form the "translational-medical humanities" (TMH). At its most general level, that "translational-" is the translationality or "carried-across-ness" discussed in section 0.1: *trans* "across" + *latus* "carried." On that level "translational" could be replaced by any number of other "trans-" adjectives: transformational, transferential, transpositional, transmutational, transfigurative, transgressive, transitive, and so on. Specifically, here, the medical phenomena I am interested in studying humanistically in this book are *in transition, in transformation:* moving through changes ("translationality"). Sense-data move through our sensory apparatus to our central nervous systems, and there are translated not only into a coherent picture of reality but a coherent picture of reality *shared by other members of our culture.* How does that happen? How does a culture shape the neural translation of sense-data into a coherent picture of reality in all or most of its member individuals? The ability to answer that question is primarily what I seek in TMH.

More narrowly, of course, "translational" also refers to the act of translating a text from one language to another, and thus indirectly to the relatively young field of translation studies (TS), or even, intersemiotically (Jakobson 1959), from one sign system to another (words to images, images to melodies, etc.), and thus to adaptation studies (AS). TS, taken bare, without the filtering of MH through it, is the interdiscipline in which I am most proficient: I have been contributing to it since *The Translator's Turn* in 1991. But then that "taken bare," when used to refer to my own work in the field, is somewhat misleading, since one of the methodological innovations that I introduced in *The Translator's Turn* was the study of the *somatics* of translation, which is to say, of how our sense of "the right word or phrase" or "equivalence" between two texts is organized neurologically through what Antonio Damasio calls "somatic markers." That was the beginning of my interest in MH – though I did not know to call it that for many years. The Damasio team in fact did not begin to publish on somatic markers in medical journals[3] until nearly a year (November 1991) after my book was published in the days between Christmas of 1990 and the new year; when I wrote that book in 1988–1989 I was working with a mostly intuitive model of somatic response, based scientifically only on the theorization of somatic response offered by Akhter Ahsen (1984) at the American Imagery conferences I attended in the mid-1980s – without the "marking" function later hypothesized by the Damasio team. Damasio's first popular treatment of the somatic-marker hypothesis, *Descartes' Error,* was published in 1994; by the end of the 1990s, I was integrating that theory with my own, and expanding it through further reading in the neurophysiology of affect and further applications to the translation process, both as I experienced it in the professional translation marketplace and as other translation scholars were theorizing it. Later studies of the medical humanities of translation (MHT) would include Robinson (1996, 2003, 2011, 2013c, 2015a, 2016b, 2016c, 2017a, and 2017b).

I have also published several books and articles on translation that do not invoke the MHT of "somatic theory" or (later) "icotic theory" (notably Robinson 1997b and 2001), and MH studies of other subjects than translation, including literature (Robinson 2008), writing (2012), postcolonial culture (2013a), the philosophy of mind (2013b), and rhetoric (2016a).

"Translational-medical" also, of course, implicitly refers to the field of translational medicine (TM), which is younger still. The interdiscipline of TM is "translational" in the broad "transitional" or "transitive" sense that it tracks the translation of [a] medical research into clinical trials, [b] clinically trialed drugs and devices into patient care, and also, increasingly, in MH (see again Morrissey 2014), [c] patient care into a phenomenology of illness and health, pain and its alleviation, treatment and healing, as organized culturally by belief and value systems surrounding the causes of and cures for illness and injury. Medical professionals tend to focus on (a) and (b); one of the things I mean by TMH would be (c) an MH approach to TM, with a focus on the narrativized phenomenology of illness, treatment, health, and dying as an embodied and situated "lived experience."

Accordingly, then, in this book I track "translational-medical humanities" through four combinatorial vectors, one each in the book's three essays, and the fourth in the Conclusion:

Essay 1. *The Medical Humanities* (MH): medical knowing and saying and understanding framed humanistically, through narrative and image. It's not just that narrative and image humanize medical knowledge; the requirements of storytelling, metaphor, and so on reshape medical knowledge. *Foci:*

- Richard Powers's 2006 novel *The Echo Maker;*
- Jean Baudrillard's theory of simulacra;
- the 2010 movie *Jackass 3D;*
- Cervantes's *Don Quixote.*

Essay 2. *The Translational Humanities of Medicine* (THM): the history of medical literature (fading gradually into the history of imaginative literature) understood humanistically through both the act and the pretense of translation. *Foci:*

- Galen translated into Arabic by the ninth-century translation team led by Ḥunayn ibn 'Isḥāq (أبو زيد حنين بن إسحاق العبادي/'Abū Zayd Ḥunayn ibn 'Isḥāq al-'Ibādī, 809–873) in the Abbasid House of Wisdom in Baghdad, and critiqued by the Persian polymath Rhazes (مح??د زکریای کر برازی/Abū Bakr Muhammad ibn Zakariyyā al-Rāzī, 854–925);
- Rhazes critiqued in Latin translation by Andreas Vesalius (1514–1564), who not only translated Galen into Latin but adapted him transformatively in *De Fabrica* (1543), the first modern anatomy textbook;
- ancient and modern accounts of melancholy/depression collected, translated, and commented upon in the great humanistic/theological compendium *The Anatomy of Melancholy* (1621) by Robert Burton (1577–1640);
- Greek originals and Latin translations of Hippocrates and Galen edited by François Rabelais (1483/94–1553), a physician who also wrote what is arguably the first modern novel, *Gargantua et Pantagruel*

(1532–1564), which also pretends to be a translation of an ancient text found in a gargantuan coffin;
- Rabelais translated and improved upon by Sir Thomas Urquhart (1611–1660), in Scots dialect (1653);
- Urquhart's translation edited and polished (made more parlor-ready, in London English) in 1693 by Pierre/Peter le Motteux (1663–1718) and in 1737 by John Ozell (d. 1743);
- the Urquhart/Motteux/Ozell Rabelais and Burton's *Anatomy* used by Laurence Sterne as inspiration for his brilliant 1759 novel *The Life and Opinions of Tristram Shandy, Gentleman;*
- Sterne's novel translated medical-humanistically into Portuguese by Manuel Portela; and
- thoughts on medical/literary history as/and translationality-as-transformation.

Essay 3. *The Medical Humanities of Translation* (MHT): the medical-humanities study of translating and interpreting, moving from brain scans of interpreters and cognitive-science studies of the translation process to the neurology of translational affect. *Foci:*

- the "neurocultural" and "neurophenomenological" complexity of textual hermeneutics, specifically what Friedrich Schleiermacher called *das Gefühl des fremden*/"the Feeling of the Foreign"; and
- the ancient Chinese (Daoist and Confucian) theories of 心/*xin*/"heart, feeling" that arguably influenced the German Romantics.

Conclusion. *The Humanities of Translational Medicine* (HTM): the humanistic study of translational medicine. *Focus:*

- the staging of phenomenologies of patient care in Margaret Edson's play *Wit* (1993).

Two definitions there: "neurocultural" and "neurophenomenological." Both are my own sociobiological coinages, based on the idea that our nervous systems are *shaped* by culture and *felt* as an experiential phenomenology – and the conviction that the cultural shaping and phenomenological feel of the nervous system should be major humanistic foci of MH. The humanities without a medical focus tend to treat culture and phenomenology as autonomous humanistic realms that can be studied in isolation from medical brain science; medical brain science without a humanistic focus tends to treat neurophysiology as an autonomous medical/scientific realm that can be studied in isolation from culture and the feeling of being alive and experiencing the world in a human body. The TMH with which I will be concerned in this book mediates between those two extremes by exploring the neurocultural organization and neurophenomenological experience of everyday life.

In fact, what is so useful about the *medical* part of MH is that medical study of various deficits and disorders has brought far greater clarity to issues like the processuality of the construction of a sense of reality than would have been possible without it – than would have been possible with only, say, metaphysical speculation. One of my research interests over the last few years has been ancient Chinese thought, Confucianism and Daoism, especially the works of Mengzi and Laozi, both of whom – as we'll see in section 3.4.2 – articulated an ecological vision of emergence of events (物/*wu*) out of feeling (心/*xin*) that is strikingly similar to the ecological vision represented by Richard Powers in *The Echo Maker*, discussed here in Essay 1; as mentioned, in Robinson (2016a) I explored a confluence of socioecological thinking in Mengzi and Aristotle. That is all metaphysical speculation – by which I do not mean to demean any of those ancient thinkers. My point is only that without confirmation from cognitive neuroscience, it is far more difficult to persuade skeptics to take that speculation seriously. (Of course dyed-in-the-wool humanistic traditionalists will reject evidence from cognitive neuroscience as well: it is, after all, *not their field*, and therefore nothing that they feel they have to take seriously.)

Each essay explores a different axis of interests in all this. Essay 1 considers the medical humanities in terms of the creation of a sense of the real and ecological emergence, without translation; Essay 2 considers translationality first in the context of the history of medical literature, then segueing into the history of imaginative literature and of literary translation, without much in the way of brain science; Essay 3 considers the brain science of translation, culminating in the social ecologies of icosis and ecosis. The Conclusion retreats from interlingual translation and brain science into the humanistic phenomenology of medical treatment, as a key concern of translational medicine. The shifting perspectives on what I'm calling the translational-medical humanities, in other words, are kaleidoscopic.

0.4 Acknowledgments

Essay 1 was born out of a chance conversation with Ivan Delazari, in which I happened to mention the Capgras delusion as an interesting neurological disorder that might shed considerable light on somatic theory; his response was to refer me to Richard Powers's novel *The Echo Maker*, which he knew I had bought but not yet read. Ivan ended up not only reading the entire manuscript and making countless transformative suggestions, but chatting with me on a weekly basis throughout the writing process of each essay. My debt to him is enormous.

From April 5 to 25, 2016, I posted an earlier and much shorter draft of Essay 2 to academia.edu for "workshopping," and the responses posted by sixteen participants over those twenty days were extraordinarily useful: Karen Bennett, Susana Valdez, Nataliya Rudnytska, Alexander Zaytsev, Aditya Kumar Panda, Jeremiah Chung, Hamid Varmazyari, Sonia Vandepitte, Kseniya Leontyev, Rodrigo Tadeu Gonçalves, Deborah Dawkin, Sean Golden, Anne Coldiron, Spencer Hawkins, James Hadley, and Outi Paloposki. As is always the case with feedback, even the misreadings and misunderstandings were highly productive, in drawing attention to the need for further clarification and even retheorization, but many of the participants also provided invaluable suggestions and examples that were incorporated into the finished paper as submitted to *Target* for publication. Thanks also to the anonymous reviewers for their helpful comments as that paper went through review and production at *Target*. Several of the participants in the academia.edu workshop complained that that original formulation (which has now been resequenced, in roughly reverse order, as section 2.3) lacked cases, examples, and illustrations, and so was more like a manifesto than a scholarly article; in response to that pushing I decided to rewrite it radically, so as to flesh it out with a history of translationality (section 2.2).

Essay 3 in its initial conception was a kind of umbrella conference paper: sometime in the late spring of 2016 I realized that I had promised to deliver six guest lectures and plenaries between June and Christmas, all on similar topics – and that I could write up a long essay that would incorporate all of them, and simply draw on sections of the omnibus write-up as I went along. Accordingly:

- At the Third Hermeneutics and Translation Studies Symposium in Cologne, Germany (June 30 to July 1), organized by John Stanley, I delivered a truncated version of section 3.4.2.
- At Chulalongkorn University in Bangkok, Thailand (August 19), invited by Phrae Chittiphalangsri, I delivered a truncated version of sections 3.2 and 3.3.
- At the symposium on Translation, Interculturality, and Hermeneutics at the University of Granada, Spain (October 13–15), hosted by the Confucius Institute and organized by Alicia Relinque, Sultana Wahnon, and Dorothy Kelly, I delivered a version of sections 3.4.1–2.
- At the symposium on Eco-Translatology at University College London (November 10–11), organized by Theo Hermans, I delivered a version of section 3.5.
- At the first World Interpreter and Translator Training Association (WITTA) Congress at Guangzhou University of Foreign Studies (November 19–20), invited by Zhu Chunshen, I delivered more or less the same version of section 3.4.2 that I had presented in Germany, with a more detailed focus on the contents of Laozi's and Mengzi's theories of 心/*xin* "heart-becoming-mind" or "feeling-becoming-thinking."
- At the Hundred Years of Ostranenie conference at the University of Erfurt, Germany (December 15–17), invited by Alexandra Berlina, I delivered a truncated version of section 3.3.

Each presentation, needless to say, involved considerable give and take first with the organizers, then with the audiences, all of which had a salutary effect on the quality of the final product. Thanks to all involved.

Larisa Cercel also asked me to contribute an article to a volume she was editing on creativity and hermeneutics, and I revised sections 3.3.1 and 3.3.2 into an article for her.

My main thanks as always go to Sveta Ilinskaya, for all the rousing conversations we've had about culture, trauma, and performativity – especially the ones where she, a cultural studies theorist, argues that culture doesn't exist.

Notes

1 I take several of these examples, with thanks, from Blumczynski 2016a and 2016b.

2 According to Tom Rockmore (2002, 184), Kant never actually used the phrase "Copernican Hypothesis" about the upheaval he engineered in philosophy; it was later applied to his thinking by others. Victor Cousin (1854, 21) explained the derivation of the metaphor a century and a half ago:

> Copernicus, seeing it was impossible to explain the motion of the heavenly bodies on the supposition that these bodies moved around the earth considered as an immovable centre, adopted the alternative, of supposing all to move round the sun. So Kant, instead of supposing man to move around objects, supposed on the contrary, that he himself was the centre, and that all moved round him.

Metaphorically, in other words, in Kant's rejection of objectivism ("supposing man to move around objects") and defense of what he called "subjective universalism," we humans are the "sun": *we* create the constructs that we take to be reality. Beginning in the twentieth century, Kant's followers have been less inclined to universalize that "subjectivism" (social constructs tend to be culture-bound), and, especially in the phenomenological/hermeneutical tradition and later cognitive science/philosophy of mind, less inclined to treat a philosophy centered on human experience as "subjective" (social constructs tend to be interactive, enactive, embodied, and embedded).

3 The Damasio team had in fact begun to move strongly in the direction of the somatic-marker hypothesis before their first publication presenting it in 1991, in three articles on the neural substrates of memory in the prefrontal cortex (Damasio 1989; Damasio et al. 1990a, 1990b); as Damasio (1994) explains in his first popular treatment of the subject, it was the team's research into the prefrontal cortex, spurred on by a series of clinical encounters with patients who could reason and remember but could not prioritize tasks, that led to the formulation of the somatic-marker hypothesis. For Damasio's other neurological research that connects up with topics covered in this book, see Damasio and Geschwind (1984) for "The Neural Basis of Language," and Tranel and Damasio (1985) for a study of face (mis-)recognition (section 1.1). For Damasio's later popular presentations of the team's research, see also Damasio (1999, 2003, 2010).

Essay 1 The medical humanities

The creation of the (un)real as fiction

The overarching question I want to ask in this essay is: where does the "reality" of the world come from? What makes other people and our own selves seem real? And, if the deterioration or outright collapse of the neurocultural support system for that seeming would appear to suggest that what we call "reality" is actually a lot more like "fiction" than we thought, *is* there a difference between fiction and reality, and if so, how is it created and maintained?

To support that overarching question I will be asking a series of subquestions, marked Q1, Q2, Q3, etc.; the direction in which I plan to move over the course of the essay is that "reality" is a production of the limbic system, especially of the emotions – our *feeling* of reality. My trigger observation for the series of explorations that follow is that some thinkers have been arguing over the last few decades that our feeling or sense of reality, our ability to "realize" the world and our selves, has just recently been depleted (over the last century or so); Jean Baudrillard (1981/1994) in particular, in his controversial notion of simulacra, has even argued that it has been lost entirely, that "reality" has been completely subsumed into virtuality. David Shields (2010) argues somewhat more moderately that we have developed a "reality hunger" – a craving for "authenticity," things and personalities that feel (more) real because they represent a nostalgic past sense of reality; but of course the Baudrillardians would insist that the "reality" of a vinyl record, a treadle sewing machine, a plank floor, or an exposed-brick wall is just a simulacrum of a different vintage (a "counterfeit"), not qualitatively different from a streaming video or an ePub whose pages rustle when you turn them. The runaway popularity of Baudrillard's "topos of simulacra" (Smith 2001, 2) among the culturati speaks to a pervasive sense that "reality" is nowadays somehow at risk, under assault, or perhaps just crumbling away into nothing. Something like this concern about the ascendancy of "fiction" – pretense, fakery, fraudulence, imposture – over "reality," authenticity, and so on, is also a key theme and structural organizer in Richard Powers's (2006/2007) novel *The Echo Maker*. How should we understand this?

What I argue in this essay is that neurological deficits and disorders – especially the famous Capgras delusion, which provides the major plot point in *The Echo Maker* – can shed some light on the question of the depletion or disappearance of "reality." I also show that two applications of the most obvious, literal, popular interpretation of Baudrillard to humanistic texts – Kevin Casper's 2015 application of simulacra to the 2010 *Jackass 3D* movie and Álvaro Ramírez's 2005 application to *Don Quixote* – reveal that interpretation as completely inadequate, and a confederation of the Capgras delusion and other neurological "misidentification" disorders in the Powers novel and subtler interpreters of Baudrillard begins to compensate for that inadequacy en route to that broader theory of human social interaction that I call "icosis."

1.1 Capgras fictions 1: *The Echo Maker*

The basic plot of the novel is that Mark Schluter, a fairly ordinary 27-year-old working-class man from Kearney, Nebraska, skids off an icy country road and flips his truck, and then hangs there unconscious for an untold period of time, slowly freezing, until someone spots the wreck and makes an anonymous call to the police. Once Mark has been found and cut out of his truck with an acetylene torch and rushed to Good Samaritan Hospital in Kearney, someone (else?), whom he comes to think of as his mysterious "guardian," leaves a mysterious note on his table:

> I am No One
> but Tonight on North Line Road
> GOD led me to you
> so You could Live
> and bring back someone else. (12)

Those five lines also become the titles of the novel's five parts:

The first part, "I AM NO ONE," tells the story of Mark's initial recovery (and diagnosis as suffering from the Capgras delusion) through the eyes mostly of his older sister Karin, who Mark thinks is a double (possibly a government spy); then Karin's boyfriend Daniel finds two books by Dr. Gerald Weber, a famous cognitive neurologist, and Karin contacts him, in the hope that he might come and cure Mark.

The second part, "BUT TONIGHT ON NORTH LINE ROAD," tells of Dr. Weber's first visit to Kearney, his interactions with Mark and Karin, Mark's two wild guy friends Duane Cain and Tom Rupp, Mark's sometime girlfriend Bonnie Travis, Mark's empathic attendant Barbara Gillespie, and the attending neurologist at Good Samaritan, Dr. Hayes.

The third part, "GOD LED ME TO YOU," tells the story of Mark's move back home, where he is initially convinced that his dog and his house are doubles, and then, gradually, that the entire neighborhood is a *Truman Show*–like production, where everyone and everything is a phony stand-in for some person or thing or place he remembers. His paranoia grows, and he begins obsessively documenting the imposture that he finds all around him. Meanwhile, Dr. Weber's reputation is unraveling, as he is accused of professional ethics violations and even, hintingly, outright fraud.

Part 4, "SO YOU MIGHT LIVE," continues the plot developments in part three – Mark's paranoia, Dr. Weber's professional meltdown, Karin's panicky attempts to remain cognitively solvent in the turbulence of Mark's paranoia – but also brings the mysteries of Mark's accident and Barbara's sinister vibe to closure. And the very brief concluding part five, "AND BRING BACK SOMEONE ELSE" – only a dozen pages long, out of nearly 600 – ties together the loose ends, drug and mild shock therapy curing Mark of his Capgras, so that he recognizes Karin as his sister again and comes out of the paranoid concoction of wild conspiracy theories.

The neurological disorder that Powers "translates" from cognitive neuroscience into the plot engine of his novel, the Capgras delusion (also called Capgras syndrome), was first diagnosed and named by Joseph Capgras (1873–1950) in 1923. The disorder typically presents as the patient's conviction that loved ones have been killed or kidnapped and replaced by doubles (see Hirstein and Ramachandran 1997; Ramachandran 1998, ch. 8; Breen et al. 2000; Ellis and Lewis 2001). Capgras sufferers are certain that their spouses, their children, their close friends, even their pets are not the "real" people or other creatures they pretend to be: Mark first believes that his sister Karin is not really his sister but an impostor – a government spy, or possibly a cleverly programmed robot – then that his house and his dog are doubles, and eventually that everything, his entire town of Farview, perhaps his entire universe, is a fake, a sham, a charade, an imposture. As they get used to the "impostors," too, Capgras sufferers typically begin to "realize" that the first-order doubles have been killed or kidnapped and replaced by doubles-of-doubles, who in turn are eventually replaced by doubles-of-doubles-of-doubles. Worse, some look in the mirror and become convinced that they themselves have been replaced by doubles. This seems to happen to Mark as well: late in the novel, he begins to suspect that he ran over himself on the highway that night, and it occurs to Dr. Weber that "he'd begun to double himself" (384).

This all sounds strikingly like (one common interpretation of) Jean Baudrillard's theory of simulacra: the loss of a sense of reality; the increasing impossibility of establishing the reality of another person, a pet, or even the self. In Baudrillard's terms, the "doubles" are simulacra who look *exactly* like the "real" people, but are manifestly not them. And doubles-as-simulacra proliferate, until it seems to the Capgras sufferer as if reality has been subsumed into diabolical simulation, is drowning in simulation.

Of course there is also a significant difference, in that Baudrillard never ventures a guess as to how this happens. His theory of simulacra is not a cognitive neuroscience model – and everything in *The Echo Maker,* including the powerful ecological subplot, is about cognitive neuroscientific explanations. Baudrillard's theory of simulacra is what Charles Levin (1996) calls a "cultural metaphysics" – either a trendy apocalyptic metaphysics of the postmodern End Times or a trenchant theory of culture *disguised* as a trendy apocalyptic metaphysics of the End Times, but in either case utterly lacking in etiological detail. How exactly do simulacra come to colonize our sense of reality? What intellectual, experiential, behavioral, neural processes enable that colonization? Baudrillard and his many followers have no idea, and don't really care. The theory is cool. That's the main thing.

What Capgras can offer us, if we're interested – and Powers is a persuasive and knowledgeable guide, if we set off on that journey – is an exploration of one possible neural etiology of the depletion of "reality," based on the interaction of two neural pathways for the recognition of faces: the analysis of visual features and emotional response. Normals use both: their brain's fusiform face area (FFA) analyzes appearances based on lines, contours, and so on, and their emotions sort the results into greater and lesser degrees of familiarity, based on the presence or absence and relative intensity of an emotional "glow" signaling the face of someone they care about. Damage to the FFA causes "face-blindness": the subject (like "Joseph N.," as reported by Dr. Weber in *The Echo Maker* (188–90)) claims not to recognize the faces of friends and loved ones, but skin-conductance tests indicate a somatic response to them. (See also the Damasio team's early work on this: Tranel and Damasio 1985; Tranel et al. 1988, 1995; Damasio et al. 1990b, 1993.) S/he recognizes them emotionally, but because s/he doesn't recognize them analytically, consciously, s/he isn't aware of recognizing them, and so claims not to.

As Powers's narrator points out (190), the Capgras delusion is the opposite of face-blindness: it is caused by damage to the emotional circuits contributing to face-recognition. Capgras sufferers have fully functional FFA capabilities. They can analyze visual features perfectly, and recognize that that man sitting across from them at the dinner table "is" their husband, or that that face in the mirror "is" the self, but they feel no emotional "glow" signaling familiarity, and so confabulate otherness – or what Baudrillard calls simulation. To them it is uncanny that that person can look *exactly* like a loved one but not *be* the loved one – which is to say, not be the *real* loved one. The somatic response, measurable by a skin-conductance test (basically a polygraph machine), generates the *feeling of reality;* damage to that neural circuit creates a sense that reality has been sucked out of the "recognized" face. As a result, the face is recognized but not real. The "simulation" theory – that the loved one (or the self) has been kidnapped and replaced with a double – is the desperate confabulatory attempt made by what Michael S. Gazzaniga (1989) calls the left brain's "interpreter" to explain the discrepancy.

Now one might want to protest that according to Baudrillard the subsumption of reality into virtuality is ubiquitous, at least in the postmodern West, while the Capgras delusion is a neurological disorder that is quite rare. The simulacra that plague Capgras sufferers are also considerably more localized than Baudrillard's: they tend to be limited to the sufferer's nearest and dearest, including pets and the self. They do not include whole cities, like Los Angeles (Baudrillard 1981/1994, 12–14), or, ultimately, everything. Mark is *one* Capgras sufferer who gradually comes to believe that everything is simulated; if applied to Baudrillard's explicit theory, this model would say that *everyone* is a Capgras sufferer for whom everything is simulated – though in Baudrillard most people aren't aware of that.

But Powers seems determined to build something like Baudrillard's universalizing claim into the very fabric of his novel. For one thing, the more tendentious Baudrillardian imagery of simulation runs like a scarlet thread through the novel: Karin thinking of the streets of Kearney that they were "a simulation more predictable than one of Mark's online games" (37); Karin saying to Daniel, "Don't you see, yet? I'm not her. I'm just a simulation. Something you invented in our head" (368); the Weber-focalized narrator describing the mirror-neuron system as "simulations simulating simulations" (485). I haven't seen Powers admitting in print that he was influenced by (or was even thinking of) Baudrillard on simulacra here, or elsewhere in his writing, but the circumstantial evidence for such influence seems quite compelling. Even more compellingly, late in the novel Karin muses that "the whole race suffered from Capgras. Those birds [the cranes that migrate every March through the Platte River area just south of Kearney, Nebraska] danced like our next of kin, looked like our next of kin, called and willed and parented and taught and navigated all just like our blood relations. Half their parts were still ours. Yet humans waved them off: *impostors*" (439).[1]

Of course the problem with that equation is that the cranes weren't yesterday our loved ones, our nearest and dearest, and do not therefore, as a result of our brain-related illness or accident, come to be experienced only today as impostors or doubles. If they ever were our nearest and dearest, they were that tens of thousands of years ago, and what our collective Capgras has "destroyed" is an emotional glow of familiarity that – if it ever existed at all – is buried deep in our race memory. The "collective Capgras delusion" that Powers puts in Karin's late revelation is either a metaphor, an analogue – our denial of kinship with the rest of nature is *like* Capgras – or, if it is "real" (whatever that means), it has plagued "us" for all of human history, and indeed may be identical to human history. The "reality" of our "collective Capgras delusion," to put that more cynically, is a tendentious interpretation, an activist construct that Arne Naess and other deep ecologists, and perhaps Powers as well,[2] are trying to *inculcate* in a transformed human consciousness – trying to *make* real. Trying to infuse with the *feeling* of reality, through powerful storytelling. That cynical reading makes the whole thing sound like a fantasy, if we proceed from the platonizing/objectivizing assumption that a thing is either "real" or "fake," simulated; but Powers emphatically rejects that Platonism/objectivism, and I want to expand on his post-Kantian model as we go along, moving in the direction of a socioecological model of reality-construction or reality-periperformance that I call "icosis."

Another way of putting that, to which I want to return in section 1.4: if we accept a post-Kantian/social-constructivist (or what I will call a "periperformativist") model of reality-creation, the difference between one person creating a reality (say, Mark believing that he is not related to the woman calling herself Karin) and an entire population creating a reality (say, humans believing that they are not related to cranes) is that *group-plausibilization* makes the latter sense of reality "sane" and the former sense of reality "crazy." There is no question but that, as the novel sees it – and we participate in that group seeing as well – Mark's Capgras delusion is crazy. As things stand today, it is equally crazy to see humans as related to cranes. The deep-ecological hope, in which the novel participates, is that that will change, in the sense that *people everywhere* will come to experience cranes and other living and natural things as related to them, and the group-plausibilization of species interrelatedness will make what now seems crazy seem sane. (What's interesting there is that Mark's denial of his sibling relationship with the woman he calls Kopy Karin or Karbon Karin begins to drive Karin krazy too. As her only surviving family member, Mark is for her the most powerful group-plausibilizer of her status as his sister, and thus of a hugely important part of her identity. As a result, his denials begin to wear away at that group-plausibilized identity – begin to deplausibilize one part of it, and thus to drive a wedge into the very core of her identity, destabilizing the whole thing.)

One might be tempted to argue, given Baudrillard's utter disregard for the neurological *how* of his topos of simulacra, and the wild hyperbolic "poetry" of the *what* in quips like "the real is no longer possible" (1981/1994, 19), that there is no connection at all between simulacra and the Capgras delusion – indeed, that his entire model is trendy speculation with no basis at all in (*umm* . . .) "reality." I propose, however, to take a different tack – or actually three:

1 *(Section 1.2)* to use the Capgras delusion to track humanistic applications of the literal reading of Baudrillard's topos to entertainment texts, in order to explore the consequences of translating the topos down from High Theory to representational practice, the better to determine what must be rethought in Baudrillard's model in order for it to work properly;
2 *(Section 1.3)* to use simulacra to track Powers's intelligent application of ecological complexity/chaos theory to Capgras and other misidentification syndromes in *The Echo Maker,* culminating in Karin's claim that the human race suffers from an ecological form of Capgras, the better to determine what must be rethought in Powers's model in order for it to work properly; and, synthesizing (1) and (2),
3 *(Section 1.4)* to build a working theory of culture around the performative collectivization and normativization of emotional reality-construction.

1.2 Capgras fictions 2: simulacra in Baudrillard and humanistic applications

Most of it what has been written about Baudrillard seems to isolate his theses about simulacra and simulation for special attention; and as one reads through that literature, one repeatedly finds the claim that "hyperreality" is an unprecedented new state of complete disconnectedness from that simple, stable ontological state called "reality." In that new state, usually called postmodernism,

> everywhere around us the real is being (re)produced and (re)processed as simulation . . . the real is now defined and delineated as that which can be represented or reproduced through these technological forms . . . the resultant "hyperreal" overcoding of the real by the processed image allows appearances to become reality . . . in the topos of simulacra, any distinction between the represented image and reality vanishes as the historical contexts in which images were produced are effaced by their (re)production and circulation.
> (Smith 2001, 2)

Levin (1996) begs to differ:

> This kind of interpretation depends upon the doubtful assumption that artificiality is the opposite of reality, as if things made are necessarily less genuine than things not made, and that some things are either less real, or not real at all. (We encounter again the Platonic ontological hierarchy of Forms, imitations of Forms, and imitations of imitations.)
>
> (190–91)

And I would agree that a big part of the attraction of Baudrillard's "topos of simulacra," as M.W. Smith puts it, is its invocation of Platonic copy theory, according to which copies are always less real than their models. Plato's mystical rationalism has, after all, served as a major founding force behind both Christianity and Western science; the notion that there is an objective state called "reality," which all right-thinking people recognize and trust, and further that that state has been undermined and perhaps even undone by the mediated artificiality of the postmodern world in which we live, is ideologically far too normative to be easy to resist. Levin's casual dismissal of "the doubtful assumption that artificiality is the opposite of reality, as if things made are necessarily less genuine than things not made, and that some things are either less real, or not real at all," deviates so egregiously from that deep-ideologically normativized topos as to be virtually incomprehensible (from within it).

What interests me about those (mis?)readings as a follow-up to Richard Powers's fictionalization of the Capgras delusion is partly that they seem to be projecting that delusion onto all of us, or at least onto all Western postmoderns: in postmodernity, experiencing the reality of the real becomes impossible! Simulacra *are* Capgras delusions! But partly also it is the fact that what Baudrillard claims he is actually theorizing is the *normal* state of experiencing the reality of the real, precisely that which Capgras sufferers are unable to achieve. As he puts it in an interview:

> If you start from the idea that the world is a total illusion, then life, thought, become absolutely unbearable. So you have to make every effort to materialize the world, realize it, in order to escape from this total illusion. And the "realizing" of the world, through science and technology, is precisely what simulation is – the exorcism of the terror of illusion by the most sophisticated means of the "realization of the world."
>
> (Gane 1993, 184; quoted in Butler 1999, 24)

If truth, reality, identity, the self, humanity, society, and so on are simulacra as materializations of the real, and those simulacra are *normal* or normative, then the inability to effect that materialization that we find in the Capgras delusion is more akin to the "the idea that the world is a total illusion," which renders life "absolutely unbearable" – the feared negative state against which simulation is, according to Baudrillard, our defense – than it is to what he calls simulation.

1.2.1 (Mis)reading Baudrillard

The two opposed readings of Baudrillard's theory, then, may usefully be taken as alternative mappings of how Capgras works, and of what Capgras tells us about how the creation of that sense of reality (truth, identity, etc.) works in normals: the *simple/superficial reading* (Reading 1: simulacra as the derealization of matter) as an approximation of the Capgras delusion, and the *complex/deeper reading* (Reading 2: simulacra as the materialization of the real) as an account of non-Capgras normality.

According to Reading 2, there are two unfortunate rhetorical strategies (URSes) in Baudrillard's development of his imagery of simulation that conduce to the misunderstandings perpetuated in Reading 1.

URS1 is his loose talk of "the real" as a kind of poetic shorthand for – well, something. He tells us in interviews that it means a social construct, in the post-Kantian sense: as Kant insists, we have never had direct access to "reality," or what Kant called the Thing in Itself *(das Ding an sich);* what we take to be "reality" is actually a socioculturally constructed/performed "simulation." In his theorizing, however, Baudrillard uses "the real" as if it referred to a stable Platonic ontology. He tells us both (in interviews) that simulation is the realization of reality and (in his theoretical works) that simulation makes reality impossible.

URS2 is his use of "no longer" as a marker of a temporal transition from what would appear to be the good old days when reality was still possible, to our post-modern world where it is no longer possible:

> Today abstraction is *no longer* that of the map, the double, the mirror, or the concept. Simulation is *no longer* that of a territory, a referential being, or a substance. . . . The territory *no longer* precedes the map, nor does it survive it. . . . It is all of metaphysics that is lost. *No more* mirror of being and appearances, of the real and its concept. *No more* imaginary coextensivity: it is genetic miniaturization that is the dimension of simulation. The real is produced from miniaturized cells, matrices, and memory banks, models of control – and it can be reproduced an indefinite number of times from these. It *no longer* needs to be rational, because it *no longer* measures itself against either an ideal or negative instance. It is *no longer* anything but operation. In fact, it is *no longer* really the real, because no imaginary envelops it *anymore.*
>
> (Baudrillard 1981/1994, 1–2; emphasis added)

Wherever could Baudrillard's critics have gotten the idea that he is nostalgic for a lost reality? What could possibly make them think that for Baudrillard things used to be very different, "real," and now that reality – "all of metaphysics" – is lost? The answer is not hard to find: because he himself says so, explicitly, over and over, in his theoretical works. "Perhaps because of his [URS2] misleading phrase 'no longer' (which does for Baudrillard what 'always already' did for Derrida)," Levin comments, "Baudrillard's neo-Borgesian image of simulation was nevertheless received with great excitement in places like New York, where it ought to have been taken for granted!" (197). But of course "always already" says expressly that there never was a temporal transition: whatever state you think is new was always already there. If Baudrillard does actually use "no longer" to mean more or less what Derrida meant by "always already," he needs to be more explicit about it: "Abstraction *has always been no longer* that of the map . . . Simulation *has always been no longer* that of a territory . . . The territory *has always no longer* preceded the map," and so on. Indeed Levin ultimately recommends that we jettison the "no longer" entirely, for "simulation has, in essence, always been like this, at least so far as social life is concerned; for society has never been anything else but a map, or more truthfully, a collection of maps, that we gradually learn to read" (196). All culture is simulation.

Rex Butler (1999, 24) adds that "the other thing to be understood about simulation, the other mistake often made with regard to it [in Reading 1], is that it is not an empirical phenomenon, something that actually happens." That is a bit confusingly written; he means that the mistake lies in thinking that it *is* something that actually happens. In other words, "the very real which we say is lost in simulation and against which we compare it is now only conceivable in simulated form. Indeed, we might even say that, insofar as we can speak of simulation at all, it has not yet occurred, that simulation is proved in its absence. Simulation is not real, then, but a kind of hypothesis." Butler quotes Baudrillard from an interview:

> To assert that "we're in a state of simulation" becomes meaningless, because at that point one enters a death-like state. The moment you believe that you're in a state of simulation, you're no longer there. The misunderstanding here is the conversion of a theory like mind into a reference whereas there should never be any references.
>
> (Gane 1993, 166; quoted in Butler 1999, 24)

Working from this passage, Butler argues, "against Lyotard and others, that Baudrillard is not merely nostalgic. He is not simply appealing to a real that might once have been. On the contrary, the problem he sets himself is how to speak against this simulation when there is nothing to which to compare it, when there is nothing outside of it or when that outside can only be imagined in its terms" (24). Butler's Reading 2 corrective is effectively a Kantian argument: since everything that we think of as "the real" is in fact a social construct, a periperformativity, a simulation, there is absolutely no way we can compare that simulation with a simulation-free reality in order to establish its degree of deviation from "true." And I think that's a useful and usable point.

The problem with Baudrillard's own statement of that point, though, is that it is just silly to claim that "there should never be any references." Clearly we refer to "real things" all the time. What he appears to mean is that when we refer to things, we mistake *constructed* or simulated things for real things – and thus that the actual Reading 1 misunderstanding is "the conversion of a theory like mind into a referential proof of the reality of reality, whereas references are always part of the simulation." Equally misleading is the cleverness of "the moment you believe that you're in a state of simulation, you're no longer there." This is more science-fiction cleverness, like playing with the famous paradoxes of time travel. It is of course absurd to suggest that believing changes your state from simulation to non-simulation: your belief, after all, is *constituted* by that collective simulation that we call society, or culture. If simulation is simply culture, as Levin argues, or a (post-)Kantian construction/performance of reality, as Butler argues, then we are *always* in a state of simulation, and believing or not believing is utterly irrelevant to our status. Baudrillard, it seems, can't resist the clever quip – and that temptation is constantly getting him into argumentative trouble. (But only with attentive readers, of course: the hordes of enamored intellectuals who have made Baudrillard a star, an iconic theorist of culture, take his cleverness-tic as a reliable sign of his vatic brilliance.)

Another way of thinking through this clash of interpretations: in Reading 1, Baudrillard wants to theorize two levels, [1] "reality" and [2] "simulation," and to read postmodern culture as foreclosing on (1) and shunting everything over into (2). Because referential signification – talking about things as if they were real – is part of (1), and (1) has been rendered inoperative by (2), it is not only impossible to talk about things in general as if they were (1) real; it is impossible to talk about (2) simulation itself as if it were (1) real. This ancient binary, which Plato inherited from the Zoroastrians and bequeathed to Christianity and Western thought at large, undoes the Baudrillard of Reading 1. Thus undone, he is ultimately forced to fall back on the age-old mystical rhetorical strategy of denying the efficacy of language to convey anything true. Use language vatically against itself; make every claim cleverly self-negating. (This rhetorical strategy remains surprisingly attractive to contemporary intellectuals.)

In Reading 2, by contrast, there are three levels: [1′] objective, pre-Kantian reality; [2′] Kantian "simulated" reality, or, as Baudrillard puts it, simulation as "realized" or "materialized" reality; and [3′] unrealized simulations, simulacra that don't feel like reality, or what Baudrillard calls the nightmare of "total illusion." The Baudrillard of Reading 2 clearly wants to foreclose on both (1′) and (3′) and analyze (2′); but because he doesn't really understand (2′), in rejecting the possibility of (1′) he keeps cleverly and counterproductively resorting to the negative theology of (3′) – and, of course, as we'll see in the next few sections, so do his Reading 1 followers, in (2). The responsible Reading 2 exfoliation of his own theory of simulation would explore the operation of *simulated reference* as a key element of (2′): we don't just (3′) simulate reality in some sort of experientially vacant way, as if we had somehow nightmarishly found ourselves in a two-dimensional world that was obviously and painfully unreal; we *realize simulated reality*. We make it real – make it *feel* real. We have not only developed a fully functional referentiality – a way of referring to things meaningfully, in the service of effective social interaction – but actually experience that referentiality *as* the real world. Foreclosing on both (1′) and (3′), the Baudrillard of Reading 2 insists that (2′) *is* what we call reality. From within Reading 2, therefore, the endless vacillations between (1/1′) and (2/3′) that characterize Reading 1 seem pointlessly silly.

As I say, however, Reading 1 has been endlessly attractive to intellectuals in the humanities as an explanatory model to apply to the texts that interest them. Let's look at two such applications: to a *Jackass* movie (section 1.2.2, followed by a corrective from a discussion of comics and cartoons in section 1.2.3) and to *Don Quixote* (section 1.2.4).

1.2.2 Jackass 3D *as "simulacra slapstick"*

The first humanistic application of Baudrillard I propose to examine is an article by Kevin Casper (2015) titled " 'I'm so glad you're fake!': Simulacra Slapstick and the Limits of the Real." Casper applies Baudrillard's theory of simulacra to the 2010 movie *Jackass 3D,* the third installment of that franchise. "Simulacra slapstick" is Casper's own coinage for "a form of slapstick comedy that upsets the stable distinction between the real and the fake that Western philosophy (and its subsidiary disciplines) is founded upon" (2015, 581–82): a kind of postmodern/Baudrillardian slapstick-plus that transgresses slapstick's traditional reliance "on a stable boundary that separates the real from the fake" (584). As Casper explains, slapstick is visual humor based on *fake* pain – pain only apparently suffered by actors and cartoon characters, which is funny because we know it's "not real." The unreality of the pain simulated in slapstick gives us license to laugh, to find the actor's/toon's distress funny. "Simulacra slapstick," by contrast, "resists confinement within the stable categories of real and fake and ultimately reveals that 'the real is no longer possible' in the era of the hyperreal (Baudrillard, [1981/] 1994, 19)" (582).

Note there not only the binary – "real and fake" – but the result of the destabilization of that binary: not (2′) a third category called simulation, which is actually the sociocultural materialization of the real, but the hyperreal impossibilization of "the real" (~~1~~>2). Casper, like Baudrillard, seems to be groping toward something like a (2′) middle ground between the real and the fake, called "simulation"; but because he can't really imagine that middle ground – and indeed because the Baudrillard of Reading 1 doesn't really give him much help in imagining it – he tends to articulate it subtractively, negatively, as "reality-minus." The Reading 2 reconceptualization of that middle ground toward which I will be working in this essay is more like "reality-plus": (2′) simulation as socially performed/constructed reality that is intensified and maintained by communally shared affect.

Let us look closely at three passages from Casper's argument.

First Passage: desiring/requiring/creating a sense of the real. As Casper glosses Baudrillard's *Simulacra and Simulation,* "a sense of the real is something that we still desire: 'We require a visible past, a visible continuum, a visible myth of origin, which reassures us about our end' ([1981/]1994, 10). But this sense is now only possible when we create it ourselves" (582).

We desire it; we require it; we create it. The plight of Capgras sufferers would seem to confirm overwhelmingly that we "require" it (life without it is well-nigh unlivable); and in that interview remark quoted just above, Baudrillard himself confirms that requirement in fairly strong terms designed to *correct* the literal Reading 1 of his theorization of simulation that Casper perpetuates: because life in "the world" as "total illusion" is "absolutely unbearable," we "realize" or "materialize" the world through simulation as a hedge against that "terror of illusion." In Reading 2, in other words, simulation is not the derealization of matter but the materialization of the real; not the impossibilization but the realization of the real. The fact that Baudrillard does also claim that "the real is no longer possible" renders his interview explanation somewhat problematic: not only is (URS1) "the real" "not possible" (whatever that might mean), but (URS2) it is "*no longer* possible." It was possible once; now, in the postmodern age of simulation, it is no longer.

The interesting questions for my purposes here, though, are:

[Q2] What does it mean to "desire" a "sense of the real"? Is "desiring" that sense like desiring food or sex? Is the "sense of the real" something that we need intermittently, the obtaining of which requires careful planning and strategizing?

[Q3] The "still" in "still desire" is obviously tied to Baudrillard's "no longer": "the real" or "a sense of the real" would appear to be something that we used to possess but that has now become a scarce commodity that we mostly lack and so endemically crave. Is that really the case? If so, when and how did this happen?

[Q4] Are the "we" who (Q3) "still desire" that (Q2) "sense of the real" [a] random individuals (who, say, possessed a sense of the real until we were 10, or 20, or whatever, and then lost it, so that we retain a nostalgic sense of what it was like to have that sense in our own individual lives); or [b] Western postmoderns (so that Western moderns still possessed it back, say, in the early twentieth century, and the rest of the world still possesses it, but "we" collectively have lost it, though most of us alive today have no memory of possessing it personally); or, say, [c] the whole human race?

[Q5] Above all, how do we create "a sense of the real"? Surely not by *wanting* to create it: the Capgras delusion is all about the inability to create it on demand, and we all know that it doesn't matter how much we *want* to create the sense that, say, we can *really* grow wings and fly to the moon, it's never going to happen. That kind of illusory/impossible "sense of the real" would be something like (2/3′) the "total illusion" that Reading 1 posits as the only possible alternative to (1/1′). It also seems to me quite problematic to suggest that our ability to "create it ourselves" only became essential recently.

I suggest the answer to (Q2) is that we "desire" that sense not because we have lost it, but because we still have it but keep getting disturbing intimations of its precarity. We desire more of it: the "reality hunger" of which David Shields (2010) writes is precisely that desire for more. But Shields's "reality hunger" is not the hunger of a starving person in a world without food; it is the hunger of a well-fed devourer of Big Macs who begins to crave "real" food, "authentic" food. We "still" desire that food (Q3) not only in the sense that we "still" remember eating homemade hamburgers, but also in the sense that the highly processed food that we mostly eat itself still retains and perpetuates the simulated image of "real" food (mass-produced hamburger patties piled high in the supermarket freezer with "Homemade!" emblazoned on the plastic bag, and advertised on TV through images of backyard cookouts). The nostalgia we feel for "real(er)" food is a simulacrum. "We" (Q4b) are postmoderns; but an indispensable Reading 2 correction to Reading 1's Baudrillard is, again, that all culture is simulation. All culture is artifice simulating/materializing "the real." "The real" is always already a cultural simulacrum. To the extent that "we" believe that " 'the real is no longer possible' in the era of the hyperreal," the "fall" or the "loss" implied by that "no longer" is itself a simulacrum. The sneaking suspicion we have that "reality" is somehow being "depleted," that there is less of it to go around today than there was in our childhood, or our parents' or grandparents' childhood, is a simulacrum. Culture is simulacra all the way down. "We" (Q4c) are ultimately the human race.

My answer to (Q5) harks back to the radical reinterpretation of Baudrillard developed by Levin (1996) and Butler (1999): *culture* creates a sense of the real. Indeed Baudrillard's own interview insistence that "the 'realizing' of the world, through science and technology, is precisely what simulation is" confirms this. His suggestion that "*you* have to make every effort to materialize the world, realize it, in order to escape from this total illusion" – as if this simulation-of-the-real were something that (Q4a) individuals did to smother their painful emotional response (existential dread) to the image of "this total illusion" – seems to feed Casper's "this sense is now only possible when we create it ourselves"; but that is silly. Reality is a collective construct – a communal periperformativity. Just how that periperformativity comes to *feel* real, though, is something that neither Levin nor Butler is able to explain. Adding that explanation to Reading 2 is the burden of this essay – and, more generally, of what in this book I am constructing/performing as TMH.

Second passage: attacking the reality principle. Casper seems to offer us a different kind of implicit definition of "the real" or "reality" by glossing another brief passage from *Simulacra and Simulation* (1981/1994, 20): "What proves most dangerous – yet also potentially productive – about the simulacra slapstick contained in *Jackass 3D,* is not that cuts and scabs and bumps and bruises befall the actors. It is that simulacra slapstick functions as simulation that 'attacks the reality principle itself' " (582).

[Q6] What is "the reality principle," and what does it mean to attack it?

Casper does not elaborate on Baudrillard's phrase there; "the reality principle" seems to function in his argument as yet another vague synonym of "the real" or "reality," and "attacking" that principle as another vague synonym of subsuming our sense of the real into virtuality. My answer to (Q6), however, would begin with the hunch that Baudrillard is specifically alluding to Freud's *Realitätsprinzip* from "Formulation of Two Principles in Mental Functioning" (1911/1957), namely the mind's ability to experience and live in accordance with the reality of the world outside it *as defined by society.* The reality principle for Freud is not "the real" or "reality" as a vague Platonic ontology; it is the individual's acquiescence to the normativization of a sociocultural periperformativity. The reality principle is specifically tied up with the ego's gradual learning to defer the gratification of the id-driven pleasure principle: it is a normative orientation to "the world" or "the real" to which the individual is incrementally socialized. To "attack the reality principle," therefore, is presumably to undermine not "reality" but society's power to socialize its members to its own *normativized* reality. That in turn would suggest that what Baudrillard calls simulation creates a state in which what is "no longer possible" is not "*the real*" as a stable ontology but that social normativization of reality that Freud calls *die Kultur* "civilization" – but also, of course, as we've seen, that (URS2) "no longer possible" is a problematic oversimplification. What the attack on the reality principle probably means is actually a *disruption* of the social normativization of reality, so that we come collectively to experience (periperform) reality differently. That is something slightly but significantly different from "but this sense is now only possible when we create it ourselves." Yes, we probably do "create it ourselves," but not "ourselves" in the sense of (Q4a) "individuals as *opposed* to society," as Casper seems to use it: "ourselves" rather in the sense of (Q4c) "individuals as *organized* by society." But, to repeat: (Q5/6) how do we do that?

Third passage: why we laugh at (simulacra) slapstick. Casper makes much of the 3D format of *Jackass 3D*, and I think rightly so. His point is a good one: that 3D supposedly enhances and heightens the "realism" of the "real" pain being experienced by the actors, but through the very artificiality of that heightened "realism" actually undermines the audience's sense of reality. But this talk of enhancing or undermining the audience's sense of reality rests implicitly on a model of how that sense of reality is created – and (Q5/6) how *does* that happen? I suspect that, like Baudrillard, Casper is content to shrug off (Q5/6) as "not my field" – to assume that it is quite reasonable to pronounce on the heightening and diminishing of an audience's sense of reality (a cultural-studies question) without needing to know anything about where that sense of reality came from in the first place (a neurocultural-studies/MH question).

The problematic of the begging of (Q5/6) is exacerbated in the central contrast Casper attempts to build between "traditional slapstick" and "simulacra slapstick." He notes that the makers of *Jackass 3D* begin the film by having Mike Judge's Beavis and Butt-head tell the audience to put on their 3D glasses, and pauses to remind us that Beavis and Butt-head represent traditional slapstick: "Butthead can beat Beavis all day and night, and, even though we might take some pleasure in watching this (partially because Beavis is a character that quickly gets under the skin), we ultimately know that no harm is ever coming to either of them" (588). A few pages later he tells us that "as [actor Dave] England flees [a battered beehive] in pain, the promise of simulacra slapstick in the skit becomes successfully realized: everyone involved is repeatedly stung. Rather than being sidestepped here, pain is celebrated, and, as a result, laughter is produced in the audience" (592). The idea seems to be that Beavis and Butt-head represent traditional slapstick because our laughter is provoked by their inability to feel pain, and *Jackass 3D* represents simulacra slapstick because our laughter is provoked by a celebration of the real pain they feel. But is this really how it works?

My answer to (Q5/6) begins experientially: whenever I've tried to watch any of the *Jackass* movies, whatever laughter they've provoked has been *painful* laughter – laughter that makes my body twist in empathic response to the pain the actors are experiencing. I was also a huge fan of MTV's *Beavis and Butt-head* in the nineties, and, *pace* Casper, often responded to them in exactly the same way as I do to the *Jackass* slapstick.

For example, episode 97 is called "Choke"; in it Butt-head gets a chicken nugget lodged in his throat, and is slowly choking to death, while Beavis walks about the house oblivious. That sequence for me was about 10% uneasy laughter and 90% vicarious empathic agony. "You idiot!" I kept wanting to scream at Beavis: "your friend is choking to death!" Finally Beavis accidentally steps on Butt-head's solar plexus and dislodges the nugget, and Butt-head is saved; but then Beavis pops the nugget in his own mouth and begins to choke and turn red and purple himself, and Butt-head is now oblivious to his friend's distress. The repetition of the gag made it funnier – as the episode ended, I was laughing appreciatively – but it was still painful laughter. I was still feeling the characters' pain.

So: what exactly is the difference between the effects on the audience's sense of reality in "traditional" and "simulacra" slapstick?

The explanatory model borrowed from Capgras-delusion neuroscience would suggest that the slapstick effects are in both cases empathic projections. It doesn't matter whether we "identify" with a loved one, a stranger whose pain we witness firsthand, a human actor in a live-action *Jackass* film, an animated cartoon like *Beavis and Butt-head,* or even a blinking blip on a computer screen: we (normals) *project* emotion onto them. Not only that: the social neuroscience of empathy has shown fairly conclusively that our bodies both project emotion onto other bodies (including soughing pines and burbling brooks, and abstract images) *and simulate* that projected emotion, through the mirror-neuron system. (Richard Powers reviews that research in some depth in *The Echo Maker,* and I return to it below; see also Robinson 2013b, 150–54, for a review of neurophysiological studies of empathy based on the mirror neurons.)[3] If we feel that a slowly blinking cursor is sad, we may begin to feel a bit melancholy ourselves; if it starts blinking faster, we may join "it" in a more upbeat feeling. It turns out that what John Ruskin (1856/1891) called the "pathetic fallacy" – projecting emotion onto nature – is normal brain function. Our ability to *share simulated affect* is at the core of our "creation" of a (shared) "sense of the real." And, conversely, the inability to experience that "fallacy" is precisely what plagues Capgras sufferers – what makes them suspect that their loved ones are not their "real" loved ones. For Mark Schluter, that inability to generate Ruskin's pathetic fallacy is what makes him suspect not only that "Kopy Karin" is not his real sister but that his dog is not his real dog, his house is not his real house, and his neighborhood is not his real neighborhood. The power of pathos to make things feel real is neither fallacious nor (in the colloquial sense) pathetic.

1.2.3 Simulacra in cartoons

For confirmation of this reading from a perhaps unexpected source, see *Understanding Comics* by Scott McCloud (1993), who argues that "WE HUMANS ARE A SELF-CENTERED RACE" (32), and goes on in Figure 1.1 to suggest that we "ASSIGN IDENTITIES AND EMOTIONS WHERE NONE

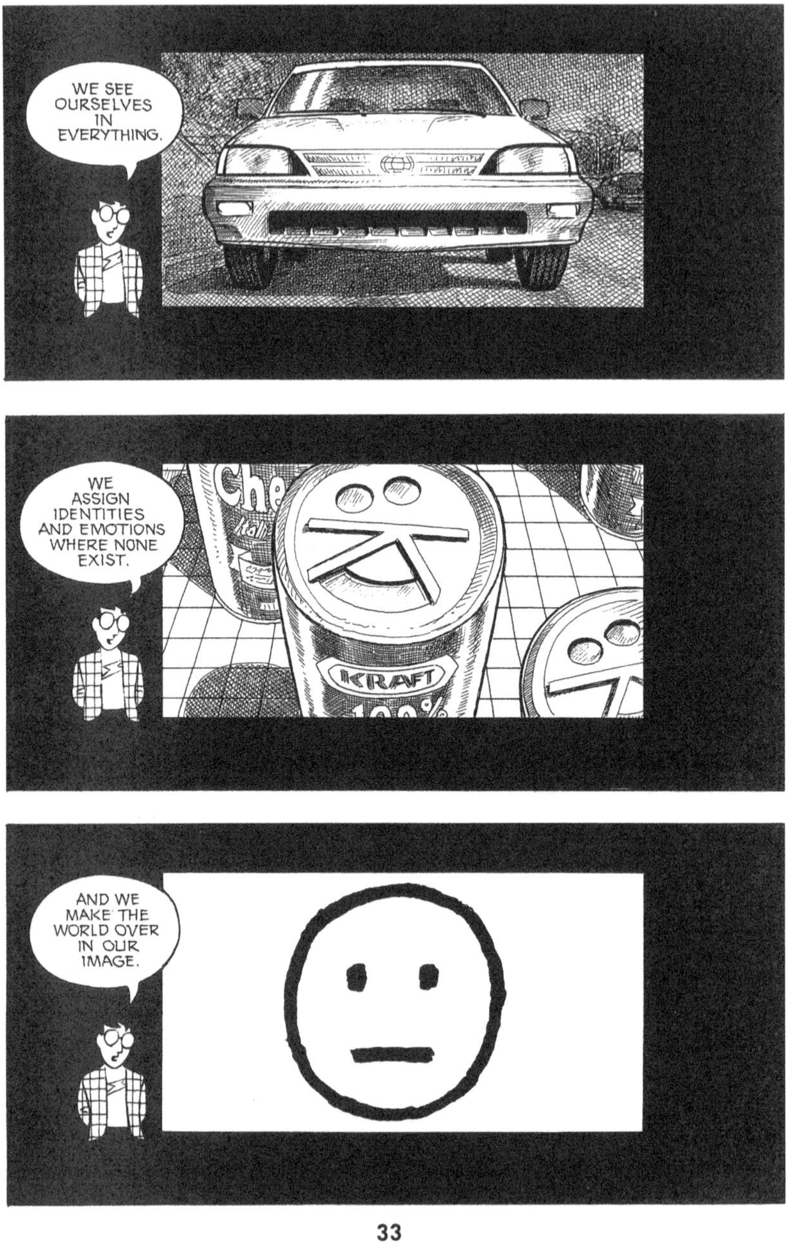
WE SEE OURSELVES IN EVERYTHING.
WE ASSIGN IDENTITIES AND EMOTIONS WHERE NONE EXIST.
KRAFT
AND WE MAKE THE WORLD OVER IN OUR IMAGE.
33

Figure 1.1 Page 33 from *Understanding Comics* by Scott McCloud, Copyright © 1993, 1994 by Scott McCloud. Reprinted by permission of HarperCollins Publishers.

EXIST" (33) not only when reading comics (or watching cartoons like *Beavis and Butt-head*) but when looking at a car's grill or a container of Kraft Parmesan cheese. He elaborates on this premise more fully in Figure 1.2, arguing that "THE CARTOON IS A ***VACUUM*** INTO WHICH OUR ***IDENTITY*** AND ***AWARENESS*** ARE ***PULLED*** . . . AN *EMPTY SHELL* THAT WE INHABIT

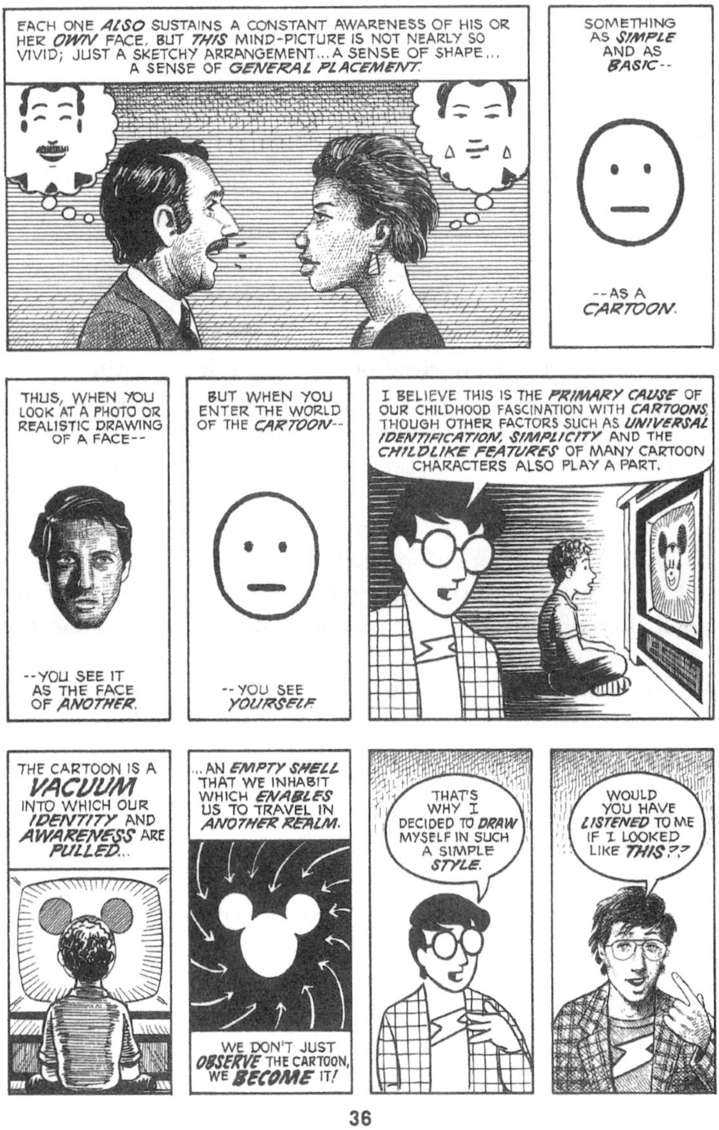
EACH ONE ALSO SUSTAINS A CONSTANT AWARENESS OF HIS OR HER OWN FACE, BUT THIS MIND-PICTURE IS NOT NEARLY SO VIVID; JUST A SKETCHY ARRANGEMENT... A SENSE OF SHAPE... A SENSE OF GENERAL PLACEMENT.
SOMETHING AS SIMPLE AND AS BASIC--
--AS A CARTOON.
THUS, WHEN YOU LOOK AT A PHOTO OR REALISTIC DRAWING OF A FACE--
--YOU SEE IT AS THE FACE OF ANOTHER.
BUT WHEN YOU ENTER THE WORLD OF THE CARTOON--
--YOU SEE YOURSELF.
I BELIEVE THIS IS THE PRIMARY CAUSE OF OUR CHILDHOOD FASCINATION WITH CARTOONS, THOUGH OTHER FACTORS SUCH AS UNIVERSAL IDENTIFICATION, SIMPLICITY AND THE CHILDLIKE FEATURES OF MANY CARTOON CHARACTERS ALSO PLAY A PART.
THE CARTOON IS A VACUUM INTO WHICH OUR IDENTITY AND AWARENESS ARE PULLED...
...AN EMPTY SHELL THAT WE INHABIT WHICH ENABLES US TO TRAVEL IN ANOTHER REALM.
WE DON'T JUST OBSERVE THE CARTOON, WE BECOME IT!
THAT'S WHY I DECIDED TO DRAW MYSELF IN SUCH A SIMPLE STYLE.
WOULD YOU HAVE LISTENED TO ME IF I LOOKED LIKE THIS??
36

Figure 1.2 Page 36 from *Understanding Comics* by Scott McCloud, Copyright © 1993, 1994 by Scott McCloud. Reprinted by permission of HarperCollins Publishers.

WHICH *ENABLES* US TO TRAVEL IN *ANOTHER REALM*. WE DON'T JUST ***OBSERVE*** THE CARTOON, WE ***BECOME*** IT!" (36).

The implication, of course, is that (Q6) our response to slapstick (or any other representation of action) does not vary significantly depending on whether we are responding to real actors who visibly suffer pain in their undeniably physical human bodies (in a live-action film like *Jackass 3D*) or cartoon characters that are only two-dimensional drawings of bodies and therefore can be presumed in some "objective" sense not to suffer pain at all (in a cartoon like *Beavis and Butt-head*). If McCloud is right, we may even empathize *more* strongly with cartoon characters than with live actors; be that as it may, it seems undeniable that the traditional definition of slapstick as funny because we know it's not "real" – we know that no one is feeling real physiological pain – is wrong. It may be that we use that reassurance as a secondary response to quell our empathic participation in the pain, along the same lines as telling ourselves that the monsters in a horror film are just CGI, or that the hero in a thriller has to survive till the end (and triumph over the bad guys), or that a nightmare is just a dream and we can wake up any time we want. But those secondary self-reassurances are responses to our primary empathic identification with the suffering hero – which is primary because that identification, that simulated oneness or sameness (identity) with other people and drawings and trees and so on, is our *only* channel for experiencing the reality of the world. This is the Kantian Copernican Hypothesis: *we do it*. The reality of the world outside our minds is a periperformativity that we build out of sense-data and organize in coherent ways. In Kant that coherence comes from God's Creation – we tend to experience "reality" in similar ways because God created us in His image. In more recent post-Kantian thought, it comes from culture, or, in MH, from "neuroculture," the cultural organization of the nervous system for interpretations of sense-data. The traditional definition of slapstick on which Casper draws is naïve pre-Kantian objectivism, which survives as common sense, of course, but is utterly discredited by modern neuroscience. More on that as we proceed.

1.2.4 Simulacra in Don Quixote

Similar Reading 1 naïveties plague Álvaro Ramírez's (2005) application of Baudrillard's theory of simulacra to *Don Quixote*. His brief is that *Don Quixote*'s pioneering role in the early history of the novel is far more radical even than it has previously been made out to be – that indeed *Don Quixote* is a "postmodern novel":

> Perhaps no other text is better suited for an analysis of this [Baudrillardian] kind than Miguel de Cervantes's *Don Quijote*[4] *de la Mancha*. I believe the orders of simulacra provide a valuable theoretical framework that allows readers to distinguish more clearly the intricate layers of meaning in the novel, thus explaining why *Don Quijote* seems to be the quintessential seventeenth-century novel, yet appears in many respects so radically

> modern, as though it were written only yesterday. In the following pages, my intention is to illustrate the way in which the three orders of simulacra – counterfeit, production, and simulation – permit this new reading of Cervantes's novel. All three orders play a central role in the text. However, for lack of space I will concentrate more fully on simulation, which is the feature of Baudrillard's theory that brings forth the radical elements of *Don Quijote*. As we shall see, this is a novel in which the author deploys a simulated world where the play of signs and images proliferate and become meaningful only in relation to other signs and images, a space where signs create a fictional reality whose referent is another fictional reality. In this simulated process, the external referent to which the sign was initially bound recedes into the background and is finally effaced until all that is left is the play of the sign, that is, the sign perpetuating the sign, the image perpetuating the image. In this respect it can be argued that *Don Quijote* is a postmodern novel.
>
> (82)

I want to return in a moment to note some serious MH dissonances in this reading; for now let me pause and review the three-stage model Baudrillard sets up for simulacra, on which Ramírez relies throughout:

- *First-order simulacra: the counterfeit.* According to Baudrillard, this first order is typical of early modernity: "The sign is no longer fixed; it is liberated and allowed to proliferate, but follows the 'natural law of value.' In other words, imitation of nature becomes the functioning paradigm in organizing the social and the representation of reality" (Ramírez 2005, 83). "Fiction paradoxically has to keep to the truth as much as possible, and this can only be accomplished by pursuing verisimilitude, which is brought about by imitation" (84). Ramírez gives the example of the canon's argument with the curate in Chapter 47 over the desirable qualities of literature: "Whether by sight or imagination[, the canon insists,] a natural simulacrum is created, for what the writer contemplates and recreates in his imagination is nature itself" (84). As examples of such "counterfeits" or first-order simulacra Baudrillard lists "the double, the mirror image, theatrical illusion," and so on (Ramírez is paraphrasing Baudrillard 1981/1994, 98), but "these cannot be exact replicas of the real. A slight difference has to be maintained between the real and its representation; otherwise, the reality principle disappears along with representation itself (*Symbolic Exchange and Death* 54–55)" (84). Note in passing there that, much like Casper, Ramírez too uses the Freudian "reality principle" ontologically, platonically, as a buttress for "the real" and "reality." The key to this order of simulacra in Ramírez's reading of Cervantes is that "appearances create an illusion of reality" (84). One of those illusions of reality, as we shall see in Essay 2 (section 2.3.2), is the pretense that *Don Quixote* is not an original novel written by Cervantes but a literary translation from a Moorish history.

- *Second-order simulacra: the production.* According to Baudrillard, this second order corresponds to late-capitalist mass production, and is typical of the nineteenth century: it "ushers in the era of the replica and serial reproduction by means of machines. Objects and reality are reproduced by technology and in doing so they obliterate the original referent of the sign. Therefore, Baudrillard affirms that at this stage the simulacra 'mask the absence of a basic reality'" (84). This "absence of a basic reality" is the first problematic claim that I want to interrogate in a moment. Ramírez's example of second-order simulacra in *Don Quixote* comes in Chapter 62, when the knight visits the printing shop where the novel he is in is being printed: "The irony of a fictional character visiting the place where he is imprinted into 'life' is worthy of notice. But we should not lose sight of the fact that the author is showing a crucial change in the process of book production. The description of what Don Quijote sees is nothing less than that of an assembly-line production" (84). Ramírez doesn't do much with this scene, except to say that "mass reproduction of images and signs with its concomitant obliteration of referent reality paved the way for the following stage in societal development, to which we turn next" (85).
- *Third-order simulacra: simulation.* According to Baudrillard, societies of first- and second-order simulacra are based on "dissimulation," in which one pretends *not* to have what one actually does have; the move to simulation in the third order is a move to pretending to have what one actually lacks (paraphrasing Baudrillard 1981/1994, 5), and thus to postmodernity. "Therefore," Ramírez glosses Baudrillard (1981/1994, 12), "in postmodern societies and their representations we find a 'transition from signs which dissimulate something to signs which dissimulate that there is nothing'" (85). This to my mind is the most problematic claim of all. What is most telling in that application, to my mind, is that every single passage and tendency Ramírez takes from the novel as an illustration of third-order simulacra in fact illustrates first-order simulacra, and so seems far more modern than postmodern; the best examples of the novel's "postmodernity" are moments over which Ramírez passes quickly, like this "irony" of Don Quixote touring the printing shop "where he is imprinted into 'life.'" He does not deal at all with the postmodern play with the illusion of reality created by the found-translation frame narrative, and the fact that the "translator" of that supposed Moorish "source text" begins to argue with its "author" in Part II, because the "translator" finds the history unrealistic.

Ramírez notes, for example, that Dulcinea is a puzzle to Sancho Panza – "the referent of Dulcinea, to whom the name refers, is to some degree ambiguous" (85) – until the moment when Don Quixote confesses that she is actually Aldonza Lorenzo, after which Sancho thinks that Dulcinea is an invented name for a real woman. This, Ramírez notes, would be a "first order simulacrum; there is still a presence behind signs, even though they may be masked over to create illusions" (85). But in fact Don Quixote also tells Sancho that "he is dissimulating and that there is nothing behind the sign," making "Dulcinea" a presence to Sancho and an absence to the knight. As Ramírez explains:

> But now the readers, unlike Sancho, realize Don Quijote is confessing a more sinister truth: there is nothing behind the image of his lady. She is, however, not a figment of the knight's imagination, which would be the narrator's way of explaining the situation. He makes it clear to his squire that Dulcinea does not refer to any specific woman they know and that there need not be any referent whatsoever. For Don Quijote, she is an unbound sign, a sign without a referent in the "real world." As a consequence, she cannot be described in such terms, but in terms of what Baudrillard calls "structural value." In other words, Dulcinea cannot be defined by referring to some external reality; she can only be defined as a sign in relation to other signs; las Dianas, las Amariles, las Galateas, etc., signs that do not have any "real" referent behind them, but who exist only by virtue of other signs.
>
> (85)

Obviously Don Quixote "perceives or constructs reality in a manner that needs explanation, and it is precisely this perception or reinvention of reality that puts him at odds with other characters in the novel" (86); this is the feature that has led most readers to attribute some form of insanity to him.

Ramírez, however, suggests that his "insanity" can be read differently, as the "situation . . . of a person slipping in and out of different levels of simulacra" (86). Note the phrasing there: Don Quixote is in a "situation"; there are these "different levels of simulacra"; and his "situation" is one of "slipping in and out" of those levels. The fulcral question is: *where are* those "levels of simulacra"? If they are in his mind only, if they are like fugue states, then he is probably insane; or, if they are in the novel only, if the ontological tensions Ramírez detects are fictional, they are what Baudrillard would call first-order simulacra: counterfeits. That reading would of course complicate Baudrillard in interesting ways, rendering simulacra recursive: a fictional first-order simulation of third-order simulacra would be a counterfeit virtuality. But it seems to me that this is not what Ramírez is claiming. As he articulates Don Quixote's "situation," the three Baudrillardian levels or orders of simulacra in and out of which he keeps slipping would appear to be *accurate depictions of real-world states of social organization* – the first order at work in the Spanish Golden Age, the real world in which Cervantes wrote, the second order kicking in some time in the nineteenth century, the third order after World War II – and therefore that Don Quixote is not crazy but *ahead of his time*. As Ramírez continues:

> At times he appears to be functioning within the logic of the first order simulacrum, dissimulating not having something. Since the rest of the characters in the novel function within this level, it is at these moments that Don Quijote is perceived by them to be in a *cuerdo* [sane] state of mind. At other times, however, he dissimulates that there is nothing behind signs, and it is at these precise moments that Don Quijote is deemed a madman.

> *Don Quijote*, then, is a novel where we find the central character negotiating his way through a simulated world, a world where the organization of social reality and its representation has undergone a critical change. In Baudrillardean terms, Don Quijote is in the reign of simulation where the play of the sign is the logic of societal construction.
>
> (86)

The generous way to read this is to understand "the organization of social reality and its representation" and "the logic of societal construction" as that system of artifice that we call "culture," or, in Charles Levin's (1996, 196) words, a "map": "Simulation has, in essence, always been like this, at least so far as social life is concerned; for society has never been anything else but a map, or more truthfully, a collection of maps, that we gradually learn to read." All culture, as I paraphrased Levin earlier, is simulation.

But it seems to me that there are two quite serious problems with that reading.

Problem 1. Don Quixote is apparently the only human being in his society that reads that cultural "map" as he does. Where then is the "map"? "In" society, "in" the "organization of social reality"? If so, why do the others not read it as Don Quixote does? If insanity is defined pragmatically as the inability to conform to current social norms, then the map is only in Don Quixote's head, and he *is* insane. Ramírez's insistence that he is not insane would seem to require, therefore, that postmodernity be a kind of parallel universe that hovers just out of reach of the other characters in the novel but is available to Don Quixote, and that his ability to access that universe of simulacra bespeaks some kind of superior-species genius on his part; but what kind of science-fiction vision is that? Ramírez nowhere even hints at how what Levin calls this Baudrillardian "cultural metaphysics" might work in the novel – how the novel might be *realistically* describing the clash between two social orders, the "modern" seventeenth-century order of counterfeits and the "postmodern" late twentieth-century order of simulacra – let alone how Don Quixote might be imagined as "slipping in and out" of that latter. Perhaps he has time-traveled back into 1605 from the future, like Hank Morgan in Twain's *A Connecticut Yankee in King Arthur's Court* (1889)? (In fact, Ramírez's Baudrillardian reading might work far better with Twain's novel: the Yankee's quixotic grandiosity/megalomania is fed by a kind of proto-postmodern advertising spin on "reality" that is remarkably reminiscent of Baudrillard's third order of simulacra, and the science-fiction time-travel premise would solve the problem of the metaphysical slippage Ramírez posits between first- and third-order simulacra in *Don Quixote*.)

Problem 2. P1 poses a conundrum only if Don Quixote is a real person in our real world – which, of course, ironically enough, would serve to restabilize Ramírez's Baudrillardian/postmodern destabilization of signs-of-reality. To stand as "proof" that Baudrillard is right about the postmodern impossibility of reality, Ramírez's Don Quixote has to be a *real postmodernist* in 1605. Why? Because if he is just a character in a novel, and specifically a character in a novel whose author is playing fast and loose with the fictional supports that prop up our sense of reality, then anything is possible. Then Don Quixote could fly to the moon, or turn into a fish. Then nothing that happens to him proves anything about the reality outside the novel – let alone about "our" "postmodern" "(hyper)reality," to which Baudrillard's theory of simulacra supposedly applies. (Nothing that happens to Don Quixote proves anything about the validity or invalidity of Baudrillard's theory of our cultural reality, certainly.) Then any application of that theory to Cervantes's novel, or any novel, is an *analogy*. Then Ramírez's idea becomes that *Don Quixote* can be *interpreted* along Baudrillardian lines – that Baudrillard offers an interesting model that, completely independently of Ramírez's claims about its "truth-value" as an account of postmodern culture, can be forcibly *adapted* to the study of Cervantes. Then, not to put too fine a point on it, Ramírez's interpretation of the novel is at best merely *ingenious* – which is to say, a good way to get an article published.

Unfortunately, Ramírez's reading of the novel is not particularly ingenious. For one thing, everything he describes as postmodern simulation collapses back into early modern counterfeiting, the creation of clever illusions of reality – something we already knew about not only *Don Quixote* but every other great novel as well. Dulcinea has no real-world referent? She is a character in a novel whose name *does not refer to a real human being in her author's world*? The obvious reason why that example seems so banal is that the same is true of every character in every modern novel, based on the "counterfeiting" (creating an illusion) of reality, the definitive pretense that the fictional narrative actually happened to real people in our world.[5] This sort of fictionalization of reality, which is constitutive of the modern novel as a realistic genre (see section 2.3.1), is really only "problematic" for real people who invent or "confabulate" realities *not accepted* by anyone around them. And, as we'll see in section 1.3, this sort of confabulation is far more common in "real life" than commonsensical constructions of "real life" would have us believe.

Indeed, as I began to suggest above, one of the discoveries Michael S. Gazzaniga (1989; 1998, passim; 2005/2006, 148–51; 2008/2009, 294–308; 2011, 96–97; 2015, 149–53) and Joseph LeDoux (2010, 92–94; 2015, 34) found in their split-brain studies was that confabulation, or what they called "the interpreter," is one of the main functions of the left brain[6] in normals:

> So when it comes to the interpreter, facts are cool, but not necessary. The left brain uses whatever is at hand and ad libs the rest. The first makes-sense explanation will do. It looks for cause and effect and creates order out of the chaos of inputs that have been presented to it by all the other processes spewing out information. This is what our brain does all day long: It takes input from various areas of our brain and from the environment and synthesizes it into a story that makes sense.
>
> (Gazzaniga 2015, 153)

Gazzaniga (2008/2009, 300; 2011, 96–97) pauses here and there to connect "the interpreter" to Capgras, but his main point is that this is something we all do, all the time – and indeed that this is the origin of "the self," our attempts to impose a narrativized sense of coherent control onto all the unfathomable things we do automatically. The key to "normality" is the normativization of confabulation/interpretation – bringing it into line with group norms. Not that we "normals" always manage to do that: we very often impose ad hoc explanations on our own actions and what is going on around us that strike the people around us as odd. All we really need is to display a willingness to adjust to group norms, and relatively regular success at that. (I will be suggesting the operation of a "collective interpreter" below, in section 1.4.)

Five quick notes to Ramírez on Don Quixote on Dulcinea:

Note 1. For real-world reference to work for a female name (or for the word "woman," or *mujer*) we don't need a single specific woman by that name; we only need a *class* of referents, women. As long as we know that Dulcinea refers to "some woman," and we know what is commonly meant by "some woman," the name has a real-world referent. The fact that there is no woman *in the novel* (let alone in real life) to whom the name Dulcinea refers is therefore an example of first-order rather than third-order simulacra.

Note 2. The (N1) problem of an absent referent for a name like Dulcinea is really only a problem when someone claims that that name refers to a real person and we begin to suspect that it doesn't – that the person is lying, or confabulating, or crazy. And this mostly applies to real people – and to fictional characters, if at all, as first-order "counterfeits" of real people.

Note 3. Baudrillard is not writing about this sort of (N2) absent-referent confabulation *in individuals:* by third-order simulacra he means that signs no longer refer to real things for *whole societies.* If Don Quixote is the only person in his society to whom the ostensible absence of referents applies (an interpretation option obviated by N1), the operative interpretation has to be insanity, not Baudrillardian simulation.

Note 4. Ramírez's denial of (N2) Don Quixote's insanity by reference to the absence of a Dulcinea-referent, and thereby his insistence that third-order simulacra are at work in the novel, collapses under the weight of (N1) and (N3).

Note 5. (N1-4) emphatically do not mean that we are forced to diagnose Don Quixote as insane. He is, after all, not a real person. Any number of other interpretations could be placed on his behavior (and of course have been). All that those points mean in the end is that Ramírez's Baudrillardian interpretation is a non-starter.

Or, in another of Ramírez's load-bearing examples: Don Quixote's apparent "insanity," he informs us, is inspired by his reading of romantic adventure books, not by anything in the social reality around him. That this is another banal example should be instantly obvious, given the fact that the view of Don Quixote that Ramírez highlights is the narrator's reading of him, and so the first thing that all readers notice. Ramírez, however, wants to spin the knight's (parodic) adherence to the code of chivalry as more evidence of third-order Baudrillardian simulation:

> Of course, he is deemed a madman by the [other characters,] for they cannot understand the world of signs which the code deploys and which serves as the organizing paradigm for the knight. For it is obvious that Don Quijote does not see people per se at the inn; he sees only signs that are meaningful to him in relation to others signs known through the code, which he has acquired through his reading of novels of chivalry. For example, the innkeeper is severed from the world of referents and gains meaning in relation to other fictional innkeepers (that is, the *castellanos*) found in chivalric literature. This is also the case with the prostitutes; they are transformed by the code into simulated women: female entities organized by a signifying process that refers only to itself, not to the real.
>
> (86)

Levin might say *yes, but then that's true of all culture;* my point here is that it's even more patently true of all fiction. Again, as in Casper's reading of *Jackass 3D,* the theoretical brick wall into which Ramírez keeps crashing is the stupid binary Baudrillard nominally sets up between (1) simple ontological "reality" and (2) reality-banishing self-referential "simulation." Simulation is a "signifying process that refers only to [2] itself, not to [1] the real." Only those two choices. No middle ground, such as the one I numbered above as (2′) Kantian "simulated" reality, simulation as what Baudrillard calls "realized" or "materialized" reality, signs that *feel real.* The fictional extreme that for Ramírez "refers only to itself, not to the real," is basically (3′) unrealized simulations, simulacra that don't feel like reality – but because it stands in no productive tension with (2′) "realized" or "materialized" reality, it has nowhere to go. It can perform no useful epistemological work. All it can do is "prove" Baudrillard "right." By contrast, Cervantes sending Don Quixote into the printing shop where the novel that is creating him is being printed *is* doing epistemological work. He is cleverly mixing (2′) the realistic *counterfeiting* of reality (our identificatory sense that Don Quixote is a real person) with (3′) the anti-realistic *undermining* of that counterfeit (our sense that Don Quixote is an impossible epistemological loop from which there is no realistic escape), in order to keep us epistemologically off balance, open to constructivist/periperformativist surprise. The playful tug-o'-war Cervantes sets up in the novel is between (2′) and (3′); the (1′) naively objectified ontological reality to which the novel's "signifying process" doesn't refer is a complete irrelevancy, a red herring that has no place at all in the discussion.

I will be exploring the complexity of fiction more trenchantly as we proceed, in sections 1.3.1 and 2.3; for now suffice it to say that what is "postmodern" about *Don Quixote* is that Cervantes weaves (3′) anti-realistic fictions in amongst his (2′) realistic counterfeits in order to suggest that everything outside the novel as well that we think of as ~~(1′) stable ontological reality~~ *is* a (2′) realistic counterfeit, which *feels* solidly real but can be (3′) disastrously undone more easily than we think. (Or at least that's how I am inclined to read *Don Quixote* in an essay organized around the Capgras delusion.)

The literal, face-value Reading 1 of Baudrillard on simulacra collapses into absurdity quickly enough when it is applied to a contemporary text like *Jackass 3D;* its silliness is even more painfully obvious when it is applied to a text written three and a half centuries before Baudrillard claims "reality" was subsumed into the virtual and became "no longer possible." Still, like Casper's Baudrillardian reading of *Jackass 3D,* Ramírez's Baudrillardian reading of *Don Quixote* is a useful kind of MH test-case for metaphysical claims about the "impossibility" of reality.

1.3 Capgras fictions 3: back to *The Echo Maker*

What makes *The Echo Maker* an even more useful MH test-case is not only that it is explicitly and even obsessively grounded in the neurological research on Capgras and other misidentification syndromes, the mirror neurons, empathy, and so on, but also that it is focused on *confabulation* as the "natural" "human" reaction of sufferers from the Capgras delusion and other misidentification syndromes to the obvious gaps in their picture of the world, relative to the neurocultural constructions shared/(peri)performed by everyone else in their world. And of course another word for confabulation is *fiction:* like Cervantes, Powers too is endlessly fascinated by the complex relationship between reality and fiction, and endlessly inclined to play with that complexity.

1.3.1 Fiction

Indeed, as Powers (2006) revealed in an online roundtable on *The Echo Maker* shortly after the novel was released, fiction was his central theme in the novel – or rather, perhaps, since this is fiction-as-the-theme-of-a-fiction, *metafiction:* "to put forward, at the same time, a glimpse of the solid, continuous, stable, perfect story we try to fashion about the world and about ourselves, while at the same time to lift the rug and glimpse the amorphous, improvised, messy, crack-strewn, gaping thing underneath all that narration."

His aim, in other words, like Cervantes's four centuries earlier, was simultaneously to (2′) *tell* and to (3′) *undermine* a traditional realistic narrative. We love traditional realistic storytelling, even when it is about monsters and witches and gods and demons and Jedis and time travel and so on, because it seems to confirm what we all work so hard (though unconsciously) to achieve: a coherent self in a coherent world. Existential coherence. Meaning. The novel's cognitive neurologist, Dr. Gerald Weber, denies early on that he is writing "fiction" (235–36) and resists being called a "writer" (286) – he is a "scientist," committed to *truth* – but as his fragile professional persona crumbles, he is increasingly forced to come to terms with the continuity between the neurological deficits he studies and his own state of mind/being, until by the end we find him reflecting on "his neurological novelistic books" (455). In his self-congratulatory persona as a celebrity author of popular books on neurology, which he and his wife Sylvie have humorously dubbed Famous Gerald, he attributes that impulse to confabulate a coherent world to the poor souls about whose brain deficits he writes; but Powers's narrator, when focalized on Weber, digs out of his deepest self-(pre-)awareness a deeper truth:

> *Personal confabulation,* the neurologist [Todd E.] Feinberg [b. 1952] called it. A story to link the shifting self back to the senseless facts. Reason was not impaired here; logic still worked on any other topic but this. Only the map of the body, the *feel* of it, had been fractured. And logic was not above redistributing its own indisputable parts in order to make a stubborn sense of wholeness true again. Lying in his rented room at 2:00 a.m., Weber could almost feel the fact in the limbs he lay numbering: a single, solid fiction always beat the truth of our scattering.
>
> (208)

All along here in Part 2, on his first visit to Kearney, he keeps getting intimations of the disintegration that lies in store for him: "Now, as he lay miles from sleep, he tried to decide whether he'd lied about not knowing it, or had just forgotten" (187); "For every story he gave Sylvie, she told him one back. But by the next morning, he felt as if he'd invented all of hers" (206). "We were not one, continuous, indivisible whole" – this is the refrain of his popular books on neurology – "but instead, hundreds of separate subsystems, with changes in any one sufficient to disperse the provisional confederation into unrecognizable new countries" (216). Or, as he rather glibly tells his editor on the next page, "we all play ourselves" (217); the only problem is that even as he says it he is already beginning to forget his lines, to forget what character he's supposed to be playing, indeed to forget what play he's in, and to be booed off the stage by an increasingly hostile audience. Having read – and obsessively reread – a bad review of his new book, he heads off on vacation to Italy with his wife, leaving the review at home, but "by the time they got to LaGuardia, he'd rewritten it in his head. He could no longer tell what he actually remembered from the evaluation and what he was fabricating" (285). The fact that he *knows* that we do this, and indeed that he has made his reputation as both a neuroscientist and as a popular science writer on that knowledge, does not prepare him for the "derealization and depersonalization" that result when his own confabulatory continuity begins to fail, leaving *him too* susceptible to "misidentification – the whole continuum of Capgras-like phenomena, phenomena that Weber had witnessed his whole life without quite noticing" (483). "It struck him that he'd invented Nebraska," the narrator reports. "The whole story: some foray into a mixed, experimental genre, a morality play masquerading as journalism. He had no reliable memory of anything that had happened there" (465). "Lying, denying, repressing, confabulating: these weren't pathologies. They were the signature of awareness, trying to stay intact. What was truth, compared to survival?" (483).

What is interesting about Weber's disintegration is not so much the irony of the neurologist experiencing what he has so famously and lucratively described in others, but the very ordinariness of his collapse. Loss of reputation is almost always devastating to us. Like his wife Sylvie, we too like to think that we are (ideally) strong, autonomous beings, gods and goddesses, individuals and individualists who care nothing for public opinion; but that is just wishful thinking. We all have recurring moments of panic when "reality" doesn't line up as neatly as we would like it to; we are all susceptible to self-doubt, self-recrimination, anxiety, depression, and other forms of collapse when our personality card castles blow over, or even when they ruffle slightly in a light breeze. The intensity with which this disintegration affects most of the characters in Powers's novel makes the narrative seem bleak; but he is really only intensifying our normal state of being just enough for us to notice it. Normally we are quite adept at hiding the precarity of our meaning-fortresses from others and ourselves.

Barbara Gillespie, with whom Weber has a brief sexual encounter at the end, tries to jolly him out of his funk:

> She leaned in and lifted his chin. "Listen to me. They're no one. They have no power over you."
>
> It took him a moment to identify *them:* the court of public opinion. "Clearly they do," he said. More power over him than he had over himself. The human cortex had first evolved by way of navigating intricate social rank. Half of cognition, the chief selection pressure now in play: the herd in the head.
>
> And shaped for it by the power of *them,* her brain read his. "What do you care about that monkey-troop stuff? Grooming and jockeying. Nothing matters but your own sense of work."
>
> (409)

Ironically, this is a replay of a very recent previous conversation in which they play the opposite roles, Weber denying that he cares about what others think of him, Barbara gently pointing out that he obviously does:

> She looked up, the pupils of her hazel eyes as large as the spots on a masquerading moth. They knew him. "It's all still about pecking order with humans, isn't it? Even when the ranking is imaginary."
>
> "Not a contest I have much interest in."
>
> She reared back, that same look of amused skepticism she'd just given Mark. "Of course you have interest. This book is you. The hunters are circling. Nothing imaginary there. What are you going to do, roll over and die?"
>
> (402)

We teeter constantly on the fulcrum between those two attitudes: between admitting and denying the power the crowd has over our self-esteem, our self-image, our identity. Dr. Weber is no less like the rest of us for being a neurologist. He knows far more about all of us than all of us do, but just as little about himself – and his knowledge cannot protect himself from the churning incoherence to which we all are prone.

The other characters provide multiple examples of this ordinary disruption of meaning-making as well:

- Karin desperately needs to be affirmed, and in search of that affirmation will become whomever she's with; as a result, her commitment to saving her brother leaves her violently susceptible to breakdown when for one entire year he keeps relentlessly insisting that she is not herself, that she is an impostor, trained by the government to spy on him. As she tells Robert Karsh, "He's decided I'm never going to be me again. And after half a year? He's right" (371).

- What Daniel wants from meditation is "Nothing!" Which does not mean that he doesn't want anything – that he's fine the way he is. He means "I want it to help me want nothing. . . . It makes me more . . . an object to myself. Disidentified" (92). His confabulatory desideratum is Nirvana – or, less mystically, the vegetative state of a tree. As Weber articulates a similar self-protective strategy, late in the novel: "*The self is a burning house; get out while you can*" (514).
- Weber's daughter Jess is diabetic, and has bought an insulin pump, but it doesn't always work: "Zuul still inhabits me from time to time. Capricious little fiend. Came and took me over in the middle of the night last week. First time in a long time. Scared the crap out of both of us" (277).
- Nor is it only the human population that faces this potential collapse: at one point Weber hears a bird crash into the window, "a large male cardinal who, for the last two weeks, had been attacking his reflection in the nook window, thinking himself an intruder on his own territory" (452). Attack as a fictional strategy.

1.3.2 The human brain as ecosystem

As in (Q4a) Baudrillard's interview remarks on our desperate reactions to the "terror of illusion," however, there would appear to be an individualizing impetus to many of these stories. Each of us, the novel repeatedly seems to suggest, struggles as an individual against the forces of disorder arrayed in the worlds both outside and inside our brains. The sense-data fed us by the world are complex and conflicting; and our brain's ability to sift through them and impose coherent "neurocultural" order is shaky, unreliable. It's each individual against the world, and that individual's only ally in the unremitting skirmish, it seems, is his or her klugey nervous system. That nervous system, and the self it mobilizes (see Damasio 2010), is multiple, to be sure – "The self was a mob, a drifting, improvised posse" (453) – but to the outside world, that self is still only one. And even from the inside, this mob metaphor makes it seem as if the self has no allies on the outside. "We think we access our own states," Weber tells his undergraduate students; "everything in neurology tells us we do not. We think of ourselves as a unified, sovereign nation. Neurology suggests that we are a blind head of state, barricaded in the presidential suite, listening only to handpicked advisors as the country reels through ad hoc mobilizations . . ." (460). There is nothing in that passage to suggest that the "advisors" are other people. They too are part of the mob that is the self, that "drifting, improvised posse" – an image that Powers admits to Stephen J. Burn he borrowed from Daniel Dennett's (1991) pandemonium model of consciousness.[7] The "advisors" are all internal "demons." They're all inside each individual brain.

In a trenchant ecological reading of the novel, Nicola Brindley (2012, 8) places particular stress on the parallels Powers draws between the brain and any ecosystem out in the world:

> Mark is seen to reconstruct his sense of selfhood in a way which supports comparisons between the structure of the brain and that of an ecosystem: rather than a single, indivisible "self" he is seen as multiple and in process, described as "piecing himself back together" [21]. While lying in his hospital bed he claims that "his parts came back to him [. . .] his body, countless microscopic creatures banded together in need." Continuing the biological analogy, Mark's pre-conscious brain is compared to "a whale in the street [. . . a] beached creature blocks long", while his interacting neurons appear as "tiny land-born lives" which drift back, gradually "reclaiming their crushed homes" [52–53]. Dr. Weber, the book's cognitive neurologist, makes clear the proposed link between human brain-function and the kinds of biological organisation found elsewhere in the natural world by suggesting that in regard to brain function, humans are "like coral reefs [. . .] complex yet fragile ecosystems" [235].

She also cites Charles B. Harris (2008, 232) on Powers's representation of the human brain as "a networked ecology that mirrors the networked ecology of all life, including birds, the core parts of whose brains are still contained in our own" (quoted in Brindley 2012, 10).[8] This is obviously a far more ecological metaphor than the mob and the blind head of state and his or her advisors – but it is structurally isomorphic with those political metaphors, in the sense of imagining the individual as internally multiple but unconnected to others. The brain-as-ecosystem and self-as-mob tropes are certainly more complex than what we might call, adapting Judith Butler (1991), Sylvie's "panicked individualism"[9]: in trying to get her husband to ignore the critics who are attacking his latest book, she repeatedly tells him that "consensus was the delusion" (341), and that "public judgment is nothing but shared schizophrenia" (451). Sylvie's implicit model is Lockean rationalism, or the Victorian triumphalism of William Ernest Henley's "Invictus": "I am the master of my fate: / I am the captain of my soul." But the self-as-mob or brain-as-ecosystem trope is only *inwardly* more complex than Henley's self-as-captain: less well protected against collapse, because less unified, less perfectly subordinated to a chain of command. Outwardly, in its engagement with the world outside the skull, it is basically the same.

For the most part, the novel's conception of the world outside the skull is equally multiple:

> Somehow, when he wasn't looking, private thought gave way to perpetual group ratings. The age of personal reflection was over. From now on, everything would be haggled over in public feedback brawls. Call-in radio, focus groups every time anyone moved. Leo Tolstoy: 4.1. Charles Darwin: 3.0.

And yet, every time he logged off, nauseated by the relentless assessments, he found himself immediately wanting to check again, to see if the next response might erase the last mindless dismissal. He compared his numbers to those of other writers he was lumped with. Was he alone in this backlash? Who was the moment's darling? Which of his colleagues had also fallen? How did the public manage to bank and wheel in such perfect synchrony, as if on signal?

(342–43)

The analogy fleshed forth in "bank and wheel in such perfect synchrony," obviously, is between "the public" and a flock of birds. "The brain" is one ecosystem; "the public" is another. The two interact, but are also structurally similar. If the public is a mob, the brain is another. If the brain is a mob, the public is another.

The two questions I want to pose to this model are: [Q7] is there any sense in which these two analogical mobs are *the same mob,* and, if so, [Q8] *how do they rule* as that same mob? Clearly, if the brain and the public are both ecosystems that operate under similar homeostatic conditions, or, to put that less politely, mobs that rule with the same kind of klugey pandemonium *tendencies* toward order, that's cute, and clever, and all, but not particularly useful in imagining a *sociology* of all this – and particularly a sociological or socioecological way forward. If the two mobs/ecosystems communicate but are not part of the same communication ecosystem, then things really are bleak.

As it happens, Powers does provide an answer to (Q7), though it comes very late in the novel, which perhaps makes it easy to miss. The answer lies in the mirror-neuron system:

A part of the brain that did physical things was being cannibalized for making imaginary representations. Science had at last laid bare the neurological basis of empathy: brain maps, mapping other mapping brains. One human wit quickly labeled the find *monkey-see monkey-do* neurons, and all others followed suit. Imaging and EEG soon revealed that humans, too, were crawling with mirror neurons. Images of moving muscles made symbolic muscles move, and muscles in symbol moved muscle tissue.

(449)

It's not just "the herd in the head" (409), in other words; it's the herd that *merges* heads. Or again:

What-if mimicking what-is; simulations simulating simulations. When his Jess was not yet a month old, he could get her to stick out her tongue just by sticking out his tongue at her. No counting the miracles involved. She had to locate his tongue relative to his body, then somehow map his parts onto the feel of hers, find and order a tongue she could not even see, could not even know about. And she did all this at the mere sight of him, this infant who had been taught nothing. Where was the end of his self, the start of hers?

> The self bled out, the work of mirror neurons, empathy circuits, selected for and preserved through many species for their obscure survival value.
>
> (485)

It's not just that the self is a mob and the public is a mob; because of the communicative action of those "empathy circuits," the boundaries between the self and the public are porous:

> To be awake and know: already awful. To be awake, know, and *remember:* unbearable. Against the triple curse, Weber could make out only one consolation. Some part of us could model some other modeler. And out of that simple loop came all love and culture, the ridiculous overflow of gifts, each one a frantic proof that *I* was not it. . . . We had no home, no whole to come back to. The self spread thin on everything it looked at, changed by every ray of the changing light. But if nothing inside was ever fully us, at least some part of us was loose, in the run of others, trading in all else. Someone else's circuits circled through us.
>
> (486)

All love and all culture are a matter of "someone else's circuits circl[ing] through us." The bleak message that Margaret Atwood extracts from the hitches in Karin's Dorothy-like return home to Kearney – that "'there's no place like home' has taken on a modern, ominous meaning: there is, literally, no trustworthy home" – here becomes a transition to a larger, more hopeful view in which the earth is our home, all nature is our home, the circling of other people's circuits and other animals' circuits and trees' and grasses' circuits and rivers' and mountains' circuits through us is our home. The "no home, no whole" that we have to come back to is a no-self as an all-self. Powers's Weber-focalized narrator makes the implications of this observation very clear in noting on that same page that "emotions moved the muscles, but merely moving the muscles made emotions. Those with damage to the insula could no longer do the imitative, integrated mapping of body-states necessary to read or adopt someone else's muscles. Then the community of self collapsed into one" (486). The *default* state of "the community of self" is societal, communal, collectivized, part of "the public"; it is only when the insula is damaged that we are unable to map and simulate other people's body states empathically, so that the self-mob is *isolated* from the public-mob. A presumption of something like that isolation seems to be the model Powers is working from throughout most of the novel; indeed he seems to adumbrate it again in the midst of this late exploration of the mirror neurons' "empathy circuits," when his Weber-focalized narrator notes, humbly, that "neurology would never grasp from without a thing that existed only deep in the impenetrable inside" (462). I suggest, however, that by "neurology" there he does not mean "the brain" or "the nervous system"; he cannot even mean the science that discovered and theorized the mirror neurons and their "empathy circuits," which obviously do grasp a thing from without *as* if it were on the inside. He must mean neurology as an objectivist/empiricist science, neurology as bounded by five centuries of "scientific method" – neurology as a principled *retreat* from connection. The adjective "impenetrable" still poses an obstacle to a mirror-neuron reading of the passage, though; to get to the neural connectivity that Powers begins to explore at the end of Part 4, we would have to revise his wording along the lines of "neurology would never grasp from *without* a thing that existed only deep in an inside taken to be impenetrable; it could only grasp it from *within*."

But love and culture are not just neural connectivity – "the extended mind"[10] – between what Andy Clark (2004, 4) calls "skinbags." They are neuroculturally *organized* channels and trajectories of neural connectivity. Cranes remember their ancestral flight paths and patterns through some sort of neural connectivity – but the mirror neurons that effect that connectivity are not enough to explain their shared memory. They need *regulatory* connectivity. Love is regulatory. Culture is regulatory. Mob rule is regulatory. Mob rule is the nightmarish kind of collectivity typically invoked by panicked individualists like Sylvie Weber – this is what happens if we don't stand firmly for our inner-directedness, for the isolated self! – but it is not random violence: it is *organized* violence. What makes mob rule so frightening is that it is not organized rationally, through calm discussion and negotiation: the regulatory forces that organize it operate mostly unconsciously, driven by animal fears that are intensified in the cauldron of mirror-neuron resonance. But it too is a kind of culture. In fact it is quite reasonable to describe what we often derogate as a "love fest" in mob-rule terms: when a new couple, or even a whole group, is possessed by a shared unconscious regulatory impetus to express "mindless" (affect-driven) love and support for each other, the result is a kind of benign mob.

The fact that Powers does not essay an answer to (Q8), *how* the larger mob or ecosystem that includes the brain/self rules or regulates its environment, is unfortunate for the rather pat ending of his novel[11] – but fortunate for my purposes here, because I have devoted the last ten years of my work to developing an answer.

1.4 Conclusion: icosis

For an ingress to that answer, let us return again to Karin Schluter's narrator-reported musing that "the whole race suffered from Capgras. Those birds danced like our next of kin, looked like our next of kin, called and willed and parented and taught and navigated all just like our blood relations. Half their parts were still ours. Yet humans waved them off: *impostors*" (439). As I began to suggest earlier, the problem with this equation is that, as Powers demonstrates over and over in the novel, there is no reliable "realistic" or "empirical" touchstone against which the "reality" of someone's relatedness can be measured. It would be easy enough to simulate the cranes' human-relatedness, say in an animatronic show at Disney World, where cranes "danced like our next of kin, looked like our next of kin, called and willed and parented and taught and navigated all just like our blood relations." In fact I would predict that hundreds of thousands of visitors to the park every year would experience a strong sense of relatedness to those cranes, because they're so *cute,* so *adorable,* so *human,* and so on. The fact that the cranes would not be "real," alive, that they would be robots programmed to *look* and *act* like real cranes, would not only not prevent audiences at the shows from relating emotionally to them; it might even *enhance* their family identification. By simplifying and intensifying our identificatory processes, art tends to feel *more* real than reality. As we shall see in Essay 3 (section 3.3.1), in fact, that was the modernist impetus behind the device of estrangement *(ostranenie, Verfremdung),* Viktor Shklovsky's claim that art "makes the stone stony."[12]

The difference between the "craziness" of Mark insisting that Karin is not related to him and the "craziness" of us insisting that cranes are not related to us is that the group of people who know both Mark and Karin know in the aggregate that Karin is Mark's sister, and the group of people who know both humans and cranes know in the aggregate that we are not related. Pragmatically speaking – to return to the question of Don Quixote's possible insanity in section 1.2.4 – that means that Mark is crazy to exclude Karin from his family and we are *not* crazy to exclude cranes from our family. That sounds flippant, perhaps; surely the seriousness of the ecological tsunami human practices are bringing down upon half of the world's species and more than half of the world's habitats warrants a more responsible answer to the question Karin poses about our relatedness to cranes and other wildlife?

The fact is, however, that the only approach that could "save" us from such apparent flippancy would be a naïvely binary pre-Kantian objectivism: there is *real* relatedness and there is *simulated* relatedness; there is *real* pain and suffering and there is *simulated* pain and suffering. And so on. Humans and cranes are either *really* related or our relatedness is only an activist simulacrum, useful for bringing political pressure to bear on polluters and consumers and development councils and chambers of commerce, etc. A strong political case can be made for that objectivism, of course – it is politically expedient to be able to claim that humans and cranes are *really* and *truly* related – but as Richard Powers knows all too well, the traditional Western philosophical loyalty to that ancient Platonizing/Christianizing/scientizing objectivism, increasingly beleaguered but far from overpowered in the two-plus centuries since Kant, has suffered what would appear to be a fatal blow from brain science. Everything we know about the brain makes it clear that nothing we believe about our access to "objective" "reality" is true:

> None of the bizarre neurological insights acquired over the course of his professional life unsettled him more than this simplest one: baseline experience was simply wrong. Our sense of physical embodiment did not come from the body itself. Several layers of brain stood in between, cobbling up from raw signals the reassuring illusion of solidity. . . .
>
> Even the intact body was itself a phantom, rigged up by neurons as a ready scaffold. The body was the only home we had, and even it was more a

> postcard than a place. We did not live in muscles and joints and sinews; we lived in the thought and image and memory of them. No direct sensation, only rumors and unreliable reports.
>
> (327, 329)

It may be politically expedient to ignore this brain science; it may even be philosophically expedient, if we wish to rest easy in the comforting arms of two and a half millennia of mainstream Western thought; certainly it still seems wildly counterintuitive to claim that we have no direct access to empirical reality. Kevin Casper's take on slapstick, namely that there is a significant difference between Beavis and Butt-head feeling pain and the *Jackass* actors feeling pain, seems to make perfect (common) sense. So does Álvaro Ramírez's take on Don Quixote's participation in third-order simulacra. The only problem, as Richard Powers dramatizes so relentlessly in *The Echo Maker* and other novels, is that according to neurologists our commonsensical notions of the real and the fake are demonstrably wrong.

That claim obviously sets up a disturbing cognitive dissonance, one that I think lies at the molten core of brain science, and especially of cognitive neuroscience: we can prove scientifically that it is impossible to prove anything scientifically. We know both that the only conceivable jury on the nature of reality is the community – culture, society, public opinion, group plausibilization, all of which may be summed up as "common sense" – and that common sense is wrong about the nature of reality. What do we do about that?

One obvious solution to that recursive loop: if enough neurologists accept the "scientific proof" that our nervous systems make "scientific proof" an epistemological quagmire, then it becomes true. If enough narrative neurologists – people like A.R. Luria, Oliver Sacks, Michael Gazzaniga, Antonio Damasio, V.S. Ramachandran, and Gerald Weber – convert what cognitive neuroscientists believe into popular narrative accounts of brain science, the intelligentsia reading those books (including Richard Powers, Charles B. Harris, and me) can form a community creating a "higher" commonsensical account of how the brain works, or Common Sense2. Common Sense2 can then freely snipe at the errors of the objectivist Common Sense1 without miring the whole enterprise in hopeless self-contradiction. And of course the narrative neurologists can form a Common Sense3 that can snipe at the errors of the humanist Common Sense2, and the neurophysiologists who don't write popular neurology books can form a Common Sense4 that can snipe at the oversimplifications of the popularizing Common Sense3 (as Gerald Weber's colleagues do in *The Echo Maker*). "Common sense" is really only common to a group – not all humans; not even necessarily an entire national culture.

Or think of it this way: Michael Gazzaniga is famous for many neuroscientific discoveries, but perhaps his most germane discovery for my present purposes is the left-brain "interpreter," which, as Gazzaniga (1998, 138) puts it, "tells us the lies we need to believe in order to remain in control." And the verb "to believe" there points us syntagmatically both forward and backward: we need to believe the lies in order to believe we are in control. Gazzaniga adds: "As the social psychologist Eliot Aronson put it, we all want to shift our beliefs so we can hang onto the proposition 'I am nice and in control'" (138).

As Aronson's job title "*social* psychologist" suggests, of course, "the proposition 'I am nice and in control'" is specifically a social proposition – one that "we can [only] hang onto" to the extent that the people around us support us in our belief. Gerald Weber's self-image begins to erode as the "crowd" that populates his professional life begins to withhold that support. And indeed Gazzaniga adds further there that "this idea grew out of Leon Festinger's work on cognitive dissonance" (138), specifically Festinger's research into the failure of prophecy (Festinger et al. 1956): what happens when an apocalyptic cult's prophecy of the end of the world fails to come true. That sort of failure would create massive *social* cognitive dissonance; "Festinger's prediction," Gazzaniga reports, "assuming the momentous event did not occur, was that the followers would attempt to reduce their dissonant state at having their beliefs disconfirmed by attempting to convince others of those beliefs" (140). (Robert Coover's first novel, *The Origin of the Brunists* (1967), was based on that research; almost a half century later he published a sequel, *The Brunist Day of Wrath* (2014), set five years after the events in the first novel.)

What that makes me wonder, however, vis-à-vis Gazzaniga's interpreter theory of consciousness, is whether there isn't a *collective interpreter* – or, rather, whether the interpreter in every human's left brain isn't (partly) neuroculturally programmed by, and interactive with, the group(s) to which each individual belongs. After all, what exactly constitutes "being nice" and "being in control"? Aren't those collective virtues that the individual learns (mostly unconsciously) from the group? And as I began to suggest above, wouldn't each individual's ability to "hang onto" the belief in his or her success at niceness and control "hang" on (mostly unconscious) group endorsement? Gazzaniga seems to enjoy exaggerating the randomness of the interpreter's confabulations, partly perhaps for rhetorical effect – to counter the rationalist/individualist bias we have inherited that tells us we *are* in control – but partly also because of his half century of working with split-brain patients, who do, like other patients with debilitating lesions, find it very difficult to "plausibilize" their confabulations. Gazzaniga claims that "the interpreter-charged left brain remembers the gist of the story line and fills in the details by using logic, not real memories" (145); but in fact isn't it the case that the "logic" the interpreter uses in us normals is a *social* logic, based on collective constructions of plausibility rather than any abstract formal logic taught in philosophy classes?[13] Wouldn't that social logic be something like the "multiple interactions of a dynamic system" that Gazzaniga (2015, 350) tells us cognitive neuroscience is currently studying, only in the context of what cognitive scientists call "extended/embedded/distributed"[14] cognition, and what I have called "sociality as extended body-becoming-mind" (Robinson 2013b)?

The professional "common sense" that "verifies" the truth of the findings of scientific experiments is another such social logic, of course, at work at a conscious level in the form of professional debate (which is ideally, but not inevitably, evidence driven) among the left-brain interpreters of the hundreds or thousands of active members of a given scientific community. Scientists do not accept new findings at face value. They have trained themselves to be rigorously skeptical of all claims – to treat new claims as confabulations until proven otherwise. And the "proof" is not mechanistic/objectivist factuality so much as communal checking and cross-checking.

I mentioned earlier that in his radical reinterpretation of Baudrillard, Charles Levin (1996, 196) insists that all culture is simulation: "Simulation has, in essence, always been like this, at least so far as social life is concerned; for society has never been anything else but a map, or more truthfully, a collection of maps, that we gradually learn to read." Now let us read on:

> There is always plenty, in everything we say and do, that doesn't get included in the map, that doesn't get converted into its terms – particularly our subjective experiences, which may include observations that cannot be located. These are real and *vital*. But from the point of view of simulation, these are totally irrelevant, because, as Richard Shweder points out, "if social actors conveyed everything they actually felt . . . the performance called society, or at least the spectacle called civilization, would be very difficult to mount." (196)

I assume there that what Shweder means by "convey[ing] what we feel" is some kind of propositional communication: explaining, analyzing, justifying, and so on. But how do we convey what we feel when we recognize a face, or a place, as familiar? How do we convey what we feel when we recognize a behavior as acceptable, approved, admirable, or as unacceptable, offensive, shocking? How does a crane convey what it feels when it recognizes a stretch of river as the usual resting place? These feelings are "subjective experiences," obviously, and "may include observations that cannot be located"; certainly they are "real and *vital*"; but are they not also simulacra relevant to "the performance called society"? Are they not in fact the building blocks of "the spectacle called civilization"? It would seem undeniable that the "subjectivity" of such social feelings is a social intersubjectivity that is not only constantly being "*converted into [the] terms*" of sociocultural simulation but always already *constitutive* of sociocultural simulation. It would seem, in other words, that that feeling-based social intersubjectivity is situationally and ethnomethodologically foundational for normative social constructions/performances of "reality." It's just that, while that social intersubjectivity is technically becoming-cognitive, and so in humans always potentially activates the (collectivized) left-brain interpreter that conveys feelings propositionally, it is neuroculturally *affective-becoming-conative*-becoming-cognitive, and doesn't always emerge into full cognitive consciousness. It is often organized "automatically," autonomically, before the interpreter has a chance to confabulate its explanation of what's going on.

The model I have developed to account for this collective creation and normativization begins with somatic response,[15] which is precisely the bioelectric surge that generates the "glow" that Capgras sufferers do not experience when they see a familiar face. Indeed the Damasio team's theorization of somatic response, which was formative for my own development of the somatic theory of human social interaction, grew out of their early studies of face misrecognition (Tranel and Damasio 1985), in which somatic response works normally but FFA functionality is impaired; by the late 1980s they had shifted to the neural substrates of memory in the prefrontal cortex (Damasio 1989 and Damasio et al. 1990a, 1990b), leading to the first postulation of the somatic-marker hypothesis (Damasio et al. 1991). As their research increasingly began to draw on the mirror-neuron research over the course of the 1990s (Adolphs et al. 1994, 1998, 2000; Adolphs 2002), their understanding of somatic response began to expand, suggesting that it is

1 stored in the autonomic nervous system as experiential learning, so that it can be remobilized in specific decision-making situations – which are pretty much constant – to guide our cognition (what Damasio calls *somatic marking*);
2 displayed in body language, where it is registered visually, aurally, tactilely, and verbally by others, whose own autonomic nervous systems simulate it in their own through the mirror-neuron system, which is incapable of distinguishing an "external" experience from an "internal" one (yours from mine, projections and introjections from idiosyncratic feelings) or a "past" experience from a "present" one (remembered feelings from new ones) (I call this the *somatic transfer*, or *somatic mimesis*); and
3 cycled through all the bodies in a group almost simultaneously, with no more than a 300-millisecond lag (I call this the *somatic exchange*).

You will note that this model is very close to the neurological model on which Powers draws in *The Echo Maker*. Certainly the focus on (2) the mirror-neuron system should be familiar. What I add to what we might call the Powers model is first of all (1) Damasio's somatic markers – though Powers is on record as a fan of Damasio's work (Powers 2007; Burn 2008, 176). For me the importance of somatic markers is that they channel *guidance*, which is to say, behavioral (self-) regulation. They guide the behavior of (1) individuals, obviously – this is the basis of Powers's tropes of the self as mob and the brain as ecosystem – but then as those somatic markers are (2) *simulated* in other bodies, and then (3) circulated through entire populations, guidance becomes collective. Powers gives us (1) and (2>3) separately: his "empathy circuits" and "someone else's circuits circled through us" are precisely the movement from (2) to (3). But he does not build (1>2>3) into a collectivizing trajectory that explains how mobs rule and how ecosystems select for desirable group (and individual) action.

The basis of this model, in other words, is *neurocultural simulation*. The somatic responses that are thus mimetically transferred and exchanged are in that sense Baudrillardian simulacra. This is not exactly what Baudrillard means by simulacra, of course, but it's pretty close, and it offers a plausible grounding of his theory in the cultural shaping of the functioning of the human nervous system. The final step in that grounding, the step that explains how the somatomimetic exchange can organize simulacra into "society" or "culture" or "civilization" – a whole unconscious socioaffective ecosystem of regulatory norms and values – is what I call [4] *icosis*. I coin that processual term from Greek *eikos*/"plausible," *ta eikota*/"the plausibilities," and Aristotle's claim in the *Rhetoric* that, given a choice between a plausible story that is untrue and a true story that is implausible, we will tend to choose the former, because it has been *vetted* as true (real, etc.) by the group. Icosis is thus group plausibilization, and forms the fourth level of somatic theory. The idea is that reality, truth, identity, the self, and so on – all those simulacra that Baudrillard claims in his theoretical works have been rendered "impossible" by simulation, but that he then insists in his interviews *are* simulation – are "plausibilized," normativized as real, by the circulation through the somatic exchange of *value*. What makes this "icotic" plausibilization ("materialization") of simulation as reality possible, in other words, is the circulation through the somatic exchange not just of shared affect, but of shared *evaluative* affect: approval and disapproval, honor and dishonor, praise and blame, pride and shame.

It is thanks to various kinds of brain dysfunction like the Capgras delusion that neurologists have been able to explore how normal nervous systems organize our lives. In *Descartes' Error* Antonio Damasio (1994, chs. 1–2) reports the work his neurological team did studying first Phineas Gage – the mid-nineteenth-century railroad foreman who had an iron tamping rod propelled though his mouth and left frontal lobe by exploding gunpowder, and survived, but lost all ability to organize his life according to social norms – and (chs. 3–4) a group of more recent (and still living) sufferers from similar dysfunctions, to determine that damage to the prefrontal ventromedial area disrupts the autonomic nervous system's ability to channel lessons learned from previous experience into guidance for decision-making. This was the origin of the team's "somatic-marker hypothesis," since repeatedly tested by them and other neurologists.

As for *neurocultural* somatic marking: a case Damasio (2003, 153) reports in *Looking for Spinoza* involved an incorrigible young woman of 20 who had been run over by a car and sustained a head injury at the age of 15 months: "She was academically capable yet routinely failed to complete her assignments. Her adolescence was marked by failure to comply with rules of any sort and frequent confrontations with peers and adults. She was verbally and physically abusive to others. She lied chronically. She was arrested several times for shoplifting and stole from other children and from her own family. She engaged in early and risky sexual behavior and became pregnant at eighteen," and so on. With the breakdown of social emotion-management (i.e., what I'm calling "neurocultural" regulation) in the ventromedial prefrontal cortices, Damasio explains, "the experience of pain, which is part of punishment, becomes disconnected from the action that caused the punishment, and thus *there will not be a memory of their conjunction for future use;* likewise for the pleasurable aspects of reward" (155;

emphasis in original). This observation leads Damasio to imagine a world without the neurocultural somatic marking of social emotions, and thus to reenvision ethics as channeled somatically:

> In a society deprived of such emotions and feelings, there would have been no spontaneous exhibition of the innate social responses that foreshadow a simple ethical system – no budding altruism, no kindness when kindness is due, no censure when censure is appropriate, no automatic sense of one's own failings. In the absence of the feelings of such emotions, humans would not have engaged in a negotiation aimed at finding solutions for problems faced by the group, e.g., identification and sharing of food resources, defense against threats or disputes among its members. There would not have been a gradual build-up of wisdom regarding the relationships among social situations, natural responses, and a host of contingencies such as the punishment or reward incurred by permitting or inhibiting natural responses. The codification of rules eventually expressed in systems of justice and sociopolitical organizations is hardly conceivable in those circumstances, even assuming that the apparatus of learning, imagination, and reasoning could be otherwise intact in the face of emotional ravages, a most unlikely possibility. With the natural system of emotional navigation more or less disabled, there would not have been a ready possibility of fine-tuning the individual to the real world. Moreover, the possibility of constructing a fact-based social navigation system, independently of the missing natural system, appears unlikely. (157)

The slight correction to add to that, of course, is that the "facts" in a "fact-based social navigation system" would all be icotic simulacra – images plausibilized and normativized and made available as facts for socially reliable "navigation," which is to say, socially guided decision-making as a process of "fine-tuning the individual to the real world." That "real world," of course, is more or less what Freud calls the "reality principle." Insofar as it is an icotic world – not just social interaction but the contexts and situations (like "home" and "work" and "school") rendered "normal" or normative through social interaction – it is made up of more simulacra. The process of "fine-tuning the individual" to that world is also a mobilization and neuroculturally regulated deployment of similar simulacra. The individual's sense of self, and of the temporal continuity of that self – who I was as a small child, an adolescent, yesterday, who I am now, who I will be tomorrow – is an infinitely fractalized series of affectively mobilized simulacra, organized socially (who I was in relation to my mother, my father, my siblings, my teachers, who I am in relation to my significant other, my ex, my children, my friends, my boss, my coworkers, etc. – see Damasio 2010).

Because all those things are simulations, of course, and because the social organization and guidance of those simulations are works in progress, and a bit klugey, we often feel uneasy about their coherence, their efficacy, their range, the extent to which they are accepted by others, and so on – and that uneasiness leaves us vulnerable to apocalyptic theories of the loss of all reality, the latter-day impossibility of "the real," and so on. That vulnerability makes us Baudrillard fans who are inclined to read him literally as nostalgic for a simpler and more stable time (our childhoods?), back when reality hadn't yet completely "disappeared" (Baudrillard 2007/2011).

But our susceptibility to such naïve readings of an extremely subtle and complex thinker does not make Baudrillard wrong. It just means that Baudrillard's thought must itself be thoughtfully fine-tuned to an icotic world. And in fact the convergence Richard Powers dramatizes between neurology and (something like) Baudrillard in *The Echo Maker* might be read as pushing that fine-tuning forward in significant ways:

> Once, he'd studied an otherwise healthy man who thought that stories turned real. People spoke the world into being. Even a single sentence launched events as solid as experience. Journey, complication, crisis, and redemption: just say the words and they took shape.
>
> For decades, that case haunted everything Weber wrote about. That one delusion – *stories came true* – seemed like the germ of healing. We told ourselves backward into diagnosis and forward into treatment. Story was the storm at the cortex's core. And there was no better way to get at that fictional truth than through the haunted neurological parables of Broca or Luria – stories of how even shattered brains might narrate disaster back into livable sense.
>
> Then the story changed. Somewhere, real clinical tools rendered case histories merely colorful. Medicine grew up. Instruments, images, tests, metrics, surgery, pharmaceuticals: no room left for Weber's anecdotes. And all his literary cures turned to circus acts and Gothic freak shows.
>
> Once, he knew a man who thought that telling other people's stories might make them real again. Then others' stories remade him. Illusion, loss, humiliation, disgrace: just say the words and they happened. The man himself had arisen from doctored accounts; Weber had invented him out of whole cloth. The complete history and physical: fabricated. Now the text unravels. Even the case's name – *Gerald W.* – sounds like the feeblest of pseudonyms.
>
> (524, emphasis in original)

Right – but that account only goes halfway, and sounds quite bleak because it does not know where to go next. As long as it is just Gerald Weber telling other people's (and his own) stories and building his reality out of all that, the resulting verbal house of cards is quite easy to topple. Then the negativity of "others' stories" about him can quite easily unmake/remake him. Rethinking his disintegration icotically, we would want to say that, yes, Famous Gerald is first made, then unmade, by icosis – the group plausibilization first of FG's brilliance, then of his callous disregard for the human suffering of his "cases" – but then so too is the "self" that is a good-enough (not perfect) husband to Sylvie and a good-enough (not perfect) father to Jess and good-enough (not perfect) teacher and so on is made by icosis as well. The solution to the negative impact of the attack on Famous Gerald has on "Gerald W." is not, as Sylvie argues, to *ignore* public opinion: it is to incorporate more of it into an expansive self, to recognize the extent to which all reality, all truth, all identity is made not by words but by *shared icotic belief* in the words, collective plausibilization of the words. To the extent that Gerald Weber shares with the key people in his personal and professional life the icotic belief that he is a good man, his goodness is real. His "midlife crisis," if that's even a reasonable term for what hits him in the novel, is precipitated by his own blindness to the collective sources of his identity – something in which he has believed professionally for his entire career, but has never given much thought to in his own personal life, his own self-image. Because he thinks he *just is* who he is, and is not *group-plausibilized* as who he is, the group-deplausibilization of his positive self-image is devastating to him.

Let me close this first essay by returning one more time to Karin Schluter's narrator-reported musing that "the whole race suffered from Capgras. Those birds danced like our next of kin, looked like our next of kin, called and willed and parented and taught and navigated all just like our blood relations. Half their parts were still ours. Yet humans waved them off: *impostors*" (439). The first time I cited this passage I mentioned Arne Naess, the Norwegian proponent of "deep ecology," which he defines as "Self-realization by all living beings" (1995, 33):

N1: Self-realization!
H1: The higher the Self-realization attained by anyone, the broader and deeper the identification with others.
H2: The higher the level of Self-realization attained by anyone, the more its further increase depends on the Self-realization of others.
H3: Complete Self-realization of anyone depends on that of all.
N2: Self-realization by all living beings!
(N=norm; H=hypothesis)

The notion that humans should *identify* with cranes, and other birds, and all living beings, but also with mountains and rivers,[16] stars and stones, is an icosis that Naess hopes to instill in the human race for the future – to group-plausibilize that identification with other living beings as *true,* as part of our identity – but it is one that he also believes is already in us, and can be dredged up from the distant past *through* our present feelings. Something like that hope also seems to fuel Powers's imagination in *The Echo Maker*. But I submit that for that hope to have any chance at all of being (Self-)realized, we need more than the bleak vision of our neural fragility, our susceptibility to breakdown in the face of public opinion and the tyranny of "common sense." We need a strongly activist sociopolitical vision and rhetoric of how public opinion and common sense can be *guided,* shaped, channeled along new pathways. And for that we need icosis.

Notes

1 As Powers (2007) reports, something like this equation lay at the beginning of his thinking about the novel: having spotted the cranes in Nebraska while driving by, he began to read about them, until they

became eerily human to me, and at the same time, totally alien. I wasn't surprised to discover stories in different folk literatures about cranes and people turning back and forth into each other. Later, when I first heard about Capgras syndrome, and how its sufferers fail to recognize only those people closest to them (while having no trouble at all recognizing everyone else), something clicked, some story about familiarity and strangeness, and the book started to take shape in me.

2 Powers (2007) does seem to suggest that Karin speaks here for him:

> So here we are, sharing the planet with these creatures who are weirdly intelligent, smart in an alien way that we're not quite smart enough to see. And yet, the core parts of their brains are still contained in ours. Our estrangement from them, then, struck me as somehow analogous to our estrangement from our own subcortical selves. Setting the story in this little town in the middle of nowhere, whose central claim to fame was this annual massing of birds, gave me a way to open up the story to all kinds of neurological and ecological traces.

3 The excitement about the mirror neurons, not only in social and cognitive neuroscience but in the interdisciplinary humanities as well, has also provoked some disgruntled backlash. Rhonda Blair (2013, 145), for example, cautions:

> Among the things those working with this material have been learning is that one must be cautious in using research on the neural level to explain anything in the realm of the experiential or conscious. For example, the discovery of mirror neurons in monkeys did not immediately mean that humans had mirror neurons or that they functioned identically in humans, or that the discovery of neural simulation in humans meant that we are intrinsically empathetic. One must be clear about what is presented as scientific theory, i.e. an explanation that accounts for observable phenomena, following processes of repeatability and falsifiability, and what is speculation, i.e. *possible* explanations for phenomena which have not yet been borne out by experimentation.
>
> (This passage also appears almost verbatim, with only a one-word edit – "We" for "One" in the last sentence – in Blair and Cook 2016a, 11.)

It is quite true that the early enthusiasm about the mirror neurons led to quick overgeneralizations, and that one must be careful to frame one's applications of such research in responsible ways. But one must also be careful *not* to read warnings like Blair's to mean that the early claims "that humans had mirror neurons or that they functioned identically in humans, or that the discovery of neural simulation in humans meant that we are intrinsically empathetic [were in 2013 still only] speculation, i.e. *possible* explanations for phenomena which have not yet been borne out by experimentation." By 2013 social neuroscientists of empathy had been testing precisely these claims for nearly two decades: see e.g. Adolphs and colleagues (1994, 1998, 2000, 2002), Keysers and colleagues (Kohler et al. 2002; Gazzola et al. 2009; Keysers and Gazzola 2009), Sonnby-Borgström (2002, 433), Wicker and colleagues (2003), Leslie and colleagues (2004, 601), Singer and colleagues (2004), Banissy and Ward (2007), and Loggia and colleagues (2008). Cf. also Gazzaniga (2015, 94): "Also at the Instituto was Giacomo Rizzolatti, a young neurophysiologist of enormous talent, who later went on to discover mirror neurons (the group of neurons we all possess that track the actions of others)."

4 Note that Ramírez published his article in *Hispania,* and that he is himself a native speaker of Spanish, in which language *Don Quixote* (as Cervantes wrote the title and the name in the first edition, and as English translations ever since have continued to title it) has been written *Don Quijote* since 1815, when the Real Academia (Royal Academy) banished the letter X from official Spanish and replaced it with J, leaving the X only in place names like México and Texas and personal names like Ximena – and in English spellings of Cervantes's knight.

5 The "obvious" (commonsensical) exception to this rule would be the "(auto-) biographical" novel, or the *roman à clef*, a fictionalized account of actual historical events. But even in such novels the generic *rule* is that the characters and events are not based on real people doing things in the real world; and interpretations that seek to establish that there are in fact real people and real events behind the narrative tend to be seen as "unmasking" the work's fictional status as a lie, as if the author had somehow cheated on the reader by cutting imaginative corners. The first-order "counterfeiting" of reality is the generic norm.

6 Gazzaniga has been telling us for years that "*Only* the left brain has an interpreter" (1998, 25 (emphasis in original); see also Gazzaniga 2005/2006, 148; 2011, 77; 2015, 114, 150–53), because only the left brain has language. In Gazzaniga (2015, 295–96), however, he reports the discovery his postdoc Paul Corballis made (see Miller et al. 1999 for the original scientific publication) that the right brain has a visual interpreter as well, "one that specialized in visual information" (2015, 295). His comment: "As is so often the case in science, while an initial observation remains true, the initial interpretation can be completely wrong" (296).

7 Here is the passage from Burn's interview (2008, 174):

> Q. Do you see affinities between your understanding of narrative and Daniel Dennett's multiple-drafts theory of consciousness?
> A. I see more than affinities: I see strong equivalences! *The Echo Maker* is in many ways a narrative working-out of those ideas.

Dennett develops that theory in *Consciousness Explained* (1991); for discussion, see Robinson (2001, ch. 5; 2013b, 118). See also Dennett's (2008) fan letter to Powers.

8 Brindley (2012, 19n41) cites this passage as "Harris, 'The Story of the Self,' 436" – a page number that does not even exist in Burn and Dempsey (2008). Harris's article is the most comprehensive introduction to date to *The Echo Maker*'s "neurological realism": he covers the origins of the novel in Powers's drive through Nebraska en route from Illinois to Arizona and serendipitous discovery of the migrating cranes, and subsequent delving into the neurological research on misidentification, especially in Ramachandran (1998) (Harris 232); his determination to undermine dualistic thinking (233); what he discovered about the simultaneous multiplicity and singularity of the self (234–37); his use of the mirror-neuron research (238); the motivational ubiquity of self-protection (239–41); the role played by "self-narration" or the fictional impulse in the maintenance of an ostensibly coherent and continuous self (241–42); and the important differences between traditional psychological realism and Powers's new neurological realism (243–52): "Whereas traditional psychological realism records the effect on the 'inner self' of external forces or deep-seated neuroses, neurological realism foregrounds the effects of largely unconscious neurological activities," and in so doing deconstructs the "dualisms – inner and outer, mind and body, reason and emotion, self and other" (243) – maintained by psychological realism. But a better term might be "neurological morality play."

9 Butler's (1991) phrase is "panicked heterosexuality"; her ingenious argument is that straight people like to believe that heterosexuality is not just "normal" (grounded in social norms) but "natural" (grounded in biological nature), and therefore calmly immutable, but the lie is given to that belief by the panic many straight people feel around gays, as if gayness might be contagious. So far from being "natural," this suggests, heterosexuality is only *naturalized* as normal/normative, and further a beleaguered naturalization, under constant threat of dissolution, and therefore a stance that requires constant ideological and behavioral vigilance. By extension, therefore, Sylvie's edgy insistence that her husband is a strong, confident individual

who doesn't need to worry about what the public says about him, and her constant railing against the encroachments of public opinion on her own individualistic peace of mind, would be "panicked individualism," suggesting that she wants to naturalize the normativity of individualism but in order to do that must constantly be shoring it up against the power of the collective to tear it down.

10 The "Extended Mind Thesis" was first proposed by Clark and Chalmers (1998); for discussion, see Robinson (2013b).

11 Admitting that the novel's ending is "tidily architectonic," that the novel comes to a close with a "comforting telos," Harris (2008, 249) insists that "the novel's orderly denouement, like the false coherence forged by the human brain, is a skillful sleight-of-hand, an attempt to pull the rug over the fractured realities we have just seen dramatized" (250). Yes, okay; but if that is true of all fiction, including the fictions we all create to maintain the illusion of an orderly self in an orderly world, it's not clear to me how just creating another "false coherence" at the end of his novel makes Powers's "skillful sleight-of-hand" any different from every other fiction we've ever experienced. Harris supports his against-the-grain reading of the ending by looking back at the narrative as a whole, arguing that "we get a hint of this instability long before the faux denouement endeavors to smooth over the plot's complications" (250). And yes, that's true, but "instability" is a feature of every plot leading up to the climax and denouement, and just calling the denouement of *The Echo Maker* "faux" does not "falsify" it – does not magically transform it into something other than a *conventional* denouement. I don't see any evidence in the text that Powers is undermining the patness of his ending, or even drawing metafictional attention to it. Mark is cured; Karin decides to stay on in Kearney and keep working to save the cranes; Weber, flying home from infidelity with Barbara, worries about how his wife will receive him. Harris – to my mind astonishingly – insists that "such open endings are staples of much Modernist and virtually all Postmodern fiction" (251); I read it as a traditional denouement from the decidedly premodern, even pre-Jamesian, tradition of psychological realism.

12 Interestingly, Powers puts the most explicit statement of modernist estrangement in the mouth of the novel's "simplest" character, Daniel: "We need something to wake sleepwalkers. To make the world strange and real again" (429). Harris (2008, 251–52) comments on this moment and provides a useful quotation from Powers (2007) supporting it; for a discussion of modernist theories of estrangement *(ostranenie, Verfremdung)* see Robinson (2008, esp. chs. 3 and 5).

13 Earlier in *The Mind's Past* Gazzaniga mentions the guidance provided by "society," but rather vaguely:

> We all have had our interest sparked by an attractive stranger. A struggle ensues as we try to override the deeply wired brain circuitry provided by evolution to maintain our desire to reproduce. Allaying possible embarrassment, the mind gets around the brain's assertion this time and managed to maintain control. Society does have an effect, through yet other brain representations, and thus we are not completely at the mercy of our brain's reproductive systems. Or at least we like to believe so.
>
> (22)

Could those "yet other brain representations" include a collectivized interpreter, the guidance provided by the group for the "logic" that the interpreter attempts to impose on the story it is telling about/as the self? I would assume that that social guidance is partly automatized as well – that the social disinclination to seek sex with that attractive stranger might kick in at some pre-conscious level, as affect-becoming-conation – but that, to the extent that such automatic guidance rises to the level of conscious cognition, it would enlist the verbal assistance of the interpreter as well: "I'm married. I'm happily married. I'm not really interested in that person. It's not worth it," etc.

14 Note that this is not the kind of "distributed" cognition that Gazzaniga (2011, 64) means when he writes of his discovery that "consciousness is distributed everywhere across the brain." For the cognitive science sense of "distributed cognition," see Hollan et al. (2001), Ross et al. (2007), Dror and Harnet (2008).

15 For the development of my somatic theory, see Robinson (1991, 1996, 2003, 2008, 2011, 2012, 2013a, 2013b, and 2015a). Icotic theory began to emerge as an extension of somatic theory in early drafts (from about 2009) of what eventually became Robinson (2016a); see also Robinson (2013c, 2016b, 2016c, 2017a, 2017b).

16 Cf. Harris (2008, 237) on *The Echo Maker:* "Within the novel, the Platte River, a 'mile wide and an inch deep' (55), functions much like a character in the novel, as much Karin's kin as the birds are. 'Water wants something from her' (408), she realizes. 'Water is up to something'" (418).

Essay 2 The translational humanities of medicine

Literary history as performed translationality

Let us begin this second essay by reflecting on the humanities for a moment.

For introductory purposes, think about them reductively, as consisting of three broad areas: philosophy, history, and literature. Each can be, and has been, defined essentialistically, categorically, based on the idea that the truth about it consists of the stable set of *things that stay the same*. Philosophy studies the true (metaphysics), the good (ethics), the beautiful (aesthetics), and the methods for knowing (epistemology) and arguing (logic) about such matters. History studies written documents about the past, seeking to establish the truth of what actually happened. Literature is an attempt to delight and instruct through invented prose, poetry, and drama. There is a philosophy of history and a philosophy of literature; a history of philosophy, a history of historiography, and a history of literature; philosophy is often written in overtly literary genres (e.g., dialogues) and history is often written in narrative. And so on. All sorts of stable, essentializing things can be said about each of the three.

But what if we take another path, and explore the humanities in terms of *things that keep changing*? At the very least, then, each of the three changes in small but significant ways every time a new work in it is published, or otherwise disseminated, not only because each new work adds minutely to the whole picture, but because each at least potentially reconceives the entire enterprise in minutely (sometimes massively) different ways. To think of philosophy as an ongoing conversation among philosophers and readers, history as an ongoing conversation among historians and readers, and literature as an ongoing conversation among writers and readers is to recognize the power each new contribution to that conversation has to derail and redirect old debates. New topics and new strategies come and go with the people who launch them, contest them, ridicule them, or reinvigorate them. Approached in this transformational or "translational" style, the humanities become far more difficult to categorize in stable ways. A given work may be productively indeterminate: a (sort of) literary work that also explores philosophical issues in a recognizable historical context (is it demonstrably *not* philosophy or history?); a (sort of) historical work that tracks a philosophical debate and is written in a brilliantly literary style (is it demonstrably *not* philosophy or literature?); and so on.

Think now of all the multifarious transformations loosely covered in that previous paragraph as "translations," and the loose category to which they belong as "translationality." As I mentioned in the Preface, the Latin word *trans-latio* morphologically means "carried across," and there are many types of translation that do not involve the rewriting of a text in another language: the *translatio imperii* (transmigration of empire), the *translatio studii* (transmigration of learning), and so on. And while I do intend to zero in on something like the interlingual rewriting of texts in this essay, I want to keep the definitional boundaries around that activity as fuzzy and blurry as possible, to allow the notion of "translationality" to expand to encompass as much "transformationality" as possible. Readers who zealously guard the imaginary boundary between "translation" and "adaptation" may feel aggrieved at this expansiveness: I want to include adaptations too in "translationality."

Along the way I will want to interrogate those boundaries, and the acts of policing that (seem to) maintain them, and the impulse to exert a controlling influence over such classificational acts. What is gained, and what is lost, when we cordon things off into such neat groupings? Why is it important to identify one class of textual rewritings as "translations," because they reproduce another text "equivalently," "faithfully," supposedly without change (though of course every word in them is changed), and to identify another class of textual rewritings as "adaptations," because they transform their models so radically that the relationship between them may not even be immediately apparent?

The traditional answer, of course, is that a clear and rigid distinction between translation and adaptation enables us to stabilize the history of philosophy, literature, and historiography (not to mention the history of medicine, with which in fact we will begin in section 2.2). Without the distinction between translation and adaptation, we could not (so this justification goes) tell the difference between English translations of Homer's *Odyssey* (all of which, presumably, are to be unified as versions of *the same text*) from James Joyce's *Ulysses,* which is a *different text.* Homer wrote the *Odyssey;* Joyce wrote *Ulysses.* Both are great literary classics. George Chapman wrote a brilliant text that might in some alternative universe be considered an original literary classic – but because it is a translation of Homer's *Odyssey* (1616), it is not a literary classic in its own right. It is an English *instantiation* of Homer's epic.

It is precisely this nervous sort of stabilization that I intend to jettison here. I am interested in translationality-as-transformationality as the shifting "foundation" of human knowledge.

This is not, to put it quite mildly, a particularly popular approach. People who approach the transmission of knowledge through stable essences don't usually like to think of knowledge as transmitted down through the centuries in this slapdash way, with the latest author *rethinking and reframing* the great classics. An extreme example that we will follow in section 2.2.1 is the clash between Andreas Vesalius (1514–1564), who reframed Galen's anatomy for modern medicine by testing Galen's claims against the evidence he found in dissected cadavers, and his teacher Jacobus Sylvius (1478–1555), who lashed out viciously at his former student for daring to claim that Galen might have made mistakes. Most historians of ideas today would of course back way off from the extremism of Jacobus's attacks, and insist only on the importance of *knowing exactly what Galen wrote*, without pretending that Galen was infallible – without wanting to deny Vesalius his own glory as the founder of modern anatomy. Just as James Joyce created a new literary classic in *Ulysses* by adapting Homer, so too did Vesalius create a new anatomical classic in *De humani corporis fabrica* (1543) by adapting Galen.

What this more "tolerant" insistence on *things that stay the same* misses, however, is the transformationality that is endemic in all translation – indeed, in all human communication. The belief that a translation can grant us reliable access to the true meaning of a text originally written in a language we cannot read is unfounded. The belief on which the disciplines of classics and comparative literature were founded, that knowledge of the original languages of classical texts can grant us reliable access to the meanings of those texts, is equally unfounded. What we inevitably do with those texts, whether we read them in the original, translate them as accurately as we can, or adapt them freely, is to *reconstruct* and *reperform* them. Every new reconstruction is a new performance: this is what I am calling translationality.

To those who cling to historical stabilities, of course, this is discouraging talk. For them it is a cold and desolate outlook indeed that would take translation as a "shifting foundation" for the transmission of knowledge, precisely because that foundation keeps shifting, and therefore to their way of thinking isn't really a foundation at all. But it is difficult for them to deny the shaping effect translation has had on philosophy, history, and literature – and of course the other disciplines as well. Not only were Greek philosophy, history, and literature translated by the Romans, and Greek and Roman philosophy, history, and literature translated by medieval European and Islamic scholars, and so on; but the *transformative* effects of those translations arguably shaped the construction of "Western culture" as much as war, money, and patrilineage did.

Everyone who has ever given a few minutes' thought to such translational transmissions of knowledge can name a half dozen examples from within Western thought; those who know the histories of such transmissions well know just how much transformationality ensued every time a text was translated. A less widely known example involves the shaping influence, beginning in the early seventeenth century, of Latin and European vernacular translations of ancient Chinese and Indian thought on the Western peripheral or dissident thought that fed esoteric, Romantic, pragmatic, and phenomenological traditions – the traditions that eventually fed Occidentalist thought in the rest of the world. In a recent book (Robinson 2017b, ch. 3) I tracked such influences through a history of intercivilizational engagements that had exercised a University of Georgia scholar of Chinese Daoism named Russell Kirkland, who was inclined to think about Daoism in terms of things that stay the same. Any Daoist contact with the West, obviously, was a corrupting influence, because it changed the true stable nature of Daoism. The epitome of that corruption for Kirkland was the huge collection of English translations of the *Laozi*/《老子》 or *Daodejing*/《道德經》 (often called the *Tao Te Ching* in earlier romanizations) by people with little or no Chinese and not the slightest interest in the "original" "true" "pure" content of Daoism, which for him was molded once and for all in around 500 BCE. Equally culpable for Kirkland, however, were translators with excellent Chinese who "distorted" what he took to be the true original meaning of Daoism – and even Chinese scholars of Daoism whose thinking had been "corrupted" by Western thought. In my reading of that history I was able to show not only how signally early missionary translations of the *Laozi,* in the seventeenth and eighteenth centuries, had influenced Western counterhegemonic thought, thus conditioning the later "mystical" translations by people like Aleister Crowley and Timothy Leary who had no Chinese, but also the extent to which those missionaries were themselves, despite their avowedly Christian goals, strongly influenced by their source text. There simply was no chasm between "true Daoism" and "non-Daoist" American mysticism. Everything was a mixture. As Laozi himself might have insisted, everything flowed out of everything else. The translational transformations ran in both directions, and had been doing so for four centuries. That was no consolation to Russell Kirkland, of course, given his need to make things stay the same. (More on this history in section 3.4.2.)

2.1 Translationality vs. cloning

In one of the essays in *Simulacra and Simulation,* Jean Baudrillard (1981/1994, 96) raises the issue of cloning:

> Dream of an eternal twining substituted for sexual procreation that is linked to death. Cellular dream of scissiparity, the purest form of parentage, because it finally allows one to do without the other, to go from the same to the same (one still has to use the uterus of a woman, and a pitted ovum, but this support is ephemeral, and in any case anonymous: a female prosthesis could replace it). Monocellular utopia which, by way of genetics, allows complex beings to achieve the destiny of protozoas.

The dream of "go[ing] from the same to the same": the dream of stopping time, preventing change, forestalling death. The clone as the perfect replica of the parent – and by extension, of course, the translation as the perfect replica of the original. An end to the Curse of Babel. Total Translatability. Sexual procreation not only mixes the genes of two parents; its uncontrolled "naturalness" leaves it vulnerable to genetic mutation. *Things can change in unexpected ways.* This is the theme I am proposing for translationality: things can change. In the dream of the clone-translation, by contrast, nothing changes. Sameness is replicated, potentially to infinity. There is no need to open the gates to alterity, alteration, adulteration, atrophy, death.

But as Baudrillard muses further, it was precisely that obsessive need to keep repeating the same thing that Freud theorized as the death drive:

> What, if not a death drive, would push sexed beings to regress to a form of reproduction prior to sexuation (besides, isn't it this form of scissiparity, this

> reproduction and proliferation through pure contiguity that is for us, in the depths of our imaginary, death and the death drive – what denies sexuality and wants to annihilate it, sexuality being the carrier of life, that is to say of a critical and mortal form of reproduction?) and that, at the same time, would push them metaphysically to deny all alterity, all alteration of the Same in order to aim solely for the perpetuation of an identity, a transparency of the genetic inscription no longer even subject to the vicissitudes of procreation? (96)

This is the death drive as Thanatos, launched in opposition to Eros, the life drive channeled through sex and other forms of creativity. As Freud theorized it in *Beyond the Pleasure Principle,* the death drive was a conservative impulse in animate life to return to a primordial state of inanimateness; he found it manifested in the compulsion to repeat traumatic events, to keep re-experiencing them as present rather than simply remembering them as past. The life drive is driven by the pleasure principle; the death drive, according to Freud, is driven by the reality principle, a "civilizational" or icotic management system for the painful experiences that escape the pleasure principle, and so resist being assimilated by the life drive. If only we could repeat those experiences *on our own terms,* exactly, with minute fidelity, we could manage our fear of dying, and perhaps, ideally, die as we choose.

On the one hand, "clone-translating" as keeping things the same, the repetition-compulsion as a thanatotic management system organized by the reality principle.	On the other hand, "translationality" as change, (pro)creativity as an erotic management system organized by the pleasure principle.

Of course there are two unfortunate facts about all this.

- *Unfortunate fact 1:* We can never really have it our way. No matter how exuberantly we gravitate toward pleasure, sex, creativity, and life, pain and trauma and death always lurk just around the corner for us. And the death drive, channeled by the reality principle – society's mandate to keep our noses to the grindstone, delay gratification, obey the rules, be good boys and girls – never really protects us from those bad things either. It only gives us the impression that we are managing decay and death. In some sense the pleasure principle and its life drive and the reality principle and its death drive are both self-protective hedges against the fear of death, and while each mostly works well enough in the short run, neither works at all in the long run.
- *Unfortunate fact 2:* For the most part we are unable to choose between these self-protective options. Our fears and needs tend to choose for us. Enough fear of change and we become rigid conservatives, terrified of change, angry at every deviation from the norms closest to our hearts. Enough fear of forced conformity and we become iconoclasts, wild hedonists, risk-takers, scofflaws, terrified of being regulated, angry at every perceived encroachment on our "freedom," our "rights."

Still, I suggest that what I am calling translationality aligns well with the inevitability of change. Nothing does stay the same. Not only does the communal dialogue in each field keep changing, but translations keep changing what people say in their contributions to that dialogue. Translation is like the game of Telephone, in which a message is passed down a line of players in whispered repetitions, and everybody has a good laugh at the end when it is revealed just how drastically it changed as it was passed along. All of the principals involved in the creation of a translation – editors, researchers, translators themselves, critics – work to manage the process so as to minimize such transformations, but translation, like all human communication, and indeed all human activity, is a kluge: a clumsy workaround that shouldn't work at all but somehow, mysteriously, does. As Gary Marcus (2008) shows at gleeful length in his book of that title – subtitled "The Haphazard Construction of the Human Mind" – the human brain itself is a kluge: jerry-rigged by *random* evolution over millions of years to do many things brilliantly but many other things badly, like remembering, believing, choosing, and imposing a logical organization on what it remembers, believes, and chooses. Human speech in a single language is klugey. Writing as a representation of human speech in a single language is klugey. And because each language is klugey in a different way, the bridges we build from one language to another are multiply klugey, which is why translation is so thoroughly klugey. Every translation, even of very simple phrases that apparently lend themselves to literal translation – like "Peter ist zu Hause" for "Peter is at home" – is a rough approximation. (German "zu" does mean "at" in that context, but in other contexts it also means "to," "toward," "for," "in," "as," and so on. Even when it is used to mean "at" home, it carries echoes of those other prepositional orientations with it.) As a result, even the most meticulously careful translation transforms the source text en route to the target language.

Because this kluginess is a *human neural* characteristic, the most obsessive perfectionists on earth are doomed to fail, always. But because we are not entirely at the mercy of our hard-wiring – because we are *neurocultural* creatures, and the cultural pressures in that mix push us toward enhanced organization – we live in a constant tension between the conditioned impulse to control and the tendency for control to fail. As my theories of icosis and ecosis suggest, our neurocultural organization pushes us to control not only our behavior and discourse but the ways we *think and feel* about our behavior and discourse. As I began to suggest in Essay 1, the traditional categories that we impose on interlingual and intersemiotic retextings are good examples of that latter kind of control: we create, and experience as a deeply felt reality, a binary opposition between [1] "translation" (which supposedly reproduces the source text accurately) and [2] "adaptation" (which supposedly transforms the source text radically), and, within "translation," between [1a] "metaphrase"/"word-for-word translation" and [1b] "paraphrase"/"sense-for-sense translation." That latter distinction allows us to determine that (1a) reproduces the source-text syntax more accurately but the source-text sentence-level semantics less accurately, and (1b) reproduces the source-text syntax less accurately but the source-text sentence-level semantics more accurately. Such binaries reassure us greatly. For the elusive "reality" of perfect equivalence they substitute the "spin" of categorization, making it possible for us to imagine that we are actually achieving the perfect "reality" toward which we strive. If the "more accurate" category is bounded on the lower end, crisply and rigidly and therefore (we hope) reliably differentiated from the "less accurate" category, we may begin to suspect that it is also bounded on the upper end at perfection: perfect reproduction of the source text. If we think about it too overtly, of course, our hopes will be dashed; but thinking is overrated. If we can only relax our tendency to overthink things, it may come to *feel vaguely* to us as if translation actually achieves the cloned perfection toward which we strive. Then maybe, just maybe, source texts may (seem to) stay the same as they cross cultural and linguistic boundaries.

My MH focus in this book is literature, medicine in literature and medical literature; here in Essay 2 my focus is literary translation, and specifically literature as what I call translationality. My argument is that literary translation is not just a unique literary genre in its own right but a *paradigmatic* literary genre, typical of the transformational currents channeled through all literature. Translationality, in other words, not as an army of clones, but as ubiquitous transformation.

But let us pause for a moment here to consider the possibility that the same is true of philosophical and historical translations as well: that philosophical translation, first of all, is a unique philosophical genre in its own right, like the treatise, the dialogue, and the numbered note, and that that unique genre is paradigmatic of the transformational currents channeled through all philosophy. No clones. This is a tough sell, perhaps, even tougher than the literary version; the counterpart argument for historiography seems to me the toughest sell of all – so tough that I propose to forego the attempt to pitch it at all. I'm thinking, however, of works like Hegel's *Die Phänomenologie des Geistes/The Phenomenology of the Spirit* as a German translation of Aristotle's ϖερι ψυχε/*peri psukhe*/*De Anima*/*On the Soul*, or Heidegger's *Der Satz vom Grund/The Principle of Ground* as a German translation of Leibniz's *raison suffisante* or *principium rationis sufficientis* from the *Monadologie*. You will no doubt want to protest that these two philosophical works are *not* translations, and indeed not even adaptations: they are "originals." After all, Hegel and Heidegger are among the most original philosophical thinkers of the last two centuries, and those two works are more original than many others. Such distinctions are important "icoses," or plausibilizations, of our definitional binaries: an original work can't possibly be a translation; a translation can't possibly be an original work.

Rather than fight you on that, then, let me shift to a different example: Alain Badiou's *La République de Platon* (2012), which he describes as a "hypertranslation" and Emily Apter (2013, 20) describes as a "true adventure in philosophy." As she continues:

> He theatricalizes the mise-en-scène of Platonic discourse (in a cross between Beckett and Brecht). He introduces French slang and he takes liberties with Plato's content to the point of introducing a new female character.

> Throughout, there is an attempt to stage an encounter with the "real" through recourse to colloquial diction; a diction contributing to the translation's political intention. Badiou valorizes equality (rather than liberty or freedom of expression, associated with "the politics of appearance and opinion") alongside the text's potential for a contemporary politics of justice.

She also quotes Susan Spitzer, who translated Badiou's translation into American English:

> "Hypertranslation" is the term Badiou has used, in *The Communist Hypothesis* and elsewhere, to describe his treatment of Plato's *Republic*. Not a "simple" translation into French of the Greek original, then, and still less a scholarly critique of it, Badiou's text transforms the *Republic* into something startlingly new by expanding, reducing, updating and dramatizing it, leavening it with humor and revitalizing its language with his own philosophical lexicon. Yet, for all the plasticity of the hypertranslation, its freewheeling appropriation of the source text, it still remains an adaptation based firmly on his painstaking translation of Plato's language into modern French.
>
> (quoted in Apter 2013, 21)

Note there the descriptors: "hypertranslation," "not a 'simple' translation," and "an adaptation based firmly on his painstaking translation." Implicit in that account would appear to be a two-stage or two-level reproduction process: "translation" as the base, the lower level or first stage, and "hypertranslation" or "adaptation" up on top, built on that base. I'm not exactly sure what that means, frankly. Does it mean that Badiou rendered the text twice, the first time translating and the second time adapting/transforming/hypertranslating? Or does it mean that "translation" is a kind of *imaginary* foundation for the radical expansion/reduction/update/dramatization that he effected just once – and that that imaginary foundation is envisioned and attributed to Badiou as a cultural warrant of textual reliability? Or is Spitzer basically just saying that Badiou's French text, despite its apparent radicalism, more reminiscent of an adaptation than a translation, is still *sort of* a translation? Is the upshot here that no one quite knows what to call it, but everyone still feels compelled to call it *something*? When in doubt, categorize. When in doubt about your categories, categorize twice, in layers. Well categorized is practically cloned.

Is there any possible world in which *precisely this generic indeterminacy,* arising out of the transformative translation (or whatever we want to call it) of a major source text, is the paradigm case of all philosophizing?

That would of course be an extreme view; but it is not my invention. It is, for example, everywhere in Derrida: translationality (though he would say "iterability") as transformationality.[1] "'The history of philosophy,' as Abdelfattah Kilito reminds us with reference to the historic importance of Averroës's translation and exegesis of Aristotle," as Emily Apter (2013, 9) reports, "'is at its core the history of translation.'" She adds: "The expression 'history of translation' from my perspective implies a decided emphasis on when and where translation happens, and, especially, on how and why it fails" (9). As we'll see below, that emphasis she puts on "translation failure" is part of her gravitation toward "the Untranslatable," including things like "'lost in translation,' the mistranslated, unreliable translation and the *contresens* [misinterpretation], an impassive condition that would seem to nest in language; sometimes discernible as a pull away from language norming" (9). As my insistence on translationality-as-transformationality might suggest, I am leery of the binary opposition "translation failure"/"translation success." The ability to recognize a translation as a "failure" requires a clear definition of "success" and a wide ditch between the two – and translation as I understand it doesn't just fall into that ditch: it lives there.

Apter's dogged insistence on the irreducibility of the (non-?)category that she calls "the Untranslatable" seems repeatedly to be arguing against the position I am exploring; but I suggest that that impression is merely an artifact of a false binary. What Apter calls "translation failure," I call translationality – but that is also "translation success." It is only when translation success is defined as cloning that a failure to clone has to be condemned as translation failure, or the Untranslatable.

On the one hand, Apter wants to back off from the notion of a stable essence that can be named as a stable category: "Perhaps it would be more accurate to understand the Untranslatable, not as pure difference in opposition to the always translatable (rightly suspect as just another non-coeval form of the romantic Absolute, or fetish of the Other, or hermeneutical inaccessibility) but as a linguistic form of creative failure with homeopathic uses" (20). Homeopathy as a life-oriented management system – but a profoundly klugey one.

On the other hand, however, it is clear from the way she writes about it that she does indeed conceive "the Untranslatable" as a stable essence and a stable category:

- "Incomparables and Untranslatables," she writes, "are thus set about in a world in which mobile social placing and terrestrial property-lines both affirm and trump national heritage claims" (16). That of course tropes "Incomparables and Untranslatables" as discrete *things* that can be set in place. It is of course entirely possible that the tenor of that trope is considerably less thing-y; but what could it be?
- "The Untranslatable emerges as something on the order of 'an Incredible,' an 'Incontournable [inevitable],' an 'Untouchable' (*L'Incorruptible* in French). There is a quality of militant semiotic intransigence attached to the Untranslatable, making it more than just a garden-variety keyword" (34). The Untranslatable "emerges" as a "something," and when it emerges, it has a "quality" of intransigence "attached" to it. This is not "pure difference," pure negativity: it is a thing with positive characteristics.
- "Words that assign new meanings to old terms, neologisms, names for ideas that are continually re-translated or mistranslated, translations that are obviously incommensurate (as in the use of *esprit* for 'mind' or *Geist*), these

> are among the most salient symptoms of the genuine Untranslatable" (35). There is not only a stable category called "the Untranslatable"; the "genuineness" of that category is attested by "salient symptoms." Like the mythical all-knowing clinician, the comparativist invariably/infallibly recognizes "the [genuine] Untranslatable" in and through a stable symptomatology. Even though Apter admits that her usage is "rightly suspect as just another non-coeval form of the romantic Absolute, or fetish of the Other, or hermeneutical inaccessibility" – the mystical strategy for talking about the transcendent, the ineffable, whatever cannot be captured in words – she can't help herself. She *wants* that "romantic Absolute." She needs it.

Or, in a more complicated trope: "With translation assumed to be a good thing *en soi* – under the assumption that it is a critical practice enabling communication across languages, cultures, time periods and disciplines – the right to the Untranslatable was blindsided" (8). The mixed metaphor there is telling: "the right" (not some person's or group's right, just "the right") apparently has eyes on "the right" side of its head (okay, that's a joke), and the attempt to privilege translation as Total Communication across boundaries sneaks up on it from the left, or from behind, surprising it from the side on which it sees nothing. If pushed, I suspect, Apter would tweak that trope a little, insisting instead that, like Lady Justice, "the right to the Untranslatable" is *always* blind, *has nothing but* that blindside, and that the charge against the privileging of translation is not that it snuck up on that right from the wrong side, but that it snuck up at all. That "right" has no "right" side for things to sneak up on it from. Its value lies precisely in its blindness – a trope, I'm guessing, for its mystical irrationality.

Historically, we might speculate, the "blindsiding" of "the right to the Untranslatable" was first undertaken by Christianity in its incursions into the mystery religions from which it took so much of its early impetus. As I showed in *Translation and Taboo* (Robinson 1996), the Christian principle of Total Translatability was a rationalist juggernaut launched against the mystery of the old ways, the closing first of the initiate's *eyes* in the darkness of the initiation ritual, to prevent light-of-day knowledge, understanding, then of the initiate's *mouth* after the initiation was over, to prevent light-of-day reporting on the contents of the ritual. The Will of the Christian God, by contrast, not only can be infinitely and perfectly expressed, in language open to everyone; it can be infinitely and perfectly translated, into every language on earth.

Ironically, the "blindsiding" of "the right to the Untranslatable" consisted in a forced opening of mystically closed eyes: "blindsiding" as a renunciation/repudiation of willed blindness. The principle of Total Translatability – the perfect international communication of verbal meanings as the earliest dream of globalization – snuck into the mystical cave and switched on the lights.

Of course, while Total Translatability was the official Christian theology from very early on, the actual ecclesiastical implementation of that theology was far messier. It didn't happen as instantaneously or as easily as "switching on the lights" makes it sound. The Protestant Reformation was still having to fight for the "right" to Total Translatability a millennium and a half in; and the expansion of Protestantism-cum-capitalism into the Total Translatability of globalization took another half millennium to take hold. The mystery religions were all about "unique" experiences that could not be cloned: the right to the Untranslatable, the Unclonable, extended from feeling to speaking (the ban on intralingual translation) and from speaking to translating (the ban on interlingual translation). The ban on vernacular translations of the Bible came out of the same impulse to protect the Unclonability of the Bible: the Holy Spirit wrote it in Latin, through Jerome, and that was that. Just that once. In defending that ban – though he hedges on the word "ban" – in his 1529 *Dialogue Against Heresies* (Robinson 1997/2002, 80–81), Thomas More specifically refers to "the great secret mysteries of scripture," "the high mysteries of holy scripture," "the high secret mysteries of God," and "God's great and secret mysteries": mysteries as unclonable unique experiences.

The Christian principle of Total Translatablity in its early mystical form would be what Epiphanius of Salamis (c. 310/20–403) and Augustine of Hippo (354–430) took to be the divine inspiration of the Seventy in the creation of a Greek translation of the Hebrew Bible (see Robinson 1997/2002, 22, 34), and what the medieval Church took to be the divine inspiration of St. Jerome (Eusebius Sophronius Hieronymus, c. 347–420) in the creation of the Vulgate Latin Bible. In its current late-capitalist/neoliberal pragmatic form, it would be the assumption that all transactions channel the Holy Dollar. In both forms, it is a principle of *Universal Equivalence* (see Liu 1999 and Robinson 2017a for discussion). What I am calling translationality churns up the variegated middle between Christian/neoliberal Total Translatability and mystical Unclonability. If it leans slightly in the direction of the former, its resemblance takes on form only once the reigning doctrine of the Universal Equivalent has been dethroned, revealed as fraudulent *ex post facto* image management. In the long history of that belief in Total Translatability, specific exemplars have repeatedly been demystified, but without ever dethroning the hegemonic Christian doctrine of the Universal Equivalent:

- In his Letter to Pammachius (Robinson 1997/2002, 23–30) Jerome showed at great gleeful length how many mistakes the Seventy had made, shocking Augustine, who could not read the Hebrew, and who therefore believed the myth of the Seventy's divine inspiration. History's revenge on Jerome was not his discrediting but his enthronement as the infallible translatorial channel of the Holy Spirit into Latin.
- In his new Greek and Latin New Testaments implicitly, and in his 1518 letter to Martin Lips explicitly (see Robinson 1997/2002, 65–75), Erasmus of Rotterdam showed how many mistakes Jerome had made, shocking the Catholic Church of his day, which had by then been locked into the myth of Jerome's divine inspiration for over a thousand years. Despite Erasmus, Jerome's Vulgate translation remained the Catholic Church's only acceptable source text for Bible translating until the early twentieth century.
- Internet journalism keeps revealing relentlessly just how riddled the neoliberal myth of Universal Capitalist Equivalences is with computer error and the

> whole range of fraud, graft, bribery, and so on, but without overturning the myth. Other forms of "human" influence-peddling and favor-currying are even harder to demystify, such as nepotism, old-boy networks, school friendships, and the "obvious" hierarchy of credibility whereby the more you're worth on paper the more your word is worth.

To put that differently: both the mystery religions' and the medieval Catholic Church's Ban on Clonability and the Christian Church's and neoliberalism's official theology of Infinite Clonability are grounded in clones and spin; my notion of translationality is grounded in an *overt* assertion of the ubiquity of change. No hiding; no spinning.

To put that still differently: the binary between Christian/neoliberal Infinite Clonability and mystical/Apterian Unclonability is hegemonic, the former as the preferred hegemony, the latter a shadow hegemony; my notion of translationality is counterhegemonic, and therefore also wildly counterintuitive, and unlikely to win many converts.

Apter tells us in her Acknowledgments (2013, vii) that her book project arose in large part out of her work with Barbara Cassin, Jacques Lezra, Michael Wood, and Étienne Balibar on an English "translation and re-edition" of Cassin's *Vocabulaire européen des philosophies: Dictionnaire des intraduisibles* (2004) – literally "European Vocabulary of the Philosophies: Dictionary of the Untranslatables," but titled in English *Dictionary of Untranslatables: A Philosophical Lexicon* (Apter 2014). She also borrowed the concept of "the Untranslatable" from Cassin and that project. And it strikes me that her account of Cassin's book is far more nuanced than the bulk of her other passing remarks on "the Untranslatable" – strikes me strongly enough, in fact, that I am inclined to quote at length, inserting bracketed numbers for ease of comment:

> Barbara Cassin's *Vocabulaire européen des philosophies: Dictionnaire des intraduisibles* produces [1] wide-span intellectual cartography without a hegemonic global paradigm; that is to say, through [2] interpretive procedures that reveal philosophical world-systems in the making. The book uses untranslatability as an [3] epistemological fulcrum for rethinking philosophical concepts and discourses of the humanities. With critical finesse, it [4] calls into question the very possibility of naming the predicates of Western thought even as it shows how such lodestones have been and continue to be actively translated. It is an exercise in [5] the reclamation of sophistry and logology over and against the Platonic tradition of positing truths in an absolute sense, as a kind of mathematical intelligence unbeholden to language. This semantic predicament is consequential for the humanities; useful in defining [6] a translational condition that complicates nation-based epistemes and literary denominations. Using the *Vocabulaire*'s construct of the Untranslatable, one can construe [7] a translational humanities whose fault lines traverse the cultural subdivisions of nations or "foreign" languages while coalescing around hubs of singularity.
>
> (31)

Comments:

1 "Wide-span intellectual cartography without a hegemonic global paradigm." The great temptation in a project like this is to impose a single pattern or explanatory model on all philosophizing everywhere: a "hegemonic global paradigm." Cassin's *Vocabulaire* avoids that temptation by focusing on local knots and nodes that nevertheless connect up to all manner of intellectual problems from various parts of the world.

2 "Interpretive procedures that reveal philosophical world-systems in the making." Rather than focusing on the "philosophical world-systems" as static products, Cassin's project zeroes in on the "interpretive procedures" by which such systems are made, and thus ultimately on the making itself.

3 "An epistemological fulcrum for rethinking philosophical concepts and discourses of the humanities." A fulcrum of course is the support for a lever – say, the hypothetical lever that, placed properly, would allow Archimedes to lift the entire planet. Here it works metaphorically to signal a radically new way of knowing-and-thinking-and-talking about "philosophical concepts and discourses of the humanities."

4 "Calls into question the very possibility of naming the predicates of Western thought even as it shows how such lodestones have been and continue to be actively translated." The terms "predicates" and "lodestones" there are roughly speaking *keywords*, like "subject," "sensation," "fate," etc., but Apter wants to stress the *interlingual networks of predication* mapped by these words as they travel from philosophical tradition to philosophical tradition, and how they change as they move. The metaphor of guidance on those travels is signaled in "lodestone," literally in Middle English a "course stone" or "leading stone" because lodestones, naturally occurring magnetized stones, were the first magnetic compasses. "Continue to be actively translated" would appear to be negatively tonalized, to indicate the distortions imposed on such concepts through translation; what is "call[ed] into question," obviously, is "the very possibility of naming the predicates of Western thought" *in one language*, without translation. The Christian tradition of the Universal Equivalent (or what Derrida calls a transcendental signified) – for Augustine a stable and timeless meaning that stands above or beyond all translational distortions – is impossible; and yet translators, it would seem, keep striving for it.

5 "The reclamation of sophistry and logology over and against the Platonic tradition of positing truths in an absolute sense, as a kind of mathematical intelligence unbeholden to language." The "Platonic tradition of positing truths in an absolute sense" is something like what I called above the quest to make things stay the same; the "mathematical intelligence unbeholden to language" hints at the scientific ideal of reducing cosmic truth to math, and so avoiding the distortions of language. Apter's point is not only that language is all we have; it is that *languages* are all we have, and individual languages don't match up. "Sophistry and logology" is an odd pairing: logology is Kenneth Burke's (1961/1970) coinage for "words about words,"

which works here, but Apter's invocation of sophistry seems to suggest not so much a reclamation of the teachings of the ancient Greek Sophists, who taught public-speaking strategies for the assembly *(ekklesia)*, as it does an overturning of the modern disparaging sense of sophistry as clever fallacious reasoning (based originally on Plato's and Aristotle's antagonism). It may be that she actually meant the reclamation of *casuistry*, or case-based reasoning – reasoning attacked by universalizing thinkers because it refuses to seek the stability of a universal principle.

6 "A translational condition that complicates nation-based epistemes and literary denominations." The Greek word ἐπιστήμη/*epistēmē* means "knowledge"; I'm guessing, however, that Apter is using the term in the specialized sense given it by Michel Foucault in *The Order of Things* and other works, as "the strategic apparatus which permits of separating out from among all the statements which are possible those that will be acceptable within, I won't say a scientific theory, but a field of scientificity, and which it is possible to say are true or false" (Foucault 1980, 197). An "episteme" in Foucault's sense is a kind of unconscious ideological orientation that undergirds and "vets" knowledge; it is close to what I call an icosis. The important point that Apter is making here is that modern translation – about which more will be said throughout this essay, especially section 2.3.3 – is traditionally thought through "nation-based epistemes," which is to say ideological assumptions about "the source language," according to which it is a single language belonging to a single nation, which speaks only that language, and about "the target language," according to which it is a single language belonging to a different single nation, which speaks only that language. Thus if one says "translation," the unconscious basis for everything we all know about that subject leads us back to verbal interaction between two unified nations with two unified cultures speaking two unified languages, which is to say, a transfer of textual meaning from nation/culture/language A to nation/culture/language B. What Apter is suggesting is that Cassin's *Vocabulaire* bespeaks "a translational condition" (more or less what I am calling translationality) that doesn't utterly and automatically lock into that episteme. It may participate in it partly, but it also complicates it.

7 "A translational humanities whose fault lines traverse the cultural subdivisions of nations or 'foreign' languages while coalescing around hubs of singularity." This is my destination in this essay: this "translational humanities" (TH) or translationality organized not around monolithic national languages and cultures mythically paired up like animals marching into Noah's Ark but around those multiple nodes or "hubs of singularity" and the complex semiotic "fault lines" traced through them. Presumably the geological metaphor "fault lines" is designed to suggest TH volatility as discontinuous nonlinear movement in and across a cultural "fault zone," or what Apter (2005) has called a "translation zone."

Above all, what pleases me in that passage is Apter's willingness to talk about (un)translatability *as* a "translational condition," or TH as an unstable planar fracture in a fault zone. Rather than contrasting the myth of Total Translatablity with some kind of mystical protected (and counter-capitalized) realm called the Untranslatable, she here seems to recognize that translation inevitably works in and through the klugey tensions of (un)translability. Not translatability *versus* untranslatability: both intertwined in the same textual engagements. Success in failure; failure in success. Translationality. She chides David Bellos in *Is That a Fish in Your Ear? Translation and the Meaning of Everything* (2011) for his hubristic opposition to the very idea of untranslatability, noting that his opposition likely "is guided by his role as a professional translator having to overcome difficult hurdles" (19); what she misses is Bellos's professional fallibilism, his acceptance of the impossibility of getting any translation to work perfectly, and thus the sense in which professional translatability *incorporates* the specter of untranslatability as its shadowy double or clone. The professional translator is hired to produce *a text*. That text is called a translation. If a text called a translation can always be produced, there is always translatability. That doesn't exclude the Untranslatable: it just lives with it.[2]

Now let us narrow our focus to literature, and literary translation-as-transformation.

2.2 Translations of medicine as/in literature

I propose to take two passes through this material: the first, here in section 2.2, a fairly straightforward history of translations and adaptations, understood loosely as translationality, in order to put some cases on the table for discussion; the second, in section 2.3, a series of retheorizations of translationality as (re)(peri-) performances of the "making-real." The history in this section moves from a history of medical translations/adaptations (of Galen into Latin in the sixteenth century) to a history of literary translations/adaptations with a strong medical theme (Rabelais into English in the seventeenth and eighteenth centuries).

2.2.1 Openness to the future: Galen>Rhazes>Vesalius

The premier authority on matters medical from late antiquity into the Renaissance was the Greek philosopher and physician Κλαύδιος Γαληνός, romanized as Claudius Galenus, usually referred to in English simply as Galen (129–c.200/216 BCE). He wrote a great many works on a great many subjects, including anatomy, physiology, pathology, pharmacology, and neurology, as well as philosophy and logic; one of his books was titled *That the Best Physician is also a Philosopher*. The usual European narrative has his hegemony unchallenged for 1300 years, until 1543 in anatomy, with the publication of *De Humani Corporis Fabrica*/"On the Construction of the Human Body" by Andreas Vesalius (1514–1564), and until 1628 in studies of the physiology of the circulatory system, with the publication of *Exercitatio Anatomica de Motu Cordis et Sanguinis in Animalibus*/"An Anatomical Exercise on the Motion of the Heart and Blood in Living Beings" by William Harvey (1578–1657), establishing that the heart is a pump that circulates blood throughout the body. But in fact Galen was challenged earlier in Persia, based on ninth-century Arabic translations, by وبكر مح??د زكرياى رازى (854–c. 925/932), variously romanized as Muhammad ibn Zakariyā al-Rāzī, just plain Razi (meaning from the town of شهر رى/[Shahr-e-]Rey), or Rhazes. In fact Rhazes wrote a book called *Doubts about Galen* (جالينوس على لشكوك/*Shukuk 'ala Alinusor*), challenging (among other things) Galen's humor theory by showing that introducing a warm drink into a body may raise the body's temperature even higher than the drink's temperature, suggesting that the drink didn't simply transfer its heat to the body but provoked a reaction. He also pioneered the study of ophthalmology, wrote a groundbreaking book on smallpox and measles (الشكوك على جالينوس/*al-Judari wa al-Hasbah*, translated over a dozen times into Latin), discovered compounds like alcohol and kerosene, developed various pieces of medical apparatus such as flasks, mortars, spatulas, and phials, and was the first to produce various acids.

Note the cautionary words of Sherwin B. Nuland (1988, 57), however:

> But there were problems, of the sort that are inherent in the transfer of knowledge from language to language and society to society. The first difficulty lay in the very act of translation, which in itself distorts greatly even when thoughts are transmitted between cultures far less dissimilar than the Hellenic and Moslem. Were this not enough, the form in which many of the ancient writings came to the translators had been already warped by several generations of compilers and epitomizers. When an Arab physician pored over Galen, he was likely to be studying not a translation from the original but the teachings as they had been interpreted by one of the small herd of self-appointed commentators who appeared in Byzantium after the master's death. Among the most prolific of these literary jackals were Oribasius in the fourth century, Aetius and Alexander of Tralles in the sixth century, and particularly Paul of Aegina in the seventh century.
>
> (57)

So significantly were the key texts transformed – "distorted" – by these many hands that the great Avicenna ('Abū 'Alī al-Ḥusayn ibn 'Abd Allāh ibn Al-Hasan ibn Ali ibn Sīnā/أبو علي الحسين بن عبد الله بن الحسن بن علي بن سينا, c.980–1037) was attacked by Arnold of Villanova (c. 1240–1311) as " 'a professional scribbler who had stupefied European physicians by his misinterpretation of Galen' " (quoted by Nuland 57).

Nuland continues:

> It was these Arabic materials then that finally found their way into Latin in the eleventh and twelfth centuries. The process began at the Benedictine abbey of Monte Cassino in the eleventh century. There, a Carthaginian-born monk known as Constantine the African, the "Magister Orientis et Occidentis," translated large numbers of Arabic medical texts into Latin. His work has been referred to by the German medical historian Karl Sudhoff as "a symptom of a great historical process," the entry of Moslem and

> Jewish thinking into western medicine, with the return to its origins of the prodigal art of healing. But although the translation of Hellenic scientific texts into Latin exerted a great energizing effect on European thought, what the Europeans were studying was Galen by way of compilers like Paul, and translations from Greek to Arabic to Latin. When to the problem of multiple translations is added the potential for error introduced by medically untutored scribes laboriously hand-printing each manuscript, it becomes obvious that it would have taken a series of miracles to prevent major distortions from appearing. Alas, no such miracles occurred, and the true revival of Greek learning had to wait until after the conquest of Constantinople by the Turks in 1453, when Greek scholars migrated to Italy, bringing with them the actual books and manuscripts of the ancients. Europeans thereupon began to learn Greek, to read Galen and Hippocrates in the original, and to translate them directly into Latin. Only then could real medical science begin again [in Europe], where Galen had left it thirteen hundred years before. It is a sad irony that his new intellectual heirs would use his experimental method to trample his reputation into the dust, his errors and the centuries of corruption of his teachings blinding them to the fact that it was he who had constructed the framework upon which they would now build.
>
> (57, 59)

The most famous of those "intellectual heirs" who used Galen's experimental method "to trample his reputation into the dust" was Andreas Vesalius (the Latinized version of Andries van Wesel), a Flemish physician and anatomist whose 1543 book *De Humani Corporis Fabrica*/"On the Construction of the Human Body" – often called simply *De Fabrica,* published when the author was 28 – is usually regarded as the founding text of modern human anatomy. (For detailed discussion, see Nuland 1988, ch. 3; Sawday 1995, passim.) Vesalius came from a long line of medical men: his great-grandfather, Jan van Wesel, taught medicine at the University of Leuven; his grandfather, Everard van Wesel, was royal physician to Emperor Maximilian; his father, Anders van Wesel, served the same emperor as apothecary. After intensive Greek and Latin studies, he matriculated in 1528 (at the age of 14) into the University of Leuven, where his great-grandfather taught, but when in 1532 Maximilian died and his father was made valet de chambre to his successor, Charles V, Andreas decided to move to the University of Paris and pursue a career in the military. There he studied Galen and developed his interest in anatomy under Jacobus Sylvius (Jacques Dubois, 1478–1555), who would later become one of his most implacable opponents on the issue of modifying Galenic principles based on experimental evidence. Returning to Leuven in 1537, he wrote his baccalaureate thesis on the ninth book of Rhazes – *Paraphrasis in Nonum Librum Rhazae Medici Arabis Clariss. ad Regem Almansorum de Affectuum Singularum Corporis Partium Curatione*/"Paraphrase of Rhazes's ninth book for King Al-Mansor" – and was immediately offered the chair of surgery and anatomy at the University of Padua.

By the 1530s, in his early twenties, Vesalius was translating Galen into Latin; by the early 1540s, in his late twenties, he was writing *De Fabrica,* in which he prominently employed Galenic models in style and form but equally prominently challenged key tenets in Galen's thinking, based on his dissection of human corpses. Galen had expressly stated that his findings were based on the dissection of monkeys, especially Barbary macaques, because human dissection was forbidden in ancient Rome, and, he claimed, monkeys were similar to humans; since human dissection was allowed in Renaissance Europe, Vesalius was able to show that humans were in fact anatomically quite different. This was a wildly controversial claim at the time, since Galen was taken to be medical gospel; challenging his veracity was as radical as Erasmus of Rotterdam daring to retranslate the New Testament into Latin, and to print the result *en face* with a newly edited Greek text (1516), and to show in the process that St. Jerome – who had supposedly been inspired by the Holy Spirit – had made mistakes.

As Hans-Georg Gadamer (1960/1990, 198; Weinsheimer and Marshall 1975/1989, 193) reminds us, "The highest aim of the humanist was not originally to 'understand' his models" – let alone to submit humbly to their authority – "but to imitate or even surpass them" ("Für den Humanisten ist, wie man nicht vergessen darf, sein höchstes Ziel ursprünglich überhaupt nicht, seine Vorbilder zu ‹verstehen›, sondern es ihnen gleichzutun, oder gar sie zu übertreffen"). Translationality as transcendent/transgressive imitation.

2.2.2 From medicine to the reading cure: Hippocrates>Galen>Vesalius>Burton

The course I chart through these waters is roughly chronological, but I propose to blend strict chronology with thematic coherence – in particular, with a gradual transition from medical literature to imaginative literature. The first three subsections here in section 2.2, therefore, all deal in a very loose sense with derivative works based on Hippocrates and Galen, beginning with a strict medical textbook like Vesalius's *De Fabrica* (1543); jumping from there eight decades forward to *The Anatomy of Melancholy* (1621) by Robert Burton (1577–1640), which is ostensibly a medical textbook on melancholia but ranges widely, with inventive abandon, through much of what was known and understood in the early seventeenth century, not only science and philosophy but poetry and everyday life, and goblins, and the geography of America, and so on; and then from there back nearly a century to *Les horribles et épouvantables faits et prouesses du très renommé Pantagruel Roi des Dipsodes, fils du Grand Géant Gargantua* (c. 1532) by François Rabelais (c. 1483/94–1553), which over the ensuing three decades eventually became what we know of today as *Gargantua et/and Pantagruel. De Fabrica* is a pioneering medical textbook on anatomy; Burton's encyclopedic work is a *literary* anatomy of a medical/philosophical/theological disorder; Rabelais's encyclopedic work is imaginative fiction.

Thanks to the popularity of Burton's title, "anatomy" has come to mean a comprehensive literary treatment of any subject, not just the human body: Northrop

Frye's (1957/1990) *Anatomy of Criticism*, for example, comprehensively anatomizes the critical study of literature, along the way characterizing both Burton's *Anatomy* (311) and Rabelais's *Gargantua and Pantagruel* (309) as Menippean satires, presumably because both are big, sprawling, encyclopedic works with satirical designs on their readers (and because Burton does explicitly write "I did sometime laugh and scoff with Lucian, and satirically tax with Menippus, lament with Heraclitus" (1621/1871, 31)). Later and more careful readers of Burton, however, have quite rightly disputed Frye's categorization:

> Burton may not be a thoroughgoing Calvinist, and he may oppose the excesses of "giddy precisians" (as well as Catholics), yet it is a serious misreading of the *Anatomy* to suggest that Burton is opposed to religious therapies, and that the main thrust of his section on religious melancholy is a satirical, polemical one. Just as it is right to see the text as having satirical elements, but a distortion to call it a Menippean satire [here she footnotes Frye], so it is also true that the work sometimes has a religiously polemical tone, but misleading to see it as a polemic.
>
> (Lund 2006, 672)

Burton's *Anatomy* is very much a mixed mode, grounded medically not only in Hippocrates, Aristotle, and Galen but in Vesalius as well, but pushing his medical concerns just as strongly in literary, philosophical, and theological directions, and weaving all his various strands together with a first-person narratorial voice that is ironic, importunate, often satirical, and – not coincidentally – deeply melancholic. If *De Fabrica* is a brilliantly illustrated medical textbook for future physicians, and *Gargantua and Pantagruel* is a brilliantly medicalized Menippean satire by a physician, *The Anatomy of Melancholy* is a brilliantly encyclopedic "reading cure" (Lund 2010) for a medical disorder by a theologian who understands his theme with radical holism.

The remaining four subsections of section 2.2, then, deal with "strictly" literary treatments of medical matters: translations of Rabelais into English in 2.2.4–5, and Laurence Sterne's *Life and Opinions of Tristram Shandy, Gentleman* (inspired by Rabelais, with repeated parodic pokes at Burton) in English in 2.2.6 and in Portuguese in 2.2.7.

In the course of his *Anatomy* Burton cites or mentions Hippocrates 96 times, Galen 158 times, Rabelais 5 times, and Vesalius 3 times – but those numbers alone give an inaccurate impression of Burton's reliance on Vesalius, whose *De Fabrica* stitches together the fabric of his "Digression of Anatomy" in Subsection I of Section 1, Member II. His references to Rabelais clearly hint at the directionality of the trajectory we are tracing, from "Physicke" to the bohemian decadence of literature, calumny, sedition, insanity, and licentious drunkenness:

> What remains then but to send for Lorarios, those officers to carry them all together for company to Bedlam, and set Rabelais to be their physician.
>
> (160)

> So they triumph in villainy, and justify their wickedness; with Rabelais, that French Lucian, drunkenness is better for the body than physic, because there be more old drunkards than old physicians.
>
> (303)

> It is an old saying, "A blow with a word strikes deeper than a blow with a sword:" and many men are as much galled with a calumny, a scurrilous and bitter jest, a libel, a pasquil, satire, apologue, epigram, stage-play or the like, as with any misfortune whatsoever. Princes and potentates, that are otherwise happy, and have all at command, secure and free, *quibus potentia sceleris impunitatem fecit,* are grievously vexed with these pasquilling libels, and satires: they fear a railing Aretine, more than an enemy in the field, which made most princes of his time (as some relate) "allow him a liberal pension, that he should not tax them in his satires." The Gods had their Momus, Homer his Zoilus, Achilles his Thersites, Philip his Demades: the Caesars themselves in Rome were commonly taunted. There was never wanting a Petronius, a Lucian in those times, nor will be a Rabelais, an Euphormio, a Boccalinus in ours.
>
> (446)

Implicit in these juxtapositions is an association of seriousness, sanity, sobriety, steadfast support for Church and State, piety, and medical probity with what I am calling verbal cloning (what Horace calls the steadfast ethos of the "fidus/ Interpres"/"faithful translator" – see section 2.4, below), and villainy, wickedness, drunkenness, scurrilous and bitter jesting, libel, "pasquilling" (lampooning), and so on with translationality. Gilles Deleuze and Fèlix Guattari (1972; see also Hurley et al. 1983) might want to associate the former with sedentary culture and the latter with the nomad; Sakai Naoki (1997) might want to associate the former with the regime of homolingual address and the latter with the attitude of heterolingual address. The danger in those juxtapositions, it seems to me, is that translationality may be assimilated to the Deleuzean mystique of the nomad or the outlaw – a lifestyle that is more exciting than the sedentary suburban morality of the law-abiding populace – or to the Sakaian notion that homolinguality is an ideological construct and heterolinguality is *reality.* While recognizing that translationality is just another construct, a periperformativity, not a pre-Kantian reality, I would want to resist the temptation to see it as a "superior" construct because it is "adventurous" or whatever. Translationality is a periperformativity that *partakes* of pervasive change.

2.2.3 From medicine to fiction: Hippocrates>Galen>Rabelais

François Rabelais (c. 1483/1494–c. 1553) is of course mainly honored today for his literary output, especially the five books published over thirty years that constitute the work – often described as the first modern novel – called *La vie de Gargantua et de Pantagruel* (c. 1532–c. 1564). What modern readers often forget is that Rabelais too, like Andreas Vesalius, was a physician and a noted promulgator of the Greek medical doctrines of Hippocrates and Galen; as Gilbert

Highet (1949/1985) puts it, after joining several religious orders and finding each too confining, "at last, finding his true career, he emerged as a physician and teacher of Greek and modern medical doctrines" (182). While that "true career" was problematic as well – the iconoclastic Rabelais getting into trouble "with the Lyons hospital (for taking absence without leave), with the Sorbonne (for publishing irreverent remarks about its doctors), and with the monks (for making fun of them and their orders)" (182) – he did play a role similar to that for which Vesalius is remembered, beginning about a decade earlier: "Rabelais himself lectured on the text of Hippocrates and Galen to a large audience at Montpellier; and in 1532 he published an edition of Hippocrates's *Aphorisms* and Galen's *Art of Medicine*" (180; see also Stone 1969, 51).

R. R. Bolgar (1940, 1954/1964) in fact takes issue with Rabelais's editorial work for that collection. In his first outing, Bolgar's reading of Rabelais's editorial work is quite negative: "In the absence of wide knowledge, such enthusiasm possesses an amateurish naïveté" (1940, 66). When he returns to the topic in Chapter VII of *The Classical Heritage,* his assessment of Rabelais is more balanced, and in the end takes a significant turn: "He tells us that when he lectured on the *Aphorisms* of Hippocrates, he corrected the standard translations after a very old manuscript in his possession. For, he says, they contained many deficiencies and unauthorized additions" (1954/1964, 290). And so when the printer Gryphius offered to publish the new edition, Rabelais readily agreed. But, Bolgar notes, while it is true that Rabelais's desire to contribute to the "advancement of medicine" by "reveal[ing] the true meaning of Hippocrates where others had been misled by incorrect readings" was "the standpoint of a strict Humanist" (290–91), a closer look at the text tells a different story. In fact he did very little to the text; the changes he made were changes he borrowed from other scholars; he missed several changes that needed to be made; and he explained none of his emendations in his notes. Bolgar concludes:

> The philologically slipshod character of his Hippocrates suggests that the real interests of the movement lay elsewhere; and we have only to glance down a bibliography of Rabelais and we shall find a clue to their orientation. For Rabelais edited also Manardi's plea for a more rational approach to medicine and was himself an advocate of dissection in the study of anatomy. Scientific advance rather than the apotheosis of Greek knowledge was the prime concern of the circles in which he moved.
>
> (291)

In other words, Rabelais was correcting Hippocrates *medically* rather than philologically. Like Vesalius, his primarily loyalty was to the advancement of medicine – or, as I would put that, to medical translationality – rather than to some stabilized "true meaning" of the Greek texts. Highet (1949/1976) applies this same principle to the writing of Rabelais's great novel as well:

> To say this is not to underestimate the essential part played in Renaissance medicine by experiment and discovery; Rabelais knew, and boasted

> of knowing, a great deal of anatomy; but he started towards his anatomical knowledge from the rediscovery of the classics. The comic over-emphasis with which medical descriptions are elaborated and medical authorities cited and multiplied in *Gargantua* and *Pantagruel* shows that for Rabelais medicine with its new discoveries was not an ordinary activity to be accepted and used like commercial law, but an exciting proof of the power of the newly awakened human mind.
>
> (180–81)

And indeed physicians are everywhere in the novel. Book I, "The Very Horrific Life of Great Gargantua, Father of Pantagruel" – written and published second, in 1534 – is in fact a disguised treatise on child-rearing, after the best medical advice from a physician named Master Theodorus; in Book II, "The Horrible and Terrifying Deeds and Words of the Very Renowned Pantagruel King of the Dipsodes, Son of the Great Giant Gargantua" – published first, pseudonymously, in c. 1533 – Pantagruel is born and raised, and wanders through France exploring the various possibilities in life, at one point considering becoming a physician, "mais il considera que l'estat estoit facheux par trop & melencolicque/& q' les medicins sentoient les clysteres comme vieulx dyables" (Rabelais 1533, n.p.)/"but he considered that that calling was too troublesome and melancholick; and that Physicians did smell of glisters like old devils" (Urquhart 1653–1693/1994, 183). Chapter 8 is a famous letter to Pantagruel from his father Gargantua, giving him advice on how best to live his life; one of the instructions he passes along is:

> Puis songneusemét revisiter les liures des medicins Grecz/Arabes & latins sans contemner les Tamuldistes [*sic*] et Cabalistes/et par frequéntes anathomies acquiers toy parfaicte congnoissance de l'autre monde qui est l'homme.
>
> (n.p.)

> Then faile not most carefully to peruse the books of the *Greek, Arabian,* and *Latine* Physicians, not despising the *Talmudists* and *Cabalists;* and by frequent anatomies get thee the perfect knowledge of the other world, called the Microcosme, which is man.
>
> (197)

When Book I was published in 1534, Vesalius's *De Fabrica* (1543) was still nearly a decade in the future, and his baccalaureate thesis on Rhazes (1538) was four years in the future; but it is tempting nevertheless to identify the "Greek physicians" as Hippocrates, Galen, and Dioscorides, the "Arabian physicians" as Rhazes, Avicenna, and Averroes ('Abū l-Walīd Muḥammad Ibn 'Aḥmad Ibn Rušd/بو الوليد محمد ابن احمد ابن رشد , 1126–1198), and the "Latin physicians" as the likes of Vesalius and perhaps Michael Servetus, whose *Christianismi Restitutio* (1553) was still twenty years in the future, published in the presumed year of Rabelais's death.

Book III, "The Third Book of the Heroic Deeds and Sayings of Good Pantagruel," published in 1546 – and, like both of its predecessors, immediately banned, though this time it continued to be sold despite the ban – tells the story of Pantagruel's friend Panurge, who makes a pilgrimage to the Oracle of the Bottle, to learn whether he should marry (though he hasn't yet picked out a bride-candidate). The resulting collection of reports back from the war between the sexes is one of the novel's most influential sequences for later writers; in section 2.2.4 we will see Laurence Sterne adapting Book III in Volume IV of *Tristram Shandy.* Stories about and advice from physicians figure prominently in the book; here for example is a longish passage from Chapter XXXIV, "How Women ordinarily have the greatest longing after things prohibited," in the famous translation by Sir Thomas Urquhart of Cromarty (1611–1660), this book left unpublished at his death and first published as edited and revised by Pierre/Peter Antoine/Anthony le Motteux in 1693:

> Welcome, in good Faith, my dear Master, welcome: It did me good to hear you talk, the Lord be praised for all. I do not remember to have seen you before now, since the last time that you acted at *Monpelliers,* with our ancient Friends, *Anthony Saporra, Guy Bourguyer, Balthasar Noyer, Tolly, Ihon Quentin, Francis Robinet, Jhon Perdrier,* and *Francis Rabelais,* the Moral Comedy of him who had espoused and married a *Dumb Wife.* I was there, quoth *Epistemon;* the good honest Man, her Husband, was very earnestly urgent to have the Fillet of her Tongue untied, and would needs have her speak by any means: at his desire some pains were taken on her, and partly by the industry of the Physitian, other part by the expertness of the Surgeon, the *Encyliglotte,* which she had under her Tongue, being cut, she spoke and spoke again; yea, within a few hours she spoke so loud, so much, so fiercely, and so long, that her poor Husband returned to the same Physitian for a Recipe to make her hold her Peace: There are (quoth the Physitian) many proper Remedies in our art to make dumb Women speak, but there are none, that ever I could learn therein, to make them silent. The only Cure which I have found out, is their Husband's *Deafness.* The Wretch became within few Weeks thereafter, by Vertue of some Drugs, Charms or Enchantments, which the *Physitian* had prescribed unto him, so *deaf,* that he could not have heard the Thundring of Nineteen hundred Canons at a *Salve.* His Wife perceiving, that indeed he was as *deaf* as a Door-nail, and that her Scolding was but in vain, sith that he heard her not, she grew stark mad.
>
> Some time after the Doctor asked for his Fee of the Husband; who answered, That truly he was *deaf,* and so was not able to understand what the tenure of his Demand might be. Whereupon the Leech bedusted him with a little, I know not what, sort of Powder; which rendred him a Fool immediately: so great was the stiltificating Vertue of that strange kind of pulverized Dose. Then did this Fool of a Husband, and his mad Wife joyn together, falling on the Doctor and the Surgeon, did so scratch, bethwack,

and bang them, that they were left half dead upon the place, so furious were the Blows which they received: I never in my Life-time laughed so much, as at the acting of that Buffoonry.

Let us come to where we left off, (quoth *Panurge*) your Words being translated from the Clapper-dudgions to plain English, do signifie, that it is not very inexpedient that I marry, and that I should not care for being a *Cuckold*. You have there hit the Nail on the Head. I believe, Master Doctor, that on the day of my Marriage you will be so much taken up with your Patients, or otherways so seriously employed, that we shall not enjoy your Company: Sir, I will heartily excuse your absence.

Stercus et urina medici sunt prandia prima.
Ex aliis paleas, ex istis collige grana.

You are mistaken (quoth Rondibilis) in the Second Verse of our Distich; for it ought to run thus:

Nobis sunt signa, vobis sunt prandia digna.

If my Wife at any time prove to be unwell, and ill at ease, I will look upon the Water which she shall have made in an Urinal-glass, (quoth Rondibilis) grope her Pulse, and see the disposition of her *Hypogaster*, together with her Umbilicary Parts, according to the Prescript Rule of *Hippocrates*, 2. *Aph.* 35. before I proceed any further in the Cure of her Distemper. No, no, (quoth *Panurge*) that will be but to little purpose; such a Feat is for the Practice of us that are Lawyers, who have the Rubric, *De Ventre inspiciendo.* Do not therefore trouble your self about it, (Master Doctor) I will provide for her a Plaister of warm Guts. Do not neglect your more urgent occasions otherwhere, for coming to my Wedding, I will send you some supply of Victuals to your own House, without putting you to the trouble of coming abroad, and you shall always be my special Friend. With this approaching somewhat nearer to him, he clapp'd into his Hand, without the speaking of so much as one word, four *Rose Nobles. Rondibilis* did shut his Fist upon them right kindly; yet as if it had displeased him to make acceptance of such Golden Presents; he in a start, as if he had been wroth, said, He he, he, he, he, there was no need of any thing, I thank you nevertheless; *From wicked Folks, I never get enough;* and *I from honest People refuse nothing.* I shall be always, Sir, at your Command. Provided that I pay you well, quoth *Panurge*. That (quoth *Rondibilis*) is understood.

(435–36)

The Latin there is Rabelais's jeering at physicians:

Sawbones will breakfast on ordure and sharp yellow rain.
Glean from all others but straw, but these yield real grain. . . .
For us they're but signs, but for you they're a clambake arcane.
(translation DR)

Scoggin (1919) tracked that second line back to an old free-floating adage, which he found in numerous versions beginning in the fifteenth century, culminating for Rabelais, he argues, in the first modern satire, the *Epistolæ Obscurorum Virorum*/"Letters of Obscure Men" (1515–1519) – a collection of pretend letters supposedly written by zealous theologians debating whether all Jewish books should be burned, basically intended to mock scholastics and monks. The collection was published anonymously, but Erasmus of Rotterdam is generally believed to have had a hand in it – as Scoggin notes, "Whenever a good joke was going the rounds, it is usually safe to assume that Erasmus speeded it with his blessing" (387). This is the form in which Scoggin suggests Rabelais would probably have found it in the *Epistolæ* (followed by my translation):

> Dat Galienus opes, et sanctio Iustiniana;
> Ex aliis paleas, ex istis collige grana. (387)
>
> Galen grants gold, and so does the Justinian Code;
> Glean from all others but straw, but these yield fine grain.

In other words, while the characters may be jeering at physicians' clinical practices, Rabelais himself, by implicitly invoking this little poem, may be jeering at physicians' reliance on Galen. Galen is shit and piss; those who rely on him are eating the shit and drinking the piss. (And of course in British slang Rabelais is also – always – *taking* the piss.)

Or, to put that in my terms here: those who worship Galen, or any other classical authority, or any other source author, as gospel, and refuse to accept translationality – new medical discoveries, new literary effects – out of veneration for an unchanging source text, are coprophages. Translationality, by contrast, is healthy, invigorating food.

2.2.4 Translation as transformation: Rabelais>Urquhart

Sir Thomas Urquhart, Laird of Cromarty in the Highland area of Scotland, was a Royalist during the volatile period of the English Civil War. After participating in the Trot of Turriff in 1639 at the age of 28, he was knighted by King Charles I for his efforts; after participating in the Royalist uprising at Inverness in 1648, he was declared a traitor by Cromwell's Parliament but otherwise unpunished; when he marched with Charles II in the battle of Worcester in 1650–1651 – the decisive victory for the Parliamentarians/Roundheads over the Royalists/Cavaliers that established the Commonwealth of England under Cromwell – he was taken prisoner and had all his property confiscated. Since his father had died in 1642 and left him with heavy debts worth more than his total assets, this was not necessarily a terrible thing; but all his manuscripts were also confiscated and destroyed, and that was a major disaster. And, of course, he was under threat of a death sentence for treason. Apparently, however, the authorities gave him a chance to prove that he was worth a pardon; as the story has it, he produced most of his brilliant literary works to that end, including the *Pantochronachanon* (a hoax genealogy of the Urquhart family back to Adam and Eve, 1652), *Eksubalauron, or The Discovery of a most Exquisite Jewel* (a grab bag of things mostly aimed at "vindicating Scotland's honor" but also proposing a universal language, 1652), the *Logopandecteision* (an expansion of the proposal for the universal language, 1653), and, most memorably, his translation of Rabelais into Scots English: Books I and II in 1653, Book III left unpublished at his death (probably in 1660) and not published until 1693, edited by Peter le Motteux (1663–1718), who added Books IV and V in his own translation to the whole in 1708. Cromwell paroled him and restored him as Laird of Cromarty in 1652, and he relocated to the Continent in 1653 – possibly as a condition of his pardon.[3]

Urquhart's Rabelais is often described as the greatest literary translation in history. As Roger Craik (1999, 163) writes, "The more of Urquhart's translation one reads, the more aware one becomes of Urquhart as translator: his unflagging exuberance makes reading Rabelais an exhilarating experience."[4] And I would suggest that "becom[ing] aware of Urquhart as translator" also means "becoming aware of the translator as a writer" – as an original creator. Urquhart's translation is to Rabelais's original as Vesalius's *De Fabrica* is to Galen: an imitation that improves on its original. Vesalius improves on Galen because he is a modern physician and medical educator who loves and admires Galen but also believes in testing scientific claims with the experimental method, and in so doing finds that Galen made many errors, and corrects them; Urquhart improves on Rabelais because he is a Scottish writer in his own right who feels a strong literary kinship to Rabelais, not only feels Rabelais's creative/performative/transformative impulse in himself but feels it *as his own,* and indulges that impulse freely. As Craik puts it, "Nowhere is he more himself and at the same time more Rabelaisian than when he exerts himself over Rabelais's lists, such as the endearments which Gargantua's governesses lavish on the young giant's penis" (163):

> Lune la nommoit ma petite dille, laultre ma pine, laultre ma branche de coural, laultre mon bondon, mon bouchon, mon vibrequin, mon poussouer, ma teriere, ma pendilloche, mon rude esbat roidde et bas, mon dressouir, ma petite andouille vermeille, mon petit couille bredouille.
>
> (Garg, ch. 11)

> One of them would call it her little dille, her staffe of love, her quillety, her faucetin, her dandilollie: Another, her peen, her jolly kyle, her bableret, her membretoon, her quickset Imp: Another again, her branch of coral, her female adamant, her placket-racket, her cyprian scepter, her jewel for Ladies: and some of the other women would give it these names, my bunguetee, my stopple too, my busherusher, my gallant wimble, my pretty boarer, my coney-borow ferret, my little piercer, my augretine, my dangling hangers, down right to it, stiffe and stout, in & to, my pusher, dresser, pouting stick, my hony pipe, my pretty pillicock, linkie pinkie, futilletie, my lustie andouille, and crimson chitterling, my little couille bredouille, my pretty rougue, and so forth . . . (l R, Ch. ll, p. 56).
>
> (quoted in Craik 163)

Note first of all, there, that Urquhart's rendition is considerably longer than Rabelais's French original: he has not only expanded the list, adding a full twenty-five synonyms to the thirteen Rabelais provides, but picked up the phrase *Lune la nommoit*/"One of them would call it" and replicated it as "another," "another again," "and some of the other women would give it these names," to flesh out the mere humorous *list of names* in the original into a round-robin *narrative of naming*. Rabelais's text is a humorous lexicon; Urquhart's translation is a humorous scene, populated with governesses standing admiringly around a giant baby.

The second thing to note in Urquhart's translation is the prosody. Even in the longer lists in that passage he isn't just listing synonyms; he's jumping from alliteration ("stiffe and stout," "pretty pillicock," "crimson chitterling") to rhyme ("placket-racket," "linkie pinkie") to consonance ("busherusher," "dangling hangers"). And note the rhythms: not "my stopple" but "my stopple too," the "too" sounding semantically out of place but giving the line a rhythmic coherence; not "my wimble, my boarer," but "my gallant wimble, my pretty boarer"; even as the rhythms shift through the list, as in "my dangling hangers, down right to it, stiffe and stout, in & to, my pusher, dresser, pouting stick, my hony pipe, my pretty pillicock," he conveys a strong sense of *poetic organization* throughout, the embodied sense that these are not just words but a coherent account of the world.

The third thing to note is, as Roger Craik details, how he did the work:

> What Urquhart deliberately omits to mention, however, is that he succeeded where his predecessors came to grief because unlike them he had at his disposal Randle Cotgrave's *Dictionarie of the French and English Tongues* (1611), a volume towering over all previous French-to-English dictionaries and, invaluably for Urquhart, translating all but 1,000 of the words that Rabelais invented. Urquhart, whose French was not expert, had Cotgrave to hand all the time that he was translating. Therefore, if we ourselves sit with the 1542 revised editions of Rabelais and with Cotgrave's Dictionarie we can place ourselves in Urquhart's mind in the mid-seventeenth century in the very process of translation.
>
> (155)

In translating the penis passage, for example, Urquhart seems to have used (at least) the following entries in Cotgrave's dictionary:

DILLE.	The Quille, or Fawcet of a Hogshead, &c.
PINE.	A bung, or stopple.
BOUCHON.	A stopple; also, a wispe of straw, &c; also the bush of a tavern, or alehouse.
VIBREQUIN.	A wimble.
TERIERE.	An Augur.
TERRIER.	The hoile, berrie, or earth of a Connie, or Fox.
TERRIERE.	A Terrier, or Augur.
PENDILOCHES.	Jugs, danglings, or things that hang danglingly.

DILLE.	The Quille, or Fawcet of a Hogshead, &c.
ESBAT.	Sport, pastime, play, recreation; delight, pleasure, dalliance, jeasting, recreation.
DRESSOUIR.	A setting yron, or poating stick, for ruffe bands; a standing thing.
ANDOUILLE.	A linke, or chitterling.
COUILLE.	A mans yard; also (but less properly) a cod, ballocke, or testicle.
MA PETITE BREDOUILLE.	My pretty rougue, my little knave (a tearme used much by the nurses of France).
	(quoted in Craik 164)

Craik notes the way Urquhart creates diminutives from those: "quillety," "faucetin," "bableret," "membretoon," "bunguetee," "linkie pinkie." He notes the way Urquhart converts Cotgrave's "things that hang danglingly" as a translation of "PENDILOCHES" into "dangling hangers," and adds the parenthetical gloss, "(with the plural giving a slight hint of testicles)" (165). He notes how "even Urquhart's errors enhance the writing. The marvelous 'busherusher,' with its twin suggestions of childish language and sexual activity, is prompted by 'the bush of a taverne,' but this is not the correct sense" (165). I would read that a bit differently: yes, "busherusher" is partly prompted by "the bush of a tavern," and yes, that is semantically the wrong direction to go with "BOUCHON," but Urquhart is looking for ideas, for inspirations, not accurate equivalents, and "bush" takes him back to the *sound* of *bouchon,* and the image of the female pubic bush, and his "childish"/poetic ear adds "rusher" to hint at sexual activity. "Another error," Craik writes, "is 'coney-borow ferret,' for Urquhart's eye mistakenly fell on this definition while seeking that of 'terriere.' This technical flaw does not matter" (165). Again, I'm not sure why Craik needs to go to "mistakenly" and "flaw," or why he needs the faint praise of "this technical flaw does not matter." There is no "mistake" or "flaw" there: Urquhart is *trans(per-)forming* Rabelais. His propagation of "ma teriere," which Cotgrave renders as "an Augur," into a full four items in his English list, "my pretty boarer, my coney-borow ferret, my little piercer, my augretine," is the explosion of his exuberant brilliance – not a "flaw" that "does not matter." The notion that segueing creatively from auger/boarer/piercer/augretine to a furry ferret that hares after a hare down its burrow is a *flaw* is predicated on a narrow, dogmatic definition of translation as the static cloning of source-text meaning. Urquhart thinks of translation differently: as the imitation not of *words* or their *meanings* but of the source writer's transformative literary strategies. His goal is not a narrativized dictionary but a work of literature. To that end he seeks to *do what Rabelais did* – not simply to translate his words.

And to his credit, Craik knows this:

> The task of translating Rabelais, then, focuses Urquhart's energetic optimism on a work of literature which is itself suited to Urquhart's temperament. Only in this translation and in none of his other works do Urquhart's

> gigantic nonce-words, lists and digressions flourish, and this is because Rabelais himself joyously indulges in the same traits. Only here, too, when transmuting the great art of Rabelais into memorable English, does Urquhart's idiosyncratic prose achieve its potential, even if sometimes at the expense of Rabelais' terser accents. Urquhart worked on Rabelais in a state of sustained rapture, with virtually every paragraph of *Gargantua and Pantagruel* sending him scurrying to Cotgrave's fascinating *Dictionarie* from which he selected and then wrote down the best synonyms. Then, his excitement and interest at high pitch, he delightedly composed his translation, viewing it both as a creative work which involved no sacrifice of originality – it reads with the swing and confidence of an original work and betrays none of the unease one often senses in translation – and as a display of all his interests simultaneously.
>
> (167–68)

It is only when he delves in greater detail into the development of specific equivalents, the transition from Cotgrave's *Dictionarie* to Urquhart's inspirations, that Craik forgets this larger principle of Urquhart "viewing it both as a creative work which involved no sacrifice of originality . . . and as a display of all his interests simultaneously" and chides him for "mistakes" and "flaws."

2.2.5 *Plagues and inoculations: Rabelais>Urquhart>Motteux>Ozell*

Shaun Regan (2001) adds to our history of translationality by commenting insightfully on the editorial contributions made by Peter le Motteux and John Ozell to Urquhart's English Rabelais: Motteux by editing both Urquhart's published Books I and II and unpublished Book III for publication in 1693 and completing the translation with Books IV and V in 1708, Ozell by further editing Motteux's edition and adding his own notes in 1737. Rather than tracking the changes in detail, however, I propose to skip over this stage in the process fairly quickly by noting that Motteux and Ozell actually edited Urquhart's text quite lightly, mainly bringing about a slight but noticeable "gentrification" or "genteelization" of Rabelais by teaching eighteenth-century readers to *understand* Rabelais more "politely":

> Moving from his initial emphasis upon the reader's internal(ized) censorship or moral self-policing, Motteux ultimately encouraged his readers not merely to moderate their (illicit) responses to the text, but to avert their eyes from the most alluring parts of the textual body (to "only admire and fix our eyes on the other parts of the piece"). Just as Rabelais himself would be intermittently blamed for the text's iniquitous wordplay, here the final responsibility for failure to perform either of these diversionary operations is located with the reader.
>
> (Regan 183)

Regan shows persuasively that Motteux and Ozell promoted "allegorical" reading strategies that made the "low" or "base" or "tavern" talk a superficial and not very serious cover for a far more respectable social and political subtext – and that it was precisely in opposition to such reading strategies that Bakhtin (1940/1984) wrote *Rabelais and his World*. Regan's argument builds intelligently on the view first advanced by Brown (1933, 152) that eighteenth-century English literature was "proportionately barren of anything like true Pantagruelism," and that "Sterne himself was tainted with the new plague, as he betrays in his devious and itching treatment of sex."

Note the medical metaphor there: apparently the "plague" of politeness is figuratively a skin disease that causes itching. Regan picks up on this medical metaphor in his double – and bidirectional – use of "inoculation": on the one hand, "for Brown, the contagion of politeness became so widespread during the eighteenth century that even Sterne himself – a writer who would be lauded by William Warburton as the 'English Rabelais' – was unable entirely to inoculate himself" (174); on the other, "in Motteux's working of this figure [of viewing naked statuary], such representations are deemed to possess an inoculatory efficacy, providing a polite audience with a familiarization which prevents shock before the public display of nakedness, both male and female" (183). For Brown, eighteenth-century gentility is a plague against which Sterne is unable to inoculate himself; for Motteux, Rabelaisian debauchery is a plague against which he seeks to inoculate the eighteenth-century reader.

Described in more neutral terms, this "plague" or "contagion" is an icosis: "As cultural historians have increasingly emphasized, moreover, for many eighteenth-century commentators the genteelization of discourse was an important part of a *national* movement toward refinement – a movement in which the civilizing role of women was frequently viewed as instrumental" (Regan 174). In that sociocultural context, for Huntington Brown, the rollicking Rabelaisian humor becomes a potential "inoculation" or countericosis that unfortunately doesn't quite "take" in Sterne; but also, for Motteux, a more "decorous manner of textual converse which might both advertise and advance the progress of English politeness" (174–75) becomes a potential "inoculation" or countericosis against the plague of Rabelaisianism that surges up out of unrefined earlier centuries.

2.2.6 *The stranger's nose: Rabelais>Urquhart>(Motteux>Ozell>)Sterne*

Our history of translations, you will have noticed, has gradually been shifting from a history of medicine to a history of literature; roughly that transition is one of the primary MH subfields, not just "medicine in literature" but "narrative medicine" as well. It is also arguably a history of great literary monsters: Rabelais's *Gargantua and Pantagruel* as not only the first modern novel but a "loose baggy monster" of a novel (in Henry James's term) that gave birth to a whole raft of other loose baggy monsters; Urquhart's Rabelais as the greatest literary translation ever, because it so exuberantly outdoes even Rabelais in literary monstrosity; and now, heavily influenced by Rabelais (and Cervantes), Laurence Sterne's *The Life and Opinions of Tristram Shandy, Gentleman* (1759–1767), often called the greatest novel ever written.[5] Sterne's novel, as Judith Hawley (1993, 84) argues, is also a kind of medical novel, steeped in medical literature and medical explanations: "It is not just that the Shandy family is frequently in need of medical attention, but also that Tristram approaches the difficult subject of himself through the medical sciences." She elaborates:

> What is distinctive about Sterne's practice is that he both plays with ideas and mimics medical vocabulary, and also doctors the books of physicians, reducing their prescriptions to abstractions. Sterne reads and misreads medical texts as works of fiction and constructs his own models of the history of medicine. He is able to assemble new formations of science because he derived much of his information from encyclopaedic works such as Robert Burton's *Anatomy of Melancholy* and Ephraim Chambers' *Cyclopaedia* where ideas are detached from context and juxtaposed in an often arbitrary and relativistic fashion. The field of medical theory in *Tristram Shandy* is wide and eccentric: it encompasses ancient humoural theory, the mixed bag of a medical practitioner's knowledge, and advanced theories from the iatro-mechanical medicine of the first decades of the eighteenth century to the most up-to-date vitalistic theories of Albrecht von Haller and Robert Whytt. Animating a grotesque Rabelaisian body with a sentimental physiology, Sterne creates an anatomy as motley as but more benign than that of Frankenstein's monster. (85–6)

It has long been recognized that Sterne drew his greatest inspiration from Rabelais and Cervantes; as Ruth Whittaker (1988, 15) writes,

> Sterne was influenced by numerous earlier writers, even though *Tristram Shandy* is so strikingly original. *Don Quixote,* the novel written by Cervantes (1547–1616) in the early seventeenth century, satirizing the chivalric tradition, was published in an English translation in 1719. Sterne loved *Don Quixote,* and compares Parson Yorick with Cervantes' creation. Part of his comic method clearly derives from Cervantes. He wrote in a letter: "I am perswaded that the happiness of the Cervantic humour arises from . . . describing silly and trifling Events, with the Circumstantial Pomp of great Ones." Another great comic writer to whom he is indebted is Rabelais (c. 1494–c. 1553), whose works were published in English between 1653 and 1694. He probably read Rabelais at Cambridge, and the library at Skelton Castle (the home of his friend John Hall-Stevenson) was stocked with the works of Rabelais and other salacious literature. *Tristram Shandy* owes a great deal to *Gargantua* and *Pantagruel,* and before *Tristram Shandy* Sterne had written a "Fragment in the Manner of Rabelais," which was not published until 1775, after his death. The influence of Rabelais shows not only in the bawdy jokes and *double-entendres* of *Tristram Shandy,* but also in its

> style. Encouraged by his example, Sterne uses language with wild extravagance, and with a total disregard for moderation or decorum. The excess, the breathless and anarchic quality of *Tristram Shandy* is highly Rabelaisian, an aspect of Sterne's work that was heavily criticized in the nineteenth century.

Tristram Shandy is not, of course, a "translation" of Rabelais; but Sterne begins Volume IV with a tale that he presents, in the tradition he borrowed from Rabelais and Cervantes (see section 2.3.2, below), *as* a translation: "Slawkenbergius's Tale" (see Lamb 1989, 12–14), supposedly translated by Tristram Shandy himself from an invented Latin text called "Slawkenbergii Fabella." Of that pretend original he provides three pages *en face* in Latin, with a footnote – a *paratext* (I will return to explore paratexts in section 2.3.5) – apparently written by a fictionalized Sterne: "As *Hafen Slawkenbergius de Nasis* is extremely scarce, it may not be unacceptable to the learned reader to see the specimen of a few pages of the original; I will make no reflection upon it, but that his storytelling Latin is much more concise than his philosophic – and, I think, has more of Latinity in it" (196). That final phrase, "has more of Latinity in it," is obviously satirical enough to suggest that Sterne is not writing seriously as himself (see González 1996, 62).

As I mentioned earlier, Slawkenbergius's Tale is a retelling/reframing of Panurge's pilgrimage to the Oracle of the Bottle in Book III of *Gargantua and Pantagruel*, from which I quoted a lengthy stretch of the story of the deaf husband and dumb wife in section 2.2.3, above, and which Sterne/Slawkenbergius/Tristram mentions explicitly on p. 211; it also alludes to "El curioso impertinente" in *Don Quixote* (variously translated as "The Novel of the Curious Impertinent" by Charles Jarvis, "The Tale of Foolish Curiosity" by J.M. Cohen, "The Story of the Man Who Couldn't Keep from Prying" by Burton Raffel, "The Novel of 'The Man who was Recklessly Curious'" by Edith Grossman, and "The Tale of Inappropriate Curiosity" by John Rutherford). Tristram, who begins his narration with his conception and ends it with his birth, relates/"translates" this particular passage as something that his father often reads to his Uncle Toby, who has proposed to the Widow Wadman, though he has a mysterious war wound that apparently makes sex problematic, a mystery that the Widow Wadman spends the entire novel feverishly attempting to unravel. Working those two layers of his narration simultaneously – the Latin text his father reads pointedly to Uncle Toby and his English "translation" of the text, which he presents to us to read – inspires him to dart back and forth, with little bracketed insertions like this:

> [– I must break off my translation for a moment; for if I did not, I know I should no more be able to shut my eyes in bed, than the abbess of *Quedlinburg* – It is to tell the reader, that my father never read this passage of *Slawkenbergius* to my uncle *Toby* but with triumph – not over my uncle *Toby*, for he never opposed him in it – but over the whole world.
>
> – Now you see, brother *Toby*, he would say, looking up, "that christian names are not such indifferent things;" – had *Luther* here been called by any other name but *Martin*, he would have been damned to all eternity – Not

> that I look upon *Martin*, he would add, as a good name – far from it – 'tis something better than a neutral, and but a little – yet little as it is, you see it was of some service to him.
>
> My father knew the weakness of this prop to his hypothesis, as well as the best logician could shew him – yet so strange is the weakness of man at the same time, as it fell in his way, he could not for his life make use of it; and it was certainly for this reason, that though there are many stories in *Hafen Slawkenbergius*'s Decads full as entertaining as this I am translating, yet there is not one amongst them which my father read over with half the delight – it flattered two of his strangest hypotheses together – his NAMES and his NOSES – I will be bold to say, he might have read all the books in the *Alexandrian* library, had not fate taken other care of them, and not have met with a book or a passage in one, which hit two such nails as these upon the head at one stroke.]
>
> (Sterne 1759/1986, 209–10)

The plot of the tale is that a stranger with a gigantic nose arrives in Strasbourg and occasions all manner of tumult; the whole town is abuzz with it, some denying its reality, others defending it ("'Tis a false nose"/"'Tis a true nose"/"'Tis made of fir-tree, said he, – I smell the turpentine"/"'Tis a dead nose"/"'Tis a live nose, and if I am alive myself, said the inn-keeper's wife, I will touch it" (201)), but the stranger protests in a manner that underscores the age-old association between the nose and the penis:

> I have made a vow to saint *Nicolas* this day, said the stranger, that my nose shall not be touched till – Here the stranger, suspending his voice, looked up – Till when? said she hastily.
>
> It shall never be touched, said he, clasping his hands and bringing them close to his breast, till that hour. – What hour? cried the inn-keeper's wife. – Never! – never! – said the stranger, never till I am got – For heaven sake into what place? said she. – The stranger rode away without saying a word.
>
> (201)

The abbess's insomnia to which Tristram refers in his insertion quoted above is also excited by sight of the stranger's nose: "The abbess of *Quedlingberg*, who, with the four great dignitaries of her chapter, the prioress, the deaness, the subchantress, and senior canoness, had that week come to *Strasburg* to consult the university upon a case of conscience relating to their placket-holes – was ill all the night" (203). Note that "placket-holes" – openings in the upper part of skirts to enable dressing and undressing – might well be an allusion to Urquhart's invented endearment for Gargantua's penis, "placket-racket," and thus indirectly to vaginas. The entire tale seethes with sex – but then, so does the entire novel. There then ensues a long account of a scholarly disputation upon the stranger's nose among the "doctors" (learned men) of Strasbourg, the physicians pronouncing upon its possible etiology (a wen? an edema?), the likely effects of such a birth defect (if such it had been) on gestation and delivery, the logicians chopping logic about blood –

> A nose, argued the logician, cannot bleed without blood – and not only blood – but blood circulating in it to supply the phænomenon with a succession of drops – (a stream being but a quicker succession of drops, that is included, said he) – Now death, continued the logician, being nothing but the stagnation of the blood –
>
> I deny the definition – Death is the separation of the soul from the body – said his antagonist – Then we don't agree about our weapon, said the logician – Then there is an end of the dispute, replied the antagonist.
>
> (207–8)

– and the "civilians" (doctors in civil law) arguing that "such a monstrous nose, . . . had it been a true nose, could not possibly have been suffered in civil society – and if false – to impose upon society with such false signs and tokens was a still greater violation of its rights, and must have had still less mercy shewn it" (208).

Sterne also drew considerable inspiration for *Tristram Shandy* from Burton's *Anatomy* – much of it parodic, whenever to Sterne's ear Burton lapsed into pomposity or solemnity of any kind. Many of Sterne's absurd chapter titles are parodies of Burton's categories, for example; and he mercilessly pillories Burton's use of extended quotations from classical authorities. Sterne's parody of the *consolatio* genre in Chapter 3 of Volume V is a mash-up of several sections of the *Anatomy,* including a near-verbatim borrowing of Burton's English translation from the Latin of the famous consolatory letter from Servius Sulpicius to Cicero upon the death of the latter's daughter Tullia (Part II, Section III, Member V, "Against Sorrow for Death of Friends or otherwise, vain Fear, &c."). So close is this parodic "borrowing" from Burton, without mentioning Burton as the source, that it is one of the plagiaristic "illustrations of Sterne" that Dr. John Ferriar adduced against him in his 1812 book by that name. As H. D. Traill (1882) reports:

> "Returning out of Asia," declaims Mr. Shandy, "when I sailed from Aegina towards Megara" (when can this have been? thought my Uncle Toby), "I began to view the country round about. Aegina was behind me, Megara before," &c., and so on, down to the final reflection of the philosopher, "Remember that thou art but a man;" at which point Sterne remarks coolly, "Now, my Uncle Toby knew not that this last paragraph was an extract of Servius Sulpicius's consolatory letter to Tully" – the thing to be really known being that the paragraph was, in fact, Servius Sulpicius filtered through Burton.

And, let us not forget, filtered through Burton as *translator*. The objectivist protocol requires clearly marked distinctions among original writing, faithful translation, and accurate quotation, with precise and reliable attributions; to the frowning dismay of Ferriar and Traill, Sterne plays fast and loose with all such distinctions, stirring all together in a rich re(peri)performative pottage onto which he dribbles his own name as Author.

2.2.7 The diagnostics of translational medicine: Sterne>Portela

We could continue: Manuel Portela (2000), for example, details his effort to reproduce the physicality of *Tristram Shandy* in his two-volume Portuguese translation (1998), including not only the look of the typeface but the marbling of the paper. "My suggestion of actually marbling the paper so that we would have different patterns in each of the 2,000 copies," he notes wryly, "raised serious doubts about my sanity as a translator" (304).

More to the point, Portela argues that Sterne uses typography and prosody to represent the death of Le Fever:

> In volume 6, chapter 10, we find one of the typographic climaxes of the novel and two of my favourite pages: pages 45 and 46. In this case page-break, catchword, page turning, line-break and long dashes seem to have been combined to recreate in image and rhythm the last palpitations of Le Fever's dying heart. Notice how the catchword gets a sound value on its own ["flut-fluttered"]; how the long dash is used both as visual marker and as notation of cardiac arrest; how a long dash is introduced at the beginning of the second line of page 46 so that the word "moved" can be hyphenated into two syllables and the word "No" can go to the last line by itself.
>
> (296)

The typographic effect on pp. 45–46 that Portela is describing is illustrated in a facsimile reproduction of those two pages from the first edition on his own p. 299:

> Nature inſtantly ebb'd again, ——— the
> film returned to its place, ——— the pulſe
> flut-
>
> [46]
> fluttered ——— ſtopp'd ——— went on ———
> ——— throb'd ——— ſtopp'd again ——— mo-
> ved ——— ſtopp'd ——— ſhall I go on? ———
> No.

This, I would argue, is *translational diagnostics:* a hyperattentive examination of the "symptomatology" of Sterne's printed page in order to develop first a diagnosis – not just of the text as "disease" but of the psychology and phenomenology behind it, the affect and conation that might have guided and shaped it – and then a translational treatment. Like a medical clinician, after all, Portela must do more than diagnose: he must devise a strategy by which the "patient" might be helped to adapt to and so enter and engage and embody a transformed future. After all, Portela's reading of Sterne diagnoses the text as a translational phenomenology: Sterne's goal, he claims, is not to *represent* Le Fever's death accurately *for* the reader but to *reenact* that death transitively or translationally *in* the reader – to "translate" the experience of dying into the phenomenology of reading. Portela's Portuguese translation, therefore, as translational medicine (TM):

- just as medical research is translated into clinical trials, and clinically trialed drugs and devices are translated into patient care, and patient care is translated into the phenomenology of being ill and injured, of living and dying,
- so too does Sterne translate his imagination of Le Fever's dying into a textual enactment that will enactively translate the phenomenology of dying to the source reader, which phenomenology Portela seeks to translate into the phenomenology of dying for the target reader.

(Does that analogy humanize the translated text excessively? Medical purists in the past have lodged similar complaints about humanistic/humane engagements with patients. Does it medicalize the translated text excessively? No more than Portela himself does.)

Rather than extending the history essayed in section 2.2 further, however, let us take this much as our evidentiary reserve and begin to reflect more thoughtfully on it.

2.3 Rethinking translationality

Stepping back from that history of translations (and adaptations, and pretend translations), from Galen to Rhazes to Vesalius to Burton to Rabelais to Urquhart>Motteux>Ozell to Sterne to Portela, then, we next need to ask about the implications of translationality – the "transitivity" or "transformationality" of this sort of textual history as a transmission not of stable propositional meanings but of *change.*

2.3.1 The modern novel

It is important to remember that the literary history sketched in here, beginning with Rabelais in section 2.2.3, is a history not of "the novel," as if that were a genre that somehow existed outside of time, as a stable Platonic Form, but of the *modern* novel, a genre emerging with the rise of the modern nation-state in Renaissance Europe – and thus what Emily Apter attributes to a "nation-based episteme." Nations, as Benedict Anderson (1983/2006) famously declared, are "imagined communities" – which is to say, epistemes. Sakai (1997) would call them "regimes of homolingual address," regimes relying heavily on the *naturalization of imagined unity* – which is to say, the generation not only of the ideological construct of the homolingual community but of the widespread belief that this is the *natural human* way people interact with each other. In other words, to connect this model back to our earlier focus, homolinguality is naturalized as *reality*. This is (purportedly) not a "model" of reality: *it is real*. The increasing stabilization/naturalization of reality-(peri)performances in the modern era of the nation-state lends an ever-sharper epistemic edge to modern ontophilic literary genres as well, especially the novel (and, as we shall see in section 2.3.3, modern translation): the more ideological baggage that is hung on normative reality-constructs, the more the creative impulse is bequeathed an intensified power to discomfit by exposing such epistemes *as* periperformativities.

But I suggest that there is at work in this history more than a single "episteme" – more than a single "icosis." One is a hegemonic Platonic/Christian/scientistic episteme that is traditionally called *objectivism;* the other is a counterhegemonic esoteric/Kantian/Romantic/pragmatistic episteme that is traditionally called "constructivism," but that I propose to reframe here as "periperformativism," to signal the embodied social inter(en)activism of "constructs." Just as a theatrical performance brings a whole "reality" into (felt) being through embodied interaction onstage, and just as the periperformative interaction between the actors and the audience mobilize that felt reality for social use (see Robinson 2016b), so too does all social interaction periperform our shared experience of people and spaces and actions as (what we take to be) reality. In an objectivist episteme, exposing literary or dramatic realities as "illusions" means exposing them as deceptions, phantasms, misimpressions; the exposé is determinedly anti-illusionistic because its impetus is toward the stability and reliability of empirically verifiable objecthood (things that stay the same). In a periperformativist episteme, denaturalizing those felt-becoming-mobilized realities as "illusions" means celebrating them as energetic inventions, as playful effects; the celebration is not really anti-anything, because its impetus is toward enhanced human effort, Aristotelian *energeia* as transformative action or work, and an intensity of novel effect (things that change). For the scientist, an illusion is confusion; for the magician, an illusion is artistic virtuosity.

Ironically, as we've seen, neuroscience leans methodologically toward objectivism but lands epistemically in periperformativism. Think back to our discussion of Richard Powers's *The Echo Maker* in Essay 1. His theme in that novel, he said, was fiction: the confabulation of a coherent self coherently connected to a coherent world, as how we all live our lives, whether we ever write a word of it down. The Capgras delusion that drives the plot of that novel is only one of a dozen or more misidentification syndromes featured in Gerald Weber's popular neurology books, showing that our performance of a coherent world that everyone else can agree is "really real" is incredibly precarious. According to the objectivist episteme that constitutes our "common sense," and that is commonsensically associated with "scientific method," everyone lives comfortably in a stable objective reality *except* those unfortunate few who "go crazy" and start hallucinating improbable CIA plots or alien mind-control or whatnot; according to the periperformativist episteme found by brain science to be operative in human neural processing of perceptual data, our stable objective reality is a neurocultural achievement that can unravel with frightening ease.

So let us map the early history of the modern novel epistemically, twice: first through objectivism, then through periperformativism.

Objectivism

To the extent that we believe commonsensically in the externality of a shared "objective" "reality," we tend to read *Gargantua and Pantagruel, Don Quixote,* and *Tristram Shandy* as clever but absurd fantasies in which characters do impossible things like chat with their authors and translators and visit the printing press where the pages they live on are being printed. All that is impossible, of course, and therefore absurd, in the commonsensical objectivist reality that we (are certain we) occupy. After all, we aren't being created by authors; we don't live on the page; we can't visit the printing press where our world is being brought into being. All this is quite obvious to us, and doesn't require reflection, let alone fancy philosophical footwork. Because we are good commonsensical objectivists, our reality is *reality* – really *real* reality – and anything that deviates from that reality is obviously sheer fantasy. The inventively convoluted and recursive realities of Rabelais, Cervantes, and Sterne must therefore be "just literature" – and indeed literature that "perversely" (though many objectivists also love that perversity) undermines the realism of the modern novel. The Realistic Novel (RN), we know – the "normal" novel – creates a deceptively accurate illusion, or what Baudrillard calls a first-order simulacrum or counterfeit, of the real world; reading it, we are caught up in that world. We come to "believe" – at least to half-believe – in its reality. Even though the RN's reality is only a simulacrum or counterfeit, it is an accurate enough analogue of the "really real" reality that we feel we can learn something about living our own lives from reading it. Our focus, after all, our center of gravity, is in external reality. The objectivist is "ontophilic": *in love with what is* (and suspicious of what isn't). The RN has only instrumental value, as a *guide* to the external objective reality of our own lives. As long as the RN serves that reality, serves it faithfully and accurately ("realistically"), we can learn something from it about our main concern, and thereby continue to respect the work it does for us. Even a fantasy novel, from say Mary Shelley's *Frankenstein* (1818) to J. R. R. Tolkien's *Lord of the Rings* (1954–1955), can still be respected as an RN because it creates a world that differs from ours in significant ways but does so with consistent fidelity to its premises, its givens, and so can still teach us important lessons about our own reality. A novel like *Gargantua and Pantagruel,* or *Don Quixote,* or *Tristram Shandy,* by contrast, turns that whole enterprise upside down. These are flagrantly Anti-Realistic Novels (ARNs) that constantly undermine our nervous need to flesh forth a coherent world. This creates a problem for objectivists. The ARNs are not obeying the rules! What can we do with them? Must we reject them, heap scorn upon them, burn them? Or can they be brought into the objectivist fold?

The usual answer is yes, we can rescue them for objectivism: we can applaud them for reminding us that novels are *not* reality. We can make a religion out of ontophilia (the exclusive love of "really real reality") and, rather than castigating

ARNs as renegades, scofflaws, apostates, we can celebrate them as whistle-blowers, priestly inquisitors who expose the false pretenses of realistic fiction. We should not be taken in by the glittering surfaces even of the RNs! We should read these "strange" and "problematic" ARNs earnestly, so as to point our way back to the reality that we love and honor most of all, the ontophilic reality of our ordinary lives.

This objectivist literary moralism has historically been quite influential. After all, it provides us a useful commonsensical management system for the problematic relations between reality and fiction, assigning the former the leading role as Stable Object-World and the latter the supporting role as Impresario. ARNs remind us that *all* fiction exists to direct our fantasies and imaginings back to the main event, the Real World. To the extent that we even notice fiction's hoots and hollers, ARNs fix our attention transitively back on our own reality.

Periperformativism

ARNs play a radically different role in the periperformativist episteme, because there they are not problems to be solved, renegades to be rescued, but the leading edge of the Kantian revolution in philosophy that informs late twentieth-century neuroscience and postmodernism. In some sense, in fact, in periperformativism the ARNs are themselves the main event. The "constructivist" (latterly periperformativist) episteme is commonly thought to originate in Kant's "Copernican Hypothesis" (1787) – the notion that we are not planets revolving around the sun of a stable external objective reality but rather the sun that *creates* (the coherence of) that external reality – but radically innovative ARN writers like Rabelais (1533), Cervantes (1605), and Sterne (1759) were arguably there first. They assigned top priority not to some stable objective "reality" but to the fictional confabulations that (meta-/anti-/counter-)periperformed novelistic counterfeits of reality as "real." This is obviously the periperformativist convergence between "fiction" and "reality" out of which Richard Powers built *The Echo Maker* – but something very like that convergence was at work in Rabelais, Cervantes, and Sterne as well. The main difference is that postmodernism has brought about social changes that have legitimized periperformativism, so that it increasingly seems *normal* to question the reality of the feeling of reality.

Note that those social changes – the wholesale neoliberal appropriation of postmodern theory's radical attempts to undermine the "confabulatory" creation of a sense of reality in premodern art, *as* what Fredric Jameson (1992) calls "the cultural logic of late capitalism" – are effectively *neurocultural* changes. Postmodern culture reprograms how our brains process and create reality. Fifty years ago, when postmodernism was young, and still confined to a few radical writers, artists, and theorists, playful invocations of the odd and the absurd could stop a conversation dead. John Barth's (1967/1984, 72) quip that the novel has always been dying, because the novel has always been playing fast and loose with the pretense that its events really happened, sounded merely ingenious – a clever riposte without the tiniest basis in (objectivist) reality. (Dismissive critics even accused him of inventing an Argentinian writer named Jorge Luis Borges. And of course there is something perversely attractive about that kind of accusation, as there is about the bishop in Swift's day accusing him of "lying" about Gulliver's travels – attractive specifically as an exposé of the torpidity of objectivism.) The (objectivist) belief that any playful ARN celebration of the illusion of reality in the novel or short story s/he was reading would *devastate his or her pleasure in the work* was widely accepted as a truism. The reader's pleasurable affect depended entirely on the serenely naturalized functioning of that illusion of reality, because "the reader" was by default an objectivist. Now, however, in "mature" postmodernism, more and more readers not only expect the undermining of the illusion of reality, in television shows and commercials as well as in experimental fiction, but are growing sick of it: more postmodernism, groan. And yet it seems there's no going back – short of joining the Tea Party or some other fiercely nostalgic cult. Irony is mandatory – especially self-irony, a constant witty reflection on the aporias in one's own reasoning. We say "life" is different now; what we mean is that our neurocultural conditioning is different. We are guided neurally in new ways by our culture.

On that head, think back to Álvaro Ramírez's reading of *Don Quixote* in section 1.2.4. One of the striking things about that reading, it seemed to me, was that Ramírez's Baudrillardian/postmodern reading of Cervantes's novel was predicated on a sense of *postmodern reality.* For him the main event was not the confabulatory (meta-/counter-)periperformance of an illusion of reality but Reality Itself. It seems oxymoronic to describe Ramírez as a postmodern objectivist, but the neurocultural transformation brought about by postmodern society has in effect made periperformativity (seem like) an objectivist "reality." To Ramírez this or that event in the novel was not simply a novelistic *representation* (counterfeit) of Baudrillard's theory of the orders of simulacra, let alone a clever critical *reading* of the novel in terms of Baudrillard's theory, but an objective correlative of the slow march of those orders through the "real world." Ramírez lives in a postmodern world today; he reads *Don Quixote* and finds all manner of surprising indications that Spanish "reality" in the early seventeenth century is/was objectively contiguous with the postmodern reality in and through which he reads. Somehow, inexplicably but wonderfully, our own postmodern reality today comes to seem to him to be *present in Cervantes's text*! Somehow, he thinks, Cervantes must have anticipated our reality; somehow Don Quixote himself must be a postmodernist simulator, the novel itself no longer an ARN but a great postmodern RN. "The knight wants to set his feet firmly in [postmodern] simulation," he writes, "but the [turn-of-the-seventeenth-century] first order simulacra are still too close at hand to leave behind" (87). This for Ramírez is not Cervantes creating a first-order counterfeit of Baudrillardian theorizing; it is a *realistic realization* of the Real-World accuracy of Baudrillard's model. Don Quixote for him is a Real Person experiencing a transitional moment from the first-order simulacra all around him to the Postmodern Reality of his own third-order simulacra. "That is to say, he lives in a world where the proliferation of signs without referent is the law, where the real loses it[s] primacy over signs, and the law of simulation is the guiding principle of society" (87) – and because that world Cervantes creates has become objectively "real" to Ramírez, Don Quixote's postmodern sensibility serves as proof that Baudrillard was right. Ironically, of course, this also means that Ramírez is reading *Don Quixote* as precisely what Baudrillard says is impossible in third-order simulation: a semiotic world with a real-world referent. It is precisely because Ramírez takes Don Quixote to be a flesh-and-blood human being living in a world contiguous with our own that he is able to make Baudrillardian claims about the impossibility of such reality-creation in the postmodern age.

But it's actually more complicated even than that. Tim Parnell (1996) notes that there is a significant difference between "a skepticism which serves faith – and hence finally religious dogma – and a skepticism which is more or less an end in itself" (150). ARNs like *Gargantua and Pantagruel, Don Quixote,* and *Tristram Shandy,* he insists, are powerful examples of the former, and that, Parnell insists, makes them quite different from anything postmodern:

> Behind the marvellous complexities of *Gargantua and Pantagruel* and *Don Quixote* lies a fideism ["faith-ism," the belief that faith is utterly separate from reason] that is closer to the conservative scepticism of St. Paul than the radical scepticism of postmodernity. It was Erasmus [1466–1536], who in the wake of the Reformation crisis employed in *The Praise of Folly* [1511] the rhetoric of Pyrrhonian [anti-absolutist] scepticism in defence of what Terence Penelhum (1983, 294) has called a "middle-of-the-road theology." After Erasmus the alliance of fideism and the Menippean form became almost exclusively associated with a sceptical interrogation of the human-based search for truth and satire on perceived abuses in religion (Kirk 1980, ix–xxxiii). Any meaningful treatment of the texts of this sceptical tradition – which includes Cervantes, Rabelais, Burton, Swift and Sterne – has to be aware of the uses to which the sceptical arguments of Sextus Empiricus [c. 160–210, first written proponent of Pyrrhonism] were put by Catholic and Anglican apologists. The Epistemological crisis of the Reformation made a purely rational defence of religious belief quite untenable, but also produced some extraordinary "literary" texts in which sceptical discourse comes to serve an artfully disguised negative dogmatism (see Popkin 1979, 1–87).
>
> (150–51)

Two more glosses there:

- *Gloss 1.* Menippean satire is a prose form, usually novel-length, that uses a variety of rapidly shifting satirical, parodic, and burlesque forms and styles, without a clear or coherent narrative, to poke fun at established mental attitudes. In addition to Rabelais's *Gargantua and Pantagruel,* classic examples include Petronius's *Satyricon* (late first century CE), Jonathan Swift's *Gulliver's Travels* (1726), Sterne's *Tristram Shandy* (1759), and Voltaire's

Candide (1759). What Parnell calls "Menippean form" is a rollicking free-form anti-form.
- *Gloss 2.* By "negative dogmatism" Richard Popkin means the philosophical position adopted by Francisco Sanches (c. 1550–1623) that moves beyond the Pyrrhonic rejection of absolute knowledge (insistence on human uncertainty) to the apophatic theology of *Quod nihil scitur* ("that nothing is known" – the title of his famous 1581 work): "A theory of the nature of true knowledge is asserted, and then it is shown that such knowledge cannot be attained" (Popkin 40). The fideist/apophatic idea behind all this is that, once one has discarded the illusory ideal of attaining rational knowledge – religious as well as scientific rationalism, political as well as economic rationalism, and so on – whatever is left is faith. (Compare this with Baudrillard's mystical – quasi-theological – negations of "reality" in his theorizing of simulacra, as discussed in section 1.2.1, above.)

Parnell's historical argument would militate against equating Cervantes's vision in *Don Quixote* with postmodernism, and thus also with Baudrillardian simulation, because what Cervantes is seeking to undermine is not *all* referentiality but rational reference alone. Another way of putting that is to note that both Romanticism and realism are rational systems of real-world reference, and both are wrong. Realism, or principled submission to skeptical empiricism – Sancho Panza's episteme, but also Vesalius's scientific method – is based rationally in empirical reference: the principle to which one submits posits a stable and accurate one-to-one relationship between signs and ordinary mundane reality. Romanticism, or principled submission to a mystified authority – Don Quixote's episteme, but also Sylvius's scientific method – is based rationally in a code of honor: the principle to which one submits posits a stable and accurate relationship between signs and a codified human behavioral ideal. Cervantes's strategy is to pit each against the other, and thus to keep sneakily revealing the extent to which each is a counterfeit – a first-order simulacrum. What is left when the "reality" behind each system of rational reference has been thoroughly undermined is not the postmodern void but faith.

To us today that sounds like a contradiction in terms, because we tend to associate "faith" with religious dogma, and thus with theological rationalism; in skeptical fideism the faith that is left is a *credo quia absurdum*/"I believe because it is absurd" kind of faith.[6] I believe not because it makes sense, but because it doesn't.

This has two important MH consequences:

- *Consequence 1.* Human beings will continue to periperform and plausibilize a coherent reality, regardless of what (one interpretation of) Jean Baudrillard says about the impossibility of such an activity. What Baudrillard is describing is not the *loss of our ability* to periperform reality but changes in the neurocultural *guidance* for such periperformativity.

- *Consequence 2.* Medical professionals, like teachers and other service workers, tend to believe in the ethos of care for the same absurdist reasons: they continue to care for people, and to believe in the importance of caring for people, even though they know that they typically have more faith in medical (or pedagogical) care than their patients (or students) do, and even though they know that their stronger faith cannot prevent illness or decay or death (or an anti-intellectual fortress mentality). Their faith is absurd – and the more valuable for that.

A rationalist faith tends to mobilize stability: because everything makes a stabilized and therefore secure and reassuring kind of sense, it is important not to mess with the system. An absurdist faith tends to disrupt stability: because established systems of thought and behavior are *false* stabilizations of reality, it is important to remain radically open to surprise and the strange (see Essay 3), indeed to keep restlessly finding the strange in the familiar.

Consider two idealized images of the medical clinician: the first is a godlike authority, an expert who serenely commands all the relevant professional knowledge and so confronts each patient with the certainty of superior knowledge; the second is a learner, a seeker, who knows from long experience that every patient is different, every symptomatology of the "same" disease or disorder differs in significant ways from every other, so that every diagnosis and every treatment has to emerge interactively out of an engagement with a unique human being in a unique situation, and will necessarily be based in trial and error. The former is rationalist science, the objectivist Enlightenment ideal; the latter is narrative medicine, the periperformativist MH ideal. The former begins with an ideal of scientific infallibility, the doctor who never makes a mistake – impossible, of course, but something to strive for. The latter begins with human fallibility, which it enshrines in an approach to life that Charles Sanders Peirce called "fallibilism" (see Bergman 2009, 34–37): the recognition that nothing not only ever *will* be perfect but *needs* to be perfect. We can live with good enough, close enough – as long as we retain an absurd faith in the ethos of care, and expect to fail at least as often as we succeed.

2.3.2 *The found-translation framing device*

One of the definitive building blocks of realism in the modern (A)RN has historically been the pretense that it is not a novel at all but a true story. It all really happened, to real people. It was not invented. It is not a fiction. The main textual signal of this pretense has traditionally been the so-called "found narrative" – a narrative that is "found" in the sense that the author claims to have happened upon the story the reader is about to read, somewhere, somehow. The found narrative is presented in a paratextual frame (a preface or afterword, an editor's/publisher's note) as an actual memoir. The author who actually wrote the words hides his or her work behind the fictional front of this other "true author," who is actually the invented narrator and main character of the story. The person who wrote the words, and whose name is listed on the front cover as author, pretends to have "found" the narrative, and edited it into its current form. Why? To make the story sound not just *realistic* but *real*. To plausibilize it as a "true story," written by the person to whom it actually happened.

When Jonathan Swift writes *Gulliver's Travels* (1726), for example, he doesn't just create a narrator named Captain Lemuel Gulliver and have him start telling his story; he provides a provenance for the story, a paratextual paper trail, as it were, that seems to authenticate it as the true story of a real person. Richard Sympson, the "publisher" of the novel, reports that Lemuel Gulliver, his old friend, left the manuscript with him, saying he could do as he liked with it; there then follows Gulliver's own letter to Sympson, relating the history of the manuscript. The found-narrative framing device is found in many novels, up to our own day, and seems to be especially popular in fantasy novels, like *Gulliver's Travels*, or Robert Louis Stevenson's *Strange Case of Dr. Jekyll and Mr. Hyde* (1886), James de Mille's 1888 novel *A Strange Manuscript Found in a Copper Cylinder*, or Edgar Rice Burroughs's 1912 novel *A Princess of Mars* – novels that seem most flagrantly to flout the genre's realistic roots, its claim to be a true story about real people in real places.

One of the interesting hinges on which the use of the found-narrative framing device turns is authorial intention – or what we take to be authorial intention. The infamous protest from a bishop in Swift's day, that he personally believed *Gulliver's Travels* to be a pack of damned lies, was obviously predicated on his belief that Swift was actually trying to *convince* him that the found-narrative frame was true. That seems funny to us today, not only because *Gulliver's Travels* is so obviously a fantasy novel, but because we tend to assign benign motives to authors of modern novels. They aren't trying to hoax us; they're just telling pleasurable stories in pleasurable ways. But that latter attitude strikes me as something of a cultural achievement, largely as a result of education about the world, and about storytelling. Icotic strategies of plausibilization are powerful; they tend to be our main source of certainty about what we take to be reality. Novelists that tap into those strategies for the purpose of *fictional* storytelling are messing with well-established regimes for the group vetting of truth. And why? Is it enough to say merely that the *genre* requires it – that the novel *just is* a realistic genre, and realism *just does* require the pretense that the story being told really happened? (Here the tensions I've been exploring between objectivism and periperformativism obviously come into play.)

From the perspective of translationality, in fact, the situation is even more complicated, and even more interesting. What the sequence tracked in section 2.2 shows is that the early history of the modern novel was actually organized not around monolingual found narratives but around *translated* found narratives:

- The provenance Rabelais provided for his "genealogy" of Gargantua and Pantagruel was that it was found buried in a huge tomb underground, in some strange foreign script carved on elm bark, which he himself translated into French.[7]

- The provenance Cervantes provided for his history of Don Quixote was that it was (based on) a translation from an Arabic text by an invented Moorish historian named Cide Hamete Benengeli – except that he isn't content to leave it at that, but plays with the found-translation frame constantly. In Chapter 8 of Part I the Cide Hamete narrative breaks off, and the narrator is frustrated – but then in Chapter 9 he is in the Jewish marketplace near the cathedral of Toledo and a finds a boy hawking an Arabic manuscript, finds a Spanish-speaking Morisco to translate a few lines of it, and discovers that it is the continuation of Cide Hamete's history. He buys the sheaf of manuscripts from the boy, hires the morisco to translate it, and the novel continues. In Part II it transpires that there are two published versions of Don Quixote's story. Don Quixote and Sancho Panza reject both versions as lies, but the narrator continues to insist that Cide Hamete's "history" is the only veracious one – except that he also begins to quibble with the Cide Hamete story, noting that the translator finds Sancho Panza's speech to be far too educated to be believable, for example, and he reports that the translator has refused to translate some parts entirely, as too silly to bother with. The other published version was the actual sequel written by one "Alonso Fernández de Avellaneda," a pseudonym for some anonymous author or group of authors that no one has been able to identify; it has been argued that Cervantes wrote Part II in order to counteract that "false" sequel. In addition to having the knight and Sancho and various others dismiss that published account indignantly as completely false – but then of course they're also dismissing the Cide Hamete version, and thus the ostensible basis of the whole novel, as false – Cervantes attacks it satirically in a mock version of the Descent to the Underworld story from the *Odyssey* and the *Aeneid*. There is a certain lusty damsel named Altisidora who has been trying to seduce Don Quixote; when he remains faithful to his Dulcinea, she pretends to die of a broken heart. When to the shock and amazement of all present, including the knight and Sancho, she returns to life, she reports that while she was dead she came to the gates of hell, through which she could see a clutch of demons playing tennis with racquets of fire, with books as balls; one book that they smashed all to hell (so to speak) was the "false" Part II, by the Aragonese "Fernández de Avellaneda," which the demons hate so much that they condemn it to the deepest pit of hell. The version originally written in Spanish is the false one; the only credible story is the translation from Arabic, but of course it's not entirely credible either; the "real characters" dispute the veracity of both.
- Laurence Sterne only used the translated framing device locally, in the beginning of Volume IV; but by using it at all he too situated his radical novelistic experiment in the same history of *fake* translationality.
- Note too, in preparation for sections 2.3.4 and 2.3.5, that these authors play with the found-translation framing device *paratextually*. Rabelais puts his explanation that a friend found the manuscript buried in a giant tomb and he translated it into French into a prologue; Sterne has Tristram tell us in a footnote that he translated Slawkenbergius's Tale from the Latin. Compare

> the publisher's note and letter from the author to the publisher in *Gulliver's Travels.* Cervantes weaves his narrator's report that *Don Quixote* is a translation of an Arabic history into the text, without additional paratexts; it is in fact difficult to say that the narrator presents the novel *as* a found translation, since while he sometimes seems to be speaking in Cide Hamete's voice, and indeed begins the novel that way, and proceeds for several chapters before telling us that we are reading a translation, at other times he is a reporter and commentator on the translator's Spanish version of Cide Hamete's Arabic text. Sterne picks this strategy up from him as well, inserting commentary on the translation into what is supposedly the text of the translation. This differs from Cervantes's practice only in that Sterne has Tristram mark off his paratextual insertions with square brackets: in Cervantes there are no such markers. The important point is that all three authors transgressively *blur* the boundaries between text and paratext, and thus between text that readers are conditioned to consider fiction and text that readers are conditioned to trust as the truth.

Nor has the original found-translation framing device faded into history: it too is still used today (see Umberto Eco's *The Name of the Rose,* for instance),[8] and has many intriguing exemplars throughout the history of modern writing,[9] such as the first edition of Horace Walpole's *The Castle of Otranto,* which was supposedly translated by "William Marshal, gentleman, from the Italian of Onuphrio Muralto, canon of the Church of St. Nicholas, at Otranto" (1764/1901, 7). The original manuscript was supposedly printed in Naples in 1529 and found in a family library in the north of England. Walpole's novel was so successful, as a purported "medieval fiction," that beginning with the second edition the author dispensed with the found-translation framing device and took full credit for authorship himself – whereupon many of its erstwhile admirers turned on it publicly, dismissing it as romantic fluff.

Gideon Toury (1995, 40), who pioneered the study of "texts which have been presented as translations with no corresponding source texts in other languages ever having existed," calls them "pseudotranslations"; his interest in them tends to be focused on the sociocultural contexts in which they arise, and the desired or actual impact they have on the target culture:

> One "big" hypothesis which has been put forward in an attempt to reconcile these two extremes claims that new models do manage to make their way into an extant cultural repertoire in spite of the system's inherent resistance to changes if and when those novelties **are introduced under disguise**; that is, as if they still represented an established option within the culture in question. Inasmuch as the cover is effective, it is only when penetration of products and production processes pertaining to the new model has been completed that the receiving culture would appear to have undergone change, often bringing it to the verge of a new (and different) state of equilibrium.
>
> (Toury 2005, 3)

The major pseudotranslational case studies to which Toury keeps recurring throughout his career include:

- Joseph Smith's *Book of Mormon* (1830), supposedly translated (with a mystical translating machine called the Urim and Thummim) from an "Old Egyptian" text written on golden plates and revealed to Smith by the Angel Moroni. A lot of the text was reworked from the King James Bible; the basic narrative may have been borrowed from a lost novel called *Manuscript Found* (which purportedly disappeared from a trunk in the author's widow's attic in 1825, while Joseph Smith was digging a well next door) by Solomon Spalding (1761–1816). Like *The Book of Mormon,* Spalding's novel was supposedly a translation of plates found buried underground, about experiences among Native American tribes during the time of ancient Rome: there was a found-translation narrative frame in both *Manuscript Found* and *The Book of Mormon,* but arguably a hoax pseudotranslation only in the latter (again, the question of authorial intention is complicated). Since the purpose of this pseudotranslation was to create a new religion, its literary pedigree was not important, at least in theory; and yet *The Book of Mormon* is far more literary in structure and style than it would technically need to be as a sacred text, with the poetry of the King James translators and the prose narrative of Spalding's novel as its backbone. Obviously for religious purposes it was absolutely essential to maintain the illusion that this was an actual translation made possible through mystical means provided by an angel (see Robinson 2001, 54–61, for discussion).
- Karen Blixen's *Gengældelsen's Veje* ("The Angelic Avengers," 1944), an allegory of Nazism disguised as a translation done by Blixen's secretary. In this case the illusion of reality was likewise essential, but this time for political reasons, to protect the author from prosecution or other retaliation by the Nazi state.
- The patriotic poems of the "Kazakh Poet" Dzhambul Dzhabayev (Джамбул Джабаев), ghostwritten and supposedly translated from the Kazakh by a whole host of Russian poets (who knew no Kazakh), until the death at the age of 99 of the "original author" Zhambyl Zhabayev (Жамбыл Жабаев [note the different spelling], 1846–1945). As Toury (2005, 14–15) puts it, "The Soviet authorities resorted to this practice in a highly calculated attempt to meet two needs at once, each drawing on a different source: the poems had to praise 'the great leader' and his deeds in a way deemed appropriate." The praise for Stalin was the political burden of the pseudotranslations; the "way deemed appropriate" was not only literature but *ethnic* literature, from the outskirts of the Soviet Union, for enhanced "authenticity." Again for political reasons the illusion of reality had to be strictly maintained – until two decades after Stalin's death, and several years after Dmitri Shostakovich's death, when Shostakovich (supposedly) revealed it in his (possibly hoax) memoir.

Toury also touches briefly (15n4) on Walpole's *Castle of Otranto.*

Let me add parenthetically, too, that the story behind Shostakovich's posthumous "memoir" is even more interesting, and even more relevant to my topic in this section. That memoir was originally published in English, "as related to and edited by" Solomon Volkov (1979), a Russian musicologist who was born in 1944 and emigrated from the Soviet Union to the United States in 1976, one year after Shostakovich's death in 1975 at the age of 68. Volkov "authenticated" the memoir by attaching a photograph of himself with Shostakovich to it and printing the ailing composer's signature on the first page of a few chapters (which in fact turned out to be previously published lectures by the composer). The Russian "original" (or notes) that Volkov supposedly wrote in Russian, from which Antonina W. Bouis translated the memoir into English, is "lost"; the only Russian document in existence turns out to be a back-translation into Russian of the English original. According to Shostakovich's widow, too, Volkov only met with her ailing husband three or four times, briefly – not nearly long enough for him to have recorded the detailed "as related to" memoir he published. The fact that the "memoir" was widely accepted in the United States as authentic may have something to do with the fact that it portrays Shostakovich as specifically anti-Stalin and more generally anti-Soviet: it seems tailor-made for Cold War politics as understood by its American target audience. The memoir may in fact *be* authentic; but so far it has not been convincingly authenticated, and most of the (circumstantial) evidence would appear to point in the opposite direction. (The authenticity of the "memoir" was first questioned by Fay 1980; for the full debate, see Brown 2004.)

Toury's work on pseudotranslations is extremely interesting and important,[10] and I do not mean to diminish its significance by shifting focus from the sociocultural impact of such pretend or hoax translations to the generic implications of the found-translation framing device. It does seem to me, however, that those latter implications, (at least) five in number, are quite different from those of pseudotranslation, and well worth a separate investigation in the context of literature *as* translationality:

1 Translation is recognized by writers in the modern era as a unique genre that can be reframed for purposes of literary innovation.
2 Translation is valued by these writers as a unique literary genre for its default invocation and deployment of foreign authorities. The authority of those foreign authors may be enhanced by great age (Greek or Roman antiquity, the Middle Ages), exoticism (Moorish North Africa and Iberia, Asia), or a reputation for great wisdom. Because the purported source cultures are typically distant in time and/or space, the authenticity of the "translated" texts is difficult to falsify.
3 The convergence of novelistic and translational norms in the use of the found-translation framing device suggests neither that the novel is the model and translation is the copy, nor vice versa, but that writers and translators collaboratively helped shape the modern forms of both original and translated literature beginning around the middle of the sixteenth century. Their

collaboration may have been inspired by, and channeled through, the generic overlap between the novel and translation, namely, the fictional illusion of "reality": the novel is a real memoir or profile, and the translation is a real original; both were "really" written by someone other than the author of the words on the page.

4 To the extent that Toury is right about the "covert" purposes of pseudotranslators – their attempt to introduce novelty into the target culture in disguise – it is quite true that the fictional pretense or illusion of "reality" serves usefully as cultural camouflage for an objectivist reality; but the same fictional camouflage is also quite often used *meta*fictionally, to draw playful/parodic/periperformativist attention to the falsity of the pretense. The fiction that a given invented story actually happened is technically a *false* premise; the illusionism of that premise can be undermined objectivistically, in order to restore the epistemological morality of realism, or periperformativistically, in order to dramatize the periperformed nature of *all* "reality." The objectivistic use of the found-translation framing device, as in *The Book of Mormon* and the first edition of Walpole's *Castle of Otranto,* seeks to *stabilize* reality, truth, history, and identity around communal plausibility; the periperformativistic use of the found-translation framing device, as in Rabelais, Cervantes, and Sterne, seeks to *destabilize* reality, etc., to show that "reality" is an artistically tricky and therefore volatile and vulnerable periperformance. The objectivist ideal for translation is semantic equivalence, the illusion that things stay the same; the periperformativist ideal for translation is what I'm calling translationality, a celebration of the fact that things inevitably change.

5 If original-fiction writers can play metafictionally with the pretense of translation, translators can also play metatranslationally with the pretense of original writing. It may be precisely because the pretend reality in novels and translations converge in (3) that the playful novelistic experiments with undermining that reality in (4) leach over into translating as well. Theo Hermans (2000) offers a useful guide to such "abusive" translations (using the term coined by Lewis 1985), from "Nabokov's recentest [novel, which] was his [1964] multivolume annotated translation of Pushkin" (Barth 1967/1984, 69), to Louis and Celia Zukofsky's Catullus (1969), to translations of Derrida into English;[11] but arguably the earlier work by playful innovators like Thomas Urquhart in his Rabelais (and George Chapman in his Homer) are precursors to this tradition as well.

2.3.3 Literary translationality

And now let us think more carefully about the implications of translationality for our understanding of literature – of literary history in the broad sense, including the history of medical literature – by asking: what kind of literature is a literary translation?

The reason I find that question a useful one to pose is that the standard (objectivist) answer to it implies stability: [1] a literary translation is exactly the same kind of literature as its source text, because the ideal is *no change.* A translation of a novel is also a novel; a translation of an epic is also an epic; a translation of a play is also a play, and so on. Since a literary translation is an interlingual imitation of a literary text, and by definition the literary translator therefore endeavors to imitate everything about the source text in the target language, in the transition from source text to target text the *kind* (or genre) of literature remains unchanged. Implicit in that answer is that [2] literary genres are stable categories that are not transformed by translation, because [3] the translated literary text is by default a bit inferior to its original, and so lacks the power to wield a transformative effect. As Platonic copy theory has taught us for nearly two and a half millennia, an imitation is inevitably worse than the thing it imitates: paler, weaker, slighter, less hearty, less robust, a mere withering shadow of its original that lurks apologetically in dark corners.

What I am exploring here in Essay 2 is a striking periperformativistic deviation from that standard view: that [1′] a literary translation is a *different kind of literature* from an original, because what the literary translator imitates is not just the source text but *the source author's strategies in creating the source text.* By becoming a *writer* of a certain sort – someone who recreates a literary text in another language – [3′] the literary translator seeks to create not just an *inferior imitation of a great text* but a *great reperformative text* that [2′] *transforms* its model. Review this series:

- Laurence Sterne is inspired by Rabelais and Cervantes in creating *The Life and Opinions of Tristram Shandy, Gentleman* (1759–1766), so that several long passages and numerous shorter passages from those models identifiably lurk somewhere behind his own work, but he is neither "translating" those models in the traditional sense nor even "adapting" them.
- G.W.F. Hegel is inspired by Aristotle's *De Anima* in writing *Die Phänomenologie des Geistes/The Phenomenology of Spirit* (1807), and even takes over a vague sense of the structure or argumentative trajectory of Aristotle's work in creating his, but again is neither conventionally "translating" nor "adapting." (When Alfredo Ferrarin (2004, 95) writes that "Hegel translates the *De Anima* into a philosophy of spirit understood in light of the superiority of spirit over nature," by "translates" he obviously doesn't mean verbal cloning.)
- Andreas Vesalius is inspired by Galen in writing *De Fabrica,* and takes over recognizable structure, form, and style from Galen in creating it, but certainly is not conventionally "translating" him – he did that earlier, in the 1530s. He is, however, arguably adapting Galen, making key changes based on his own experimental work.
- Martin Heidegger is inspired by Leibniz's *Monadologie* in writing *Der Satz vom Grund/The Principle of Ground* (1955–1956), and conceives of the text as a kind of engaged translation-cum-adaptation-cum-commentary of/on key concepts in Leibniz's French original and its Latin translation, but does not set out to translate or adapt the whole work into German.

- In writing *Ulysses* (1922), James Joyce is explicitly and demonstrably adapting Homer's *Odyssey*. Like Hegel "adapting" Aristotle and Vesalius "adapting" Galen, he takes over structure and form – the novel's chapter sequence follows the books of the *Odyssey* meticulously, and each chapter is keyed in hundreds of minute ways to its model – but, unlike Vesalius, he writes in a radically different style (or collection of styles), and in almost every possible way repurposes Homer's epic.
- Alain Badiou claims that he is not "translating" Plato's *Republic* in *La République de Platon* (2012) – it's a "hypertranslation" somehow mysteriously *based on* a translation – but that is only because his translation is so radically transformative that it seems to defy traditional narrow definitions of translation as timidly submissive.
- Thomas Urquhart's *Works of Rabelais* (1653, 1693) is explicitly a translation of Rabelais, but it too is so transformative that some would deny the title of "translation" to it. (In the preface to his own 1955 translation, for example, J.M. Cohen describes Urquhart's translation as "more like a brilliant recasting and expansion than a translation" (31).)

Now you may protest that this series (see Table 2.1) stacks the deck unfairly: not only is Urquhart's translation one of the boldest, most ambitious, and most innovative literary translations ever published, but it is the *tamest* exemplar in that list!

But that is part of my point. As long as literary translation is defined objectivistically as a timid and slavish clone that effects the illusion of stable equivalence by positioning itself as slightly worse than its original (not just often unfortunately worse, but definitively worse) – as long, in other words, as that is how we recognize a translation, by its submissive inferiority to its original – then yes, the items in that list are bad examples of translation(ality).

But if we start at the other end, and take translationality to be a transformative potential that is *endemic* to literature, the *core impulse* of literature – say as a stylized artistic escalation of what Sakai Naoki calls the attitude of heterolingual address – things begin to look a bit different. Then those translations that are content to live down to the standard inferiorizing definition must be seen as

Table 2.1 Progressive translationality in seven writers

	Global translation	*Local translation*	*Global adaptation*	*Local adaptation*
Sterne	-	-	-	✓
Hegel	-	-	?	✓
Vesalius	-	-	?	✓
Heidegger	-	✓	-	✓
Joyce	-	-	✓	✓
Badiou	?	✓	✓	✓
Urquhart	✓	✓	✓	✓

falling short of full creative translationality. Then in fact the standard inferiorizing definition of literary translation (call it SIDOLT) itself stands revealed as an attempt either to *justify* inferior literary productions after the fact or, more radically, to *train* translators to be inferior to their source authors before they even take up the task – or possibly even both, cyclically. Then a literary translator that, rather than striving to imitate the source author's strategies in creating the source text, seeks instead to imitate only source-textual features, and in so doing, rather than creating a great text that is qualitatively different from its original, creates an inferior imitation of a great text, would be guilty of taking SIDOLT's path of least resistance. The result would not be a *standard* type of literary translation that standardly fell short of its original, and so achieved its safely inferiorized aim, but a lackluster performance – something that is all too common, of course, and therefore arguably mainstream, and by extension a "good" example of the way things usually go.

If the SIDOLT/objectivist episteme would enforce stability across time by confining translations to slavishly inferiorized clones of existing texts confined to existing genres, the translationality/periperformativity episteme would celebrate genre-busting by recognizing that every new text transforms its model(s) in new ways. One way to stabilize that translationality would be to say that literary translation is a literary genre in its own right – one that is often mobilized for transformative purposes by other genres, through the found-translation framing device and hoax pseudotranslations – but historically translationality tends to bust that genre-stabilization too. Another way of putting that: literary genres are stabilizing performativities that may seem objective but are constantly being destabilized as well. Because stabilization is useful – a reality-construct with no stability at all would be impossible even to understand, and useless for the social management of identity and relationality – we work hard in groups to plausibilize performed stabilities as objective realities; but it is only the faint of heart who cling desperately to the objectivist illusion, and ignore the ubiquity of change.

To bring this theorization back to the history of medical literature: the classic exemplar of objectivism/SIDOLT in sixteenth-century medicine would be the French anatomist Jacobus Sylvius, Andreas Vesalius's teacher and later implacable opponent, who in *Ordo et ratio ordinis legendis Hippocratis et Galeni libris*/"Order and Plan for Reading the Books of Hippocrates and Galen" argued that Galen's anatomy was infallible, indeed that Galen's Περὶ χρείας μορίων/*Peri khreias moriōn*/*De usu partium corporis humani*/"On the Uses of the Different Parts of the Human Body" was divine. Galen spoke the last possible word on human anatomy; no further progress was possible. It was not only pointless to study the dissected human anatomy, therefore: it was an outrage. It implied that medical science might still be able to learn something not already taught by Galen. If any anatomist dissecting a human corpse found anything that deviated from Galen, the only possible explanation was that that particular corpse was an anomaly – or else, more radically, that the human body had changed in the millennium-plus since Galen wrote.

Every possible "translation" of Galen, in other words – into Latin, in the Translation Studies sense of "translation," or into clinical practice and medical education, in the translational medicine sense of "translation" – must therefore be *definitively* inferior to Galen's Greek original. As for Vesalius, in a book titled *Vaesani cuiusdam calumniarum in Hippocratis Galenique rem anatomicam depulsio/* "A Refutation of a Certain Madman's Calumnies Against the Anatomy of Hippocrates and Galen" (with a pun on Vesalii as *vaesani/*"madman" – 1551, when its author was 73), Sylvius urged readers "to pay no attention to a certain ridiculous madman, one utterly lacking in talent who curses and inveighs impiously against his teacher," and demanded that he be "heavily punished and in every way restrained, lest by his pestilent breath he poison the rest of Europe" (quoted in Finger 1994/2001, 23; see also Nuland 1988, 87).

This, we are tempted to say today – with Vesalius, Loys Vassé (Ludovicus Vassaeus, 1500–1580), Charles Etienne (Carolus Stephanus, 1504–1564), and others of the time – is just bad science. It sounds more, in fact, like Sir Thomas More's characterization of the Catholic Church in the 1528–1529 *Dialogue Concerning Heresies,* according to which (contrary to popular belief, as articulated by More's Lutheran interlocutor, whom he calls the Messenger) the Catholic Church did not forbid the vernacular translation of the Bible or persecute those who undertook such translations, but simply prescribed the rigid subordination of Bible translations to the authority of a source text imagined to be universal and unchanging, as interpreted by the Church (see Robinson 1997/2002). Had it been historically accurate, this characterization would have aligned the Catholic Church of the early sixteenth century very closely with the "cloning"/SIDOLT/objectivist school of translation, as indeed also with Sylvius's dogmatic "scientific" rigidity. In actual fact throughout most of the sixteenth century the Catholic Church did indeed ruthlessly suppress vernacular translations of the Bible, confiscated and burned those that did get printed, and hounded the great Protestant Bible translator William Tyndale (c. 1494–1536) across Europe, arresting him, trying him for heresy, and putting him to death.[12] The translational practices of the Catholic Church did not come into close alignment with what I am calling SIDOLT/objectivism until late in the century, when it did finally agree to allow the translation of the Bible into the vernacular – but not from the original Hebrew, Aramaic, and Greek. Rather, until the early twentieth century all Catholic Bible translations took as their source text the Latin Vulgate translation created by St. Jerome, the Catholic Church's Galen, who was supposedly inspired by the Holy Spirit and therefore perfectly stabilized as infallible.

But note two points.

- *Point 1.* Sylvius did not think of himself as a bad scientist. Nor did his defenders among his former students, including Michel de Villeneuve (Michael Servetus, c. 1509/1511–1553), who was himself arrested, tried, and burned at the stake for heresy, at around the same age as William Tyndale. The willingness to test established views empirically, and overturn them if the evidence so decrees, is supposedly a mandate for scientists; but

Thomas Kuhn (1962/1970) makes a strong case for the historical existence of two different epistemes for scientific research, one of which, the radically open-minded quest for new paradigms, he calls "revolutionary science," the other, the timid, conservative attempt to keep seeking out experimental evidence that will protect the sanctity of established paradigms, "normal science." The history of science does show a shifting tension between self-inferiorizing respect for authorities (what Jacques Lacan calls the Discourse of the Master) and a transformative receptivity to new evidence and new theories (for Lacan the Discourse of the University). And, given that the ideological roots of modern science are in Christianity, and the ideological roots of Christianity are in Platonism, and thus in Mastery, it is unlikely that that tension will ever be broken in favor of what I am calling translationality – let alone in favor of the kind of playful, self-recursive kind of translationality that we have found in Rabelais, Cervantes, and Sterne (which Lacan would probably call the Discourse of the Hysteric, and align with his own approach to philosophy).

- *Point 2.* There is such a thing as "the science of translation," which historically has tended toward the conservative pole in that tension: controlled variables and empirical testing aimed to determine what Juliane House (1977, 1996) calls Translation Quality Assurance, which is to say, a given translation's degree of stabilized submission to source-textual meaning (commonly called "equivalence"). For a quite impassioned defense of that explicitly universalizing objectivistic science of translation, contra the "cultural relativists" who would accuse such approaches of Eurocentrism, see Chesterman (2014); for discussion, see Robinson (2014, 2015b, 2017b). That, I would argue, is the modern Translation Studies version of Jacobus Sylvius's dogmatic "scientific" submission to Galen: science in the service of authority-worship. In normal science, the willingness to explore deviations from institutional norms is always a rebellious move; and the willingness to reframe institutional norms as myopically local is too preposterous for words. (My satirical characterization of normal science in that previous sentence is steeped in the Discourse of the Hysteric.)

2.3.4 Categorizing literary translation as literature

Now take one further step, and consider the translationality of these historical transformations as endemic not just to translation (and adaptation), but to literature in general. This is where things really get interesting.

In *Fiction et/and Diction,* Gérard Genette (1991; Porter 1993) seeks to consolidate all the competing definitions of literature into an overarching theoretical model that will account for the whole field – except, as if by sheer oversight, literary translation, which he never even mentions. I assume that is because he simply accepts the standard objectivizing/SIDOLT view that a literary translation is just an imitation of an existing literary original, and therefore falls into the same generic category as the source text. He is, after all, a literary theorist, not a translation theorist.[13] Tellingly, however, he also ends up leaving in his "comprehensive" tabulation a gap that he is simply unable to fill – and I want to suggest that literary translation fills that gap perfectly. Let's see how that works.

Genette takes as his task the condensation of a massively complex collection of distinctions and definitions into a single coherent and comprehensive model – a task that he himself confesses is probably impossible:

1 Traditional stabilizing (objectivist) definitions of literature fail because
   a while it is conventional to assume that there are three literary modes, prose fiction, drama, and verse, each reliably characterized by stable (objective) criterial textual structures,
   b (1a) fails to account for the oft-claimed literary qualities of nonfictional, nondramatic, and nonverse writing, like autobiographies, histories, essays, philosophical works, and the like.

2 Destabilizing (periperformativist) definitions of literature also fail because
   a while the traditional solution to (1b) is to define literature "subjectively," pragmatically, rhetorically, periperformatively, as whatever my friends and I *call* literature,
   b (2a) fails to account for (1a) the patent fact that there are indeed stable textual structures that reliably define vast reaches of work that seem relatively immune to subjectivization, like a narrator telling a story (fiction), characters interacting in scenes without a narrator (drama), or versification (poetry).

Genette's solution (see Figure 2.1) is to build these tensions into his model. The distinction he draws there between "thematic" and "rhematic" criteria is his expansion and complication of the standard distinction between "content" and "form": the "theme" of a discourse, he insists, is *what it's about;* the "rheme" is "the discourse considered in and of itself" (22). What he calls "constitutive" literariness is the product of (1a, 2b) the essentializing/objectivizing approach

<table><tr><th>Régime / Criterion</th><th>Constitutive</th><th>Conditional</th></tr><tr><td>Thematic</td><td>FICTION</td><td></td></tr><tr><td rowspan="2">Rhematic</td><td colspan="2">DICTION</td></tr><tr><td>POETRY</td><td>PROSE</td></tr></table>

Figure 2.1 Genette's schema of literature (Porter 1993, 22)

that identifies stable textual structures or features as reliable constraints on literariness; "conditional" literariness is the product of (1b, 2a) the perspectivizing/performativizing approach that makes literariness an audience effect, a categorization that is conditional upon audience recognition.

What I like about Genette's approach is that he is willing to stretch that elusive aesthetic category/quality of "literariness" across the abysm between rigidly essentializing/objectivizing "constitutive" definitions and flexibly perspectivizing/performativizing "conditional" definitions – and that he is content to live with the abysmic classificational instability that results. In the workshop session I organized for this paper on academia.edu, that *mise en abyme* bothered a lot of participants, some because it was too slippery, others because it was too rigid. To my mind that kind of split objection is precisely right for Genette's model, and its main attraction.

His use of the two terms in his book title, "fiction" and "diction," is somewhat problematic:

> According to the traditional categories, the constitutive governs two broad types, or sets, of literary practices – fiction (narrative or dramatic) and poetry – without excluding their potential collusion in fiction that is poetic in form. Since no language, to my knowledge, provides us with a convenient positive word (that is, apart from the very awkward term *nonfiction*) to designate the third type, and because this terminological gap is a constant problem, I propose to christen this third type *diction,* a choice that at least has the advantage, assuming it is an advantage, of symmetry. The literature of fiction is literature that imposes itself essentially through the imaginary character of its objects. The literature of diction is literature that imposes itself essentially through its formal characteristics – once again, without excluding amalgams and blends. But it seems useful to me to maintain the distinction on the level of essences, and the theoretical possibility of pure states.
>
> (21)

This is of course quite clearly stated; the problem is that "diction" already has a well-established usage in literary studies, in French meaning "way of speaking" (enunciation or elocution), in English that plus the clarity of word choice – and a whole category of writing ("the literature of diction") in neither. But Genette clearly recognizes the problem and takes the necessary steps to avoid definitional confusion.

Note also that in the DICTION box at the bottom right there is no "impenetrable boundary" (21) between poetry and prose. Genette's idea is that poetry is traditionally defined more constitutively, based on finely differentiated verse forms, and prose is traditionally defined more conditionally, as writing that more or less reproduces the rhythms of speech – however we choose to define those rhythms and the manner of their literary representation – but that that distinction cannot be rigidly maintained:

> It has indeed become increasingly obvious, over the last century, that the distinction between prose and poetry may be based on other, less categorical

> criteria than that of versification, and that these criteria, which are moreover heterogeneous and more or less cumulative (for example, privileged themes, tenor in "images," graphic arrangement), leave room, under the heading of "prose poem," "poetic prose," or some other rubric, for intermediate states that make their opposition not categorical but polar, a matter of degree. (23–4)

In other words, we can – and often do – talk about "poetic prose" and "prosaic poetry," based on the situated adjustments our "conditional" performances of literariness lead us to make in the established "constitutive" definitions. We can describe even nonfictional prose – say, Julia Kristeva's theoretical writings – as poetic; and we may take it as high praise to say of Pushkin's verse (in Russian) that it adheres to strict verse forms but reads like prose.

The box of primary interest to me there, however, is the one that remains empty. For Genette that would be "a story that others take to be true[, which] may leave us wholly incredulous while appealing to us as a kind of fiction: here there is indeed a sort of conditional fictionality, a true story for some and a fiction for others" (24). He considers the possibility that myth might work there: the Bible, for example, is the literal truth for believers but (at best) literature for nonbelievers. He resists the temptation to fill the box in this way, however, "for that box is reserved not for conditionally fictional texts but for conditionally literary fictions – a notion that strikes me as passably contradictory" (24). That is, what would go in that box would not be a text that some readers consider true and others consider invented, but an obviously invented fiction that some readers consider literary and others consider nonliterary. To read the Bible as fiction, he insists, *is* to read it as literary.

But I submit that Genette is complicating things unnecessarily here. I see at least two plausible objections to his claim that the box must be left empty.

- *Objection 1.* On the one hand, the emptiness of that box is clearly predicated on his assumption that FICTION has to appear in both of the boxes in the "thematic" row, under both "Constitutive" and "Conditional" – and to me there seems to be no pressing reason why that must be the case. He could, for example, fill the Constitutive box with FICTION and the Conditional box with NONFICTION. That would make the empty box the perfect place for (1b, 2a) those nonfictional texts that large numbers of readers have (conditionally) found to be literary, such as Burton's *Anatomy of Melancholy,* Montaigne's *Essais,* or Michelet's *Histoire de France.* As the table stands now, there is no place on it for such works – the existence of which was in fact one of his most compelling early confirmations of the need for the category of "conditional" literariness, and thus the need to transgress the bounds of conventional "constitutive" definitions of literature. If thematic contents are the defining criterion for that first row, and FICTION is defined constitutively as literary by the invented nature of those contents, Genette's own argumentation would appear to require that NONFICTION be at least one type of writing defined conditionally as thematically literary.

One might want to argue, of course, that the conditional criteria for this sort of literariness in nonfictional works are intrinsically rhematic rather than thematic – that what constitutes them as nonfictional is factuality but what conditionally prompts readers to call them literary is style. But that objection, if taken seriously, would undermine the entire architecture of his table. If conditional literariness is always rhematic, the effect of that on the table's rows-and-columns binary structure is far more devastating than can be solved by the simple ruse of leaving one box empty.

- *Objection 2.* On the other hand, there are fictions that are so pedestrian, so lame, so unimaginatively and uninspiringly written that we might (conditionally) not want to glorify them with the honorific of "literature" at all. Surely, for example, what makes the Bible literature to those of us who do not believe in its literal truth is the fact that it is not just fiction but powerfully *imaginative* fiction. *Pace* Genette, to read the Bible as fiction is not necessarily to read it as literature. Or, to split that hair more finely, we might want to say that the myths in Genesis and Exodus are literature but the laws in Leviticus are not; or that the histories in the books of Joshua, Judges, and Kings are literature but the histories in the two books of Chronicles are not; or that Ruth, Job, the Psalms, Proverbs, Ecclesiastes, the Song of Songs, Isaiah, Jeremiah, Lamentations, Ezekiel, Daniel, Hosea, and Jonah are all decisively literary in ways that more "boring" parts of the Bible are not. We might want to argue over whether the lurid sensationalism of the Book of Revelation – bad genre fiction at best – should disqualify it from the exalted ranks of "Literature." One could also argue that this is really another case of the FICTION/NONFICTION argument in Objection 1: unlike the long middle section of Job, the Psalms, the prophetic works, the Song of Songs, and a few other "poetic" texts, the myths in Genesis, the laws in Leviticus, and the histories in Chronicles, Joshua, Judges, and Kings are all marked *constitutively* as nonfictional texts; what *conditionally* renders some of them literary is not our belief that they are actually invented, but our experience, reading them, that they are exciting, imaginative, colorful, aesthetically satisfying, etc. By the same token, what renders the laws in Leviticus and the histories in Chronicles nonliterary is not our belief that those events actually happened as reported, but our experience in reading them that they are boring.

So we could conceivably overturn Genette's arguments regarding that empty box. But I want to take another tack here: I suggest that we provisionally accept Genette's insistence that "that box is reserved not for conditionally fictional texts but for conditionally literary fictions," and fill it with *literary translations*. It seems to me that two things qualify them to fill that box.

- *Qualification 1.* Literary translations are arguably *fictions* insofar as they are "passed off" as originals. By "passed off" I mean a specific kind of conditionality that is imposed on translations by some readers and not by others: some accept that fiction as truth, and read *The Trial* or *The Castle* as if Kafka had originally written it in English; others read those novels in English with full awareness of the fictionality of the pretense that they were written by Kafka. This conditionality would in a sense turn Objection 1 on its head, and reinvoke my discussion in section 2.3.2, above: like the bishop who complained of *Gulliver's Travels* that he believed all the stories in it were damned lies, it would be the less sophisticated readers who (conditionally) read literary translations as true originals, and complain if the translation they happen to read isn't as good as the author's reputation, and the more sophisticated readers who understand from the start that translators don't seriously intend for their work to *be* the source text. The "imposture" decried by the former (objectivist) group is recognized by the latter (periperformativist) group as an aesthetic pretense, an illusionistic fiction, a literary strategy. The impulse arising in TS around the turn of the millennium to read translators as "narrators," and to study translator styles in terms of "narratoriality" (Hermans 1996; Shiavi 1996; Baker 2000; see Robinson 2011, ch. 5, for discussion), is clearly predicated on the *conditional* tendency to analyze translations as fictions.[14]
- *Qualification 2.* Literary translations may be read as *literary* when they are (found by readers to be) "good" and *nonliterary* when they are (found by readers to be) "bad." There is a certain joyless style of literary translation that is the human equivalent of Google's Statistical Machine Translation: each word and phrase is replaced by its statistically most frequently used target-language equivalent. If the source author refers to blood, for example, the translator doesn't need to consider visuals (is it blood-soaked? blood-spattered? bloodstained?), or rhythm and alliteration and assonance and other prosodic features (is it grisly gore? is it crimson cruor?), and so on: it's just blood. And the adjective is just bloody. And the body, if cut, just bleeds. (Note that I'm not implying that the most obvious TL equivalent is necessarily weak: what is weak is *always automatically* opting for the most obvious equivalent, using "obviousness" as the only criterion for choice, with no ear for the sound, eye for the scene, feel for the fit.) Even when this sort of "weak" or "pedestrian" translation reproduces a *constitutive* regime for literariness, therefore – it looks like a novel or a poem, for example – it may fail to reproduce a widely accepted *conditional* regime, making some readers reject it *rhetorically* as literature. This conditionality would effectively assimilate literary translation to Objection 2, above: the literariness of a given literary translation would be the translational version of the literariness of a nonfictional text like an essay, a history, or a philosophical treatise. Like the literary nonfictional text, the brilliant literary translation exceeds the conventional remit for humdrum writing.

Two notes on those qualifications.

- *Note 1:* Qualification 1's "conditional literariness" is no random predilection upon which some readers accidentally stumble; it is culturally organized, and indeed *neuroculturally* organized. It is what I call an "icosis" (see sections 1.4, 2.4, and 3.5), my coinage from Aristotle's *eikos*/"plausible," *ta eikota*/"the plausibilities," and his observation that, given a choice between a plausible story that is untrue and a true story that is implausible, we will tend to prefer the former, precisely because it has been vetted or "plausibilized" (icotized) by the community. The implication of an *icosis* of conditional literariness would be that the fictional illusion that a translation is its original is neither a phenomenality that must be consciously intended by its target author (translator), nor just a random audience effect that is occasionally imposed on a translation by individual readers, but a *normative social construct/periperformative* with lots of room for slippage built into it. The fact that some readers do take a translation to have been originally written in the target language does not establish the fiction, and the fact that some readers readily perceive the translation as a translation does not overturn it.
- *A Corollary to Note 1:* what Genette calls "constitutive literariness" is icotic as well. When in literature courses we are taught to recognize the constitutive elements of literariness, those lessons lay down neural tracks that stabilize the constitution of literariness not only in the individual but in the group of all people who have been similarly trained. The neurocultural organizing effect is a product not only of parallel teaching but of shared group affect, which organizes group conation: groups put *pressure* on their members to feel the same way about things, and by that means to constitute not just literature but everything else as well in culturally convergent ways.
- *Note 2:* Qualification 2 does not entail that "literary translation" as a unique genre consists only of that set of "good" translations that readers (or, worse, scholars) take to be literary. The genre, like any of the genres Genette considers, is a *constitutive/conditional hybrid* that exists in a productive tension between formal characteristics and audience evaluation. And the inescapable conclusion that I draw from that observation is that we need to rub out the middle bar between the "constitutive" and "conditional" boxes in the thematic row as well (see Figure 2.2) – that, very much like the difference between "poetry" and "prose" in the rhematic row, the boundary between "literary originals" and "literary translations" in the thematic row is porous. As we've seen, there are original works that are presented as, and may be mistaken for, translations: pseudotranslations and the found-translation framing device. And there are translations that are so brilliant that they are mistaken for (or recategorized as) originals.[15] By the same token, as per Objection 1, there are nonfictional works that are so brilliantly literary, like Burton's *Anatomy of Melancholy*, and, as per

Criterion \ Régime	Constitutive		Conditional
Thematic	FICTION AESTHETIC ORIGINAL	 "LITERATURE" "ILLUSIONISM"	NONFICTION RELIGIOUS TRANSLATED
Rhematic	POETRY	DICTION	PROSE

Figure 2.2 Genette's schema of literature, modified

Objection 2, mythical texts that are so brilliantly literary, like the Book of Genesis or Job, that one would be hard put to maintain a DMZ between the two categories. The three lines in the modified THEMATIC row are, respectively, the products of Objection 1, Objection 2, and the two Qualifications. ("ILLUSIONISM" is shorthand – completely inadequate, I know – for "the fictional pretense/illusion that the text was written by someone other than the actual author.")

- *A Corollary to Note 2:* There are cases where the only indication that a given text is a translation is a paratext: a title, a "translation by" attribution, a translator's preface, or the like. But as we've seen, that paratextual indication has often been playfully or deceptively manipulated by authors who for whatever reason want to *pretend* that the text they have written is actually a translation. In such cases our ability to distinguish between a translation and an original is "purely" conditional; indeed we might want to suggest that paratextual indicators should be included among a literary text's "constitutive" features, which are necessary but not sufficient criteria for generic discrimination. There are also translations like John Fowles's *Eliduc* (the second part of *The Ebony Tower*) whose status as translations is easy to miss, because the author is best known as an original author rather than a translator, and because they appear in collections of original writing and are only minimally labeled paratextually as translations. (Fowles writes a preface to *Eliduc* that begins with his experience of reading French literature at Oxford, but is mostly about Marie de France, and only at the very end of that preface – not on the book cover, nor in the table of contents – in a prepositional phrase does he identify the work as a translation: "I have attempted to convey at least a trace of this living, oral quality in my translation . . ." (Fowles 1974/1984, 121). We will return to consider the problematic nature of Genette's remark about the usefulness of paratexts in clearing up misidentifications of fiction as reality in section 2.3.5; is it possible that Fowles *wants* his readers, at least some of them, to mistake his translation for original writing?)

Based on these observations, we might want to define the "kind" or genre of literature that a literary translation is along these lines: *a literary translation is a target-language rewriting of a source text that is normatively understood in terms of the fictional illusion not only that it is* equivalent *to the source text but that it* is *the source text, and that achieves literariness not (solely) by imitating the textual contents of the source text but by imitating the literary strategies employed by the source author or similar authors in the target culture.*

Literary translation, in other words, is a *reperformative genre*. Like the adaptation, it is a discrete literary genre that seeks to create a new literary work by imitating what literary authors do in writing; but unlike the adaptation, it also impersonates the source text.

2.3.5 Speech acts

But what then are those literary strategies? What does the "original writer" *do* in writing originally, and what does the translator seek to *do* in imitating that doing?

Asking the question about literary strategies in terms of *doing* obviously situates the problem in the realm of the literary speech act, one that has attracted considerable critical attention since J. L. Austin (1962/1975), in performing the act of creating the concept of the speech act, declared that a performative is "*in a peculiar way* hollow or void if said by an actor on the stage, or if introduced in a poem, or spoken in soliloquy" (22), and thus *as literature* is "parasitic" upon its "normal" or "serious" use *in real life*. The American philosopher Stanley Cavell (b. 1926) – who in fact was present as a grad student at Austin's 1955 William James lectures at Harvard, which later, after Austin's death in 1960, were published as *How To Do Things With Words* – tried to rescue him from the apparent solecism in that claim by insisting (Cavell 1995) that, in "excluding" the literary/dramatic performance of performatives as "parasitic" upon "serious" uses, Austin was actually only temporarily setting them aside in this particular context, because he had dealt with that complexity elsewhere, in Austin (1961). What Cavell neglects to mention, however, is that Austin returns to restate that exclusion later in his lectures, along lines that seem more permanent and categorical than temporary and pragmatic:

> To take this farther, let us be quite clear that the expression "use of language" can cover other matters even more diverse than the illocutionary and perlocutionary acts and obviously quite diverse from any with which we are here concerned. For example, we may speak of the "use of language" *for* something, e.g. for joking; and we may use "in" in a way different from the illocutionary "in," as when we say "in saying 'p' I was joking" or "acting a part" or "writing poetry"; or again we may speak of "a poetical use of language" as distinct from "the use of language in poetry." These references to "use of language" have nothing to do with the illocutionary act. For example, if I say "Go and catch a falling star," it may be quite clear

> what both the meaning and the force of my utterance is, but still wholly unresolved which of these other kinds of things I may be doing. There are aetiolations, parasitic uses, etc., various "not serious" and "not full normal" uses. The normal conditions of reference may be suspended, or no attempt made to make you do anything, as Walt Whitman does not seriously incite the eagle of liberty to soar.
>
> (Austin 1962/1975, 104)

There it does seem clear that Austin is categorically dismissing the "literary speech act" as an attempt "to make you do anything." It also seems very clear that Austin is wrong here – that he simply hasn't thought the matter through properly. For of course one can perform illocutionary acts in or by joking, acting a part, or writing poetry! Whitman may not be seriously inciting the eagle of liberty to soar, but he is doing *something* – for example, inciting the citizens of a democratic country to behave democratically, to expand the behavioral role of democratic ideals and values in their own lives. The illocutionary acts performed in or by joking or acting a part or writing poetry may be implicit or indirect, but they are illocutionary acts nonetheless. I can hint at some error a friend has made by joking about it, or joking around it, joking past it, or even joking irrelevantly, or by imitating some moment in a movie or popular TV show, replaying the part of some character, so that my friend will recognize the allusion and understand it to be an *invocative implicature* or *invocature* (for which see Robinson 2003, ch. 13).

And in his crushing 100-page rejoinder to the 15 pages of condescension that make up Searle (1977), Jacques Derrida (1977/1988) pauses briefly to offer the obvious commonsensical solution to the "problem" Austin sees in the reperformance of the performative utterance onstage. In response to Searle writing that "we do not, for example, hold the actor responsible today for the promise he made on stage last night the way we normally hold people responsible for their promises" (204), Derrida replies by rolling his eyes *(duh)* and explaining heavily that "it would not be the actor who should be held responsible but rather the speaker committed by the promise *in the scene,* that is, the character" (89). Simple: the minister *in the play* says "I now pronounce you man and wife" and the bride and groom *in the play* are thereby married. The performative isn't hollow or void; it just operates in its own fictional frame.

Out of this engagement with the reperformability of the performative, Derrida develops his (arche)concept of iterability. Austin's "structural parasitism," he argues – the performability of any performative – is part of the "general iterability" of all language and thus the "internal and positive condition of possibility" of any speech act: "For, ultimately, isn't it true that what Austin excludes as anomaly, exception, 'non-serious,' *citation* (on stage, in a poem, or a soliloquy) is the determined modification of a general citationality – or rather, a general iterability – without which there would not even be a 'successful' performative?" (17). Reperformances of performatives *in a new frame,* in other words, are ultimately just a special case of reperformances in general. And without reperformances, Derrida insists, nothing would make sense. Nothing would be communicable. Utterances accrete understandability, communicability, by being reuttered, performances by being reperformed. Iterability is the "againness" of all language.

But – and this brings us back to what I am calling translationality – iterability is specifically reperformability *as change*. "Let us not forget," Derrida writes, "that 'iterability' does not signify simply, as Searle seems to think, repeatability of the same, but rather alterability of this same idealized in the singularity of the event, for instance, in this or that speech act" (119). What is iteratively accreted is not a vast collection of identical units or perfect clones of the same thing; rather, every (re)iteration of "the same" introduces some slight difference or deviation. There is no "pure" performative because in order for an utterance to "perform" meaningfully it must have been repeat-performed over and over, each time slightly differently. (Even when the words are exactly the same, as Jorge Luis Borges demonstrates in "Pierre Menard, Author of the *Quixote*," the passage of time brings about slight but significant changes in intention and interpretation.)

Oddly, when Gérard Genette picks up the thread of the literary speech act in Chapter 2 of *Fiction et Diction* (1991: a decade and a half after the Searle-Derrida debate), he cites neither Austin nor Derrida – his references are all to Searle (1969 and 1975/1979) – and yet, while claiming to read Searle in a Searlean spirit, he comes to conclusions that are much closer to Derrida than to Searle. He begins by noting that the primary literary speech act is one of *pretending:*

> "Marcel," the narrator of *À la recherche du temps perdu,* addresses his prospective reader as seriously as Marcel the character addresses the Duchess of Guermantes. The person whose "seriousness" – that is, whose illocutionary engagement – could be problematic is not Marcel the narrator but Proust the author. But I say "*could* be problematic," in the conditional, for in fact here (in the text of *À la recherche du temps perdu*) *no* speech acts belong to Marcel Proust, for the good reason that Marcel Proust never takes the floor; he is always "pretending," as Plato had already put it, to be Marcel or someone else, no matter how the narrative content may happen to relate to the biography, the life and opinions, of its author.
>
> (Porter 1993, 34)

This brings us into the "illusionistic" realm of both literary originals and literary translations: just as François Rabelais pretends to be translating a true story, and in translating him Sir Thomas Urquhart pretends to be Rabelais pretending to be translating a true story, Marcel Proust the author pretends to be Marcel the narrator remembering being Marcel the character. Note also that Genette is *not* saying that Marcel Proust the author is not performing any speech acts at all: he is saying that Marcel Proust the author is not performing any speech acts *inside the narrative.* The narrative itself, the narration of Marcel the narrator, *is* Proust-the-author's speech act of pretending.

In fact where Genette deviates significantly from Searle is in this understanding of pretending *as* a speech act. For Searle, following Austin, pretending is parasitic on "serious" speech acts:

> Comparing a fragment of an Iris Murdoch novel, then, with a fragment of a factual (journalistic) narrative, Searle readily shows that fictional utterances in the form of assertions meet none of the conditions (sincerity, commitment, verifiability) that characterize authentic assertions. He also demonstrates – in my opinion beyond doubt – that these utterances cannot be taken as *literal* illocutionary acts of some type other than assertion. From this twofold negative observation he draws two conclusions that he views as linked but that I should like to separate: first, that fictional utterances, which take the form of assertions but which do not fulfill the conditions of assertions, are pretended assertions; second, that to produce a fiction (to "write a novel") is not a specific illocutionary act.
>
> (Porter 1993, 35–36)

Note Genette's sneaky rhetorical strategy: by *pretending* to agree with Searle, he actually turns Searle on his head. By agreeing that "fictional utterances . . . are pretended assertions" but "separating" that claim from the insistence "that to produce a fiction (to 'write a novel') is not a specific illocutionary act," Genette manages to use Searle to refute Searle: "I am contending, then, that to call fictional utterances pretended assertions does not preclude, as Searle claims it does, their being something else at the same time" (36–37), namely, "by pretending to make assertions (about fictional beings), the novelist is doing something else, namely, creating a *work* of fiction" (37). "The possibility of such a concurrence," Genette adds, "does not seem to me to exceed human capabilities, and it is after all part of the definition of pretense that while pretending to do one thing, we are in reality doing another" (37).

This, however, is where Genette really needs Derrida's iterability, which radically transforms the terms of the argument. Without iterability, or some other channel of radical periperformativism, Genette somewhat facilely lapses back into objectivist thinking:

> The statement "The meeting is in session," or "You're fired," describes the institutional state of affairs brought about by its very enunciation; the statement "Once upon a time there was a little girl . . ." describes the mental state of affairs brought about in the mind of its hearer by its very enunciation, and the difference is finally quite small, for institutional states of affairs are collective mental states – as are, frequently, the mental states provoked by fictional utterances. Taken to an extreme, these assertive forms might be described as literal formulations and true assertions: fictional utterances would simply be descriptions of their own mental effect. But the disadvantage of such a definition is self-evident: the definition is far too broad, since it applies to all utterances, fictional or not. The statements "Napoleon died at St. Helena"

> and "Water boils at 100°C" describe equally well (or equally badly) the state of consciousness of their speakers and their hearers. The specific feature of fictional utterances is that, contrary to utterances of reality, which describe in addition (!) an objective state of affairs, the fictional utterance describes nothing but a mental state. The complete assertive formulation of an utterance of reality might be something like this: "It is a fact that water boils at 100°C, and by saying so I am informing you or reminding you of that fact." The complete assertive formulation of a fictional utterance would be, rather: "It is not a fact that once upon a time there was a little girl, and so on, but by pretending that it is a fact, I am getting you to think of it as an imaginary state of affairs." Obviously one cannot say that the sentence "Once upon a time there was a little girl . . ." is by itself a literal translation of that utterance, nor, a fortiori, of its directive or declarative counterparts. It is thus more accurate to consider that nonserious assertion the nonliteral (but customary) expression of one of the literal (but noncustomary) formulations mentioned earlier.
>
> (42–43)

That last part refers to Genette's earlier question of "whether fictional utterances should not be included among 'nonliterary' utterances, either *figurative,* as when, saying 'You're a lion,' I signify metaphorically 'You're a hero' (or perhaps, ironically, 'You're a coward'), or *indirect,* as when, asking if you can pass me the salt, I express my wish for you to pass me the salt" (38). Fiction, in other words, as a special case of Gricean (1975/1988) implicature – another theoretical contribution that Genette really should have consulted. What both Grice and Genette are groping toward, without quite being able to get us there, is a periperformativistic understanding of verbal communication in which "institutional states of affairs are collective mental states – as are, frequently, the mental states provoked by fictional utterances," so that, as Genette says specifically, "the difference is finally quite small."

The problem he faces, however, is that it seems inadequate to say that any statement "*describes* the mental state of affairs brought about in the mind of its hearer by its very enunciation." The manifest inadequacy of that account drives him to modify it by saying that "utterances of reality . . . describe in addition (!) an objective state of affairs" but "the fictional utterance describes *nothing but* a mental state." I'm not quite sure why he inserts that parenthetical exclamation mark after "in addition," but I would like to think that it indicates his dissatisfaction with his own tentative objectivist formulation, contrasting "utterances of reality" with "the fictional utterance" in terms of objectification: the former "describe" (objectify) external reality *and* internal mental states, while the latter describes (objectifies) *only* mental states.

Paul Grice explores a tentative periperformativist path out of this objectivism by arguing that the "meaning" of any utterance, and thus the "reality" it creates, is performed by the interpreter, through what Austin calls "uptake" – and that to be understood the utterer must therefore attempt to control uptake by manipulating socially organized expectations. For example, when in "saying 'You're a lion,' I signify metaphorically 'You're a hero' (or perhaps, ironically, 'You're a coward')," my ability to *signify* "You're a hero" metaphorically or "You're a coward" ironically depends on *your and my* (and our witnesses') participation in the group regulation of communicative acts. Grice tries to impose a rigid formalism on that regulation – what he calls "the Cooperative Principle and its maxims" – but his critics have quite rightly pointed out that communicative acts are regulated differently in different cultures, and it is just silly to universalize that regulation as a stable abstraction (see Robinson 2003, Part III, for discussion).

In other words, [1] it is not true that conversational implicatures (as Genette suggests) simply objectify things like factual realities, institutional states of affairs, and mental states: they are performative acts that depend on social interaction to *transform* what we take to be reality *(not objectivist but performativist)*. But [2] it is also not true that conversational implicatures (as Grice suggests) perform reality by reference to a single stabilized and universalized social regime like "the Cooperative Principle and its maxims." Jacques Derrida would add to (1>2) that the stabilization of such social regimes in specific cultures is effected through the repeat performances of speech acts that he calls iterability, and that the massive reiteration/alteration-of-the-same that seeks to stabilize or regiment social interaction also serves to destabilize it (it's a kluge). *Not just performativist but repeat-performativist.*

But then [3] it is further not true that conversational implicatures and other speech acts (as Derrida suggests) incrementally stabilize and destabilize social regulatory regimes simply by being reperformed. That is too vague. As we've seen, Eve Sedgwick (2003, 67–91) adds specificity to the Austinian discussion of the performative with her concept of the periperformative: a performative like "I dare you to jump off this wall" requires for its social efficacy the periperformativity of *witnesses,* who ratify that the dare was made and accepted and whether it was successfully completed. *Not just repeat-performativist but periperformativist.* Periperformativity is/shapes/wields collective guidance for performativity and for the social regulatory regimes that, as Derrida insists, are built and maintained through reperformativity/iterativity.

To illustrate the importance of that guidance, let us return one last time to Genette, inserting bracketed numbers for ease of commenting:

> Finally, we need to specify that an illocutionary definition of the discourse of fiction can in principle reach only the *intentional* aspect of that discourse, and [1] its felicitous outcome, which consists at least in achieving recognition of its fictional intent. Now, just as [2] a figure of speech or an indirect speech act may fail because its receiver is unable to decode it ("Me, a lion? You're crazy!"; "Yes, I can pass you the salt: what a stupid question!"), in the same way [3] an act of fiction may fail as such because its hearer does not perceive its fictionality, like Don Quixote getting up on Master Peter's stage to do in the bad guys and rescue the good guys. [4] Wholesale recourse to the resources of the paratext is sometimes welcome if it wards off such

> misunderstandings. But it also happens, as we know, that [5] a single story may change status according to its cultural context: produced by (and for) one group as truth, it is received by others as a false belief and reinterpreted, "recycled," as fiction. [6] Myths thus illustrate an *involuntary* state of fiction, whose illocutionary formula is not the same at the two ends of the chain. And [7] this sort of quid pro quo can affect not only "representation" but reality itself, taken as fiction, as when one pinches oneself to wake up while being all too wide awake already. The opposite of Don Quixote's error is nicely illustrated by Robert Day in an old *New Yorker* cartoon. A car has broken down in a driving rain. The driver, soaked to the bone, is struggling to change a flat tire. His two children, inside the car, are watching him impatiently and no doubt incredulously, if we are to judge by the unfortunate father's response: "Don't you understand? This is *life*, this is what is happening. We *can't* switch to another channel."
>
> (50–51, emphasis in original)

The (1) "felicitous outcome, which consists at least in achieving recognition of its fictional intent," obviously depends on the writer's ability to participate effectively in the periperformative ratification of his or her literary implicatures among the reading public. I say "participate in" rather than simply "manipulate" because to manipulate uptake effectively one has to participate in it, *feel* it from within as a periperformative engine with many moving (human) parts. This collectivistic take on the literary speech act has, I suggest, at least three significant implications, all of which Genette seems to miss:

- *Significant Implication 1.* While it's true that (2) "a figure of speech or an indirect speech act may fail because its receiver is unable to decode it," it is also a bit simplistic to suggest that the ability or inability to decode such a speech act is a matter of individual agency. In fact that (in)ability is periperformed and continually reshaped by the group. Genette's examples of that inability – "Me, a lion? You're crazy!" and "Yes, I can pass you the salt: what a stupid question!" – are deliberately humorous, because he knows how unlikely it is that adult speakers will fail to understand the implicatures of "You're a lion" or "Can you pass me the salt?" That failure is unlikely, of course, because the uptake of such implicatures is socially guided through the regulatory processes that Derrida calls iterability and Sedgwick calls periperformativity. (Only small children and intellectually disabled adults – adults with a generalized neurodevelopmental disorder that impairs their adaptive functioning – are likely to take such implicatures literally, because the children have not yet been fully socialized to conventional implicatures, and the ID adults are unable to respond adequately to those socialization pressures.)
- *Significant Implication 2.* Another thing that Genette doesn't seem to notice about the collectivized/participatory speech act is that in the modern novel it is definitively bidirectional, or bipolar, aimed at evoking audience belief *and* disbelief in the pretense. Yes, it is true that (3) "an act of fiction may fail as such

because its hearer does not perceive its fictionality, like Don Quixote getting up on Master Peter's stage to do in the bad guys and rescue the good guys" – or, in the example I have used, like the bishop who publicly denounced *Gulliver's Travels* as a pack of damned lies. We find such examples humorous because we treat them as the equivalent in adults of small children's incomplete socialization. But of course modern fiction is far more complex than what Grice calls conventional implicatures like "Can you pass the salt" for "Please pass the salt," precisely because writers have had so much fun *playing* with the periperformative complexity of the "realistic" or "illusionistic" speech act of pretending that this all really happened. It's not, as Genette seems to suggest, that fiction writers all work hard to signal the fictionality of their writing, but some readers are too stupid to notice. RN writers encourage readers to suspend disbelief – to sort-of-believe the pretense – so that the "act of fiction may [teeter on the dirty edge of] fail[ing] as such" because that's what the writer *hoped* would happen. Swift not only tells us that Lemuel Gulliver actually did travel to Lilliput, Brobdingnag, Laputa, Balnibarbi, Luggnagg, Glubbdubdrib, and the country of the Houyhnhnms; he provides extensive documentary "evidence" of those travels. And yes, those documents are all invented, but Swift makes them sound eminently plausible.[16] And ARN writers like Rabelais, Cervantes, and Sterne produce documents that deliberately put readers at sixes and sevens with the whole issue of "reality" and fictionality – that trap readers in self-recursive as-if loops from which there is no commonsensical escape.

- *Significant Implication 3.* Finally, those "documents" that "prove" or "verify" the pretense are typically paratexts, which renders Genette's aside that (4) "Le recours massif aux ressources du paratexte est parfois le bienvenu pour éviter de telles méprises" (1991, 60)/"Wholesale recourse to the resources of the paratext is sometimes welcome if it wards off such misunderstandings" quite problematic. The "ressources du paratexte"/"resources of the paratext" are icotic – organized and plausibilized by the group – and would include at least the communal belief that a paratext is a reliable source of "truth" that surrounds and frames the fictional text. If the fictional text is designed to deceive – to *pretend* to be a true story – the authorial paratext is designed to envelop that pretense in a safe and sheltered packet of truth. The title really is the title. If the subtitle is "A Novel," then the text inside the covers really is a novel. (If Swift had titled his novel *Gulliver's Travels: A Novel,* the bishop would not have been as likely to call it a pack of lies.) The jacket copy accurately describes the contents. If the author writes a preface, that preface is nonfiction – and thus completely reliable. If Genette's casual remark about "ward[ing] off such misunderstandings" is any indication, he is quite comfortable with such icotic plausibilizations, accepts them, takes them at face value: if only Don Quixote had been paratextually warned that the events he saw transpiring on Master Peter's stage were a play, he would not have climbed up on it "to do in the bad guys and rescue the good guys"!

But of course the modern novel mobilizes "the resources of the paratext" in at least two different ways that complicate Genette's talk of "[l']éviter de telles méprises"/"ward[ing] off such misunderstandings."

- *Mobilization 1:* The default genre-defining strategy of the modern RN is to *rely* on the pretense or illusion that all this really happened, and to that end to mobilize the paratexts so as strategically to *incite* "telles méprises"/"such misunderstandings." I mentioned above that "an act of fiction may [teeter on the dirty edge of] fail[ing] as such" because that's what the writer hoped would happen: the RN writer who standardly has no intention of hoaxing or tricking the reader into actually believing that the novel is a true story still definitively needs for the reader to *sort of believe*. That's what a realistic novel conventionally is: a story that readers *sort of believe* actually happened. The most "benign" version of this generic mandate – benign from an objectivist perspective – is that the author wants readers to *sort of believe and sort of not believe:* the willing suspension of disbelief as a kind of homeostasis of (dis)belief, a feeling strategically stranded between belief and disbelief, perhaps on an affective-becoming-conative-becoming-cognitive scale, where the binary decision between belief and disbelief hovers endlessly just shy of becoming cognitive. The "méprise"/"misunderstanding" of which Genette writes would be an affective-becoming-conative-becoming-cognitive belief in the objectivist pretense/illusion of reality: the bishop full-on cognitively *believes* that Swift is trying to convince him that Gulliver went to all these unlikely places and had all these unlikely adventures, and brings the full-on affective-becoming-conative weight of moral disapproval to bear on what he takes to be the imposture, to warn others against it. The problem with Genette's formulation, in other words, is that it is too categorically binary: the desired state is somewhere in between "méprise"/"misunderstanding" and "prise"/ "understanding"; and what should be "évité"/"avoided" is only the most extreme reach of "méprise"/"misunderstanding," that which propels one into real-world action. Readers should hang just slightly back from full-on belief, and the full-on belief-driven activation of moral rescue.
- *Mobilization 2:* An "act of fiction" may also *succeed by pretending to fail* "as such" (as fiction) by successfully persuading its hearer/reader to misprise its fictionality and so to become trapped in kaleidoscopic epistemologies. The modern writer of ARNs mobilizes what Genette calls "le recours massif aux ressources du paratexte"/"wholesale recourse to the resources of the paratext" precisely in order to *invite* "telles méprises"/"such misunderstandings" for use in epistemic play. The periperformativists who write ARNs know, after all, that the reliability that Genette trusts is just a periperformative reality-construct – and indeed the fact that it is a fiction that *feels* like reliable reality makes it even grittier grist for the periperformativist mill. (An obviously made-up fiction that lacked that feeling of reality would be mere chaff, easily dispersed. The epistemic playthings of choice for fiction-writing periperformativists are not mere random fictions but icoses,

> periperformative constructs icotized as objective realities.) ARN writers mobilize “les ressources du paratexte”/“the resources of the paratext” in order to inject playful confusion into the objectivist regime, which, precisely because it is hegemonic, is often superimposed onto the RN, stirred up together with the RN, mistaken for the true nature of the RN.

In the modern novel, in other words, “pretending” is a bifurcated speech act, deploying illusionistic paratexts and other infrastructural feints and bluffs to split the readership, to “hoax” some readers and delight others with the transparency of the hoax – and indeed in some sense to engineer that split pleasurably in individual readers as well, who thus come to believe and disbelieve simultaneously, and to enjoy both the illusion of reality and the undermining of that illusion. (My model here is borrowed from theories of irony hinged on a binary gate between believing and not believing the literal claim – “not getting” and “getting” the irony.)

That Genette is (at least sometimes) aware of the cultural performativity of these matters becomes clear when he notes that (5) “nous le savons, que la même histoire change de statut selon le contexte culturel: produite par (et pour) les uns comme vérité, elle est reçue par d’autres comme croyance fausse et réinterprétée, « recyclée « en fiction” (60)/ “a single story may change status according to its cultural context: produced by (and for) one group as truth, it is received by others as a false belief and reinterpreted, ‘recycled,’ as fiction.” Unfortunately, he doesn’t consider the broader implications of this “change de statut”/“status change” for the socio(neuro)cultural priming of literary speech acts. And indeed the phrase (6) “le mythe illustre ainsi un état *involontaire* de la fiction” (60–61)/“myths thus illustrate an *involuntary* state of fiction” would appear to collapse a whole series of collective performative transformations into a stable “état . . . de la fiction”/“state . . . of fiction” that ostensibly did not will itself into that state. The collective performances elided in his formulation would include not only the shift tracked in (5), “produced by (and for) one group as truth, it is received by others as a false belief and reinterpreted, ‘recycled,’ as fiction,” but the fractal icotic transformations that first recycle myth-as-sacred-story *(-as-true)* as myth-as-someone-else’s-sacred-story *(-as-true-for-them),* then as myth-as-superstition *(-as-falsehood),* and finally as myth-as-fiction *(-as-literature)*. Part of the problem is that his formulation elides the human groups and individuals that perform these actions: people *take* or *use* myth as sacred story; people *take* or *use* myth as fiction; people *take* or *use* myths to illustrate the “involuntariness” of that state, etc. This is an excellent example of icotic translationality – but Genette doesn’t think it through clearly enough to present it as such.

Still, Genette comes remarkably close to a periperformativist rethinking of his whole model here: (7) “Et ce genre de quiproquo peut affecter non seulement la « représentation «, mais la réalité même, prise pour fiction, comme lorsqu’on se pince pour se réveiller alors qu’on ne l’est déjà que trop” (61)/“This sort of quid pro quo can affect not only ‘representation’ but reality itself, taken as fiction, as when one pinches oneself to wake up while being all too wide awake already." First, a quibble: a French *quiproquo* (*mistaking* one thing for another, especially in the transcribing of a text) is not the same thing as an English "quid pro quo" (*exchanging* one thing for another, especially as a balancing of favors). Catherine Porter's translation "quid pro quo" is a *quiproquo* in the French sense: a mistranslation. The weightier question is, however: if the reader's mistaking of a truth for a fiction or a fiction for a truth "*peut* affecter . . . la réalité même"/"*can* affect . . . reality itself," does that mean it affects reality only intermittently, at odd moments? If so, what might make the difference between a periperformativist moment and an objectivist moment? Or are we to think that we live in objective reality *except* at those sudden moments of insanity (see section 3.3.3) when the moorings of "reality," or of our grasp on reality, come loose? Essay 1's foray into the Capgras delusion and other misidentification syndromes would prompt one to ask whether, if those moorings *can* come loose at odd moments, and may even disintegrate entirely, perhaps we should rethink the ontology behind the objectivist belief in a stable external reality that is immune to human craziness.

2.4 Conclusion: icosis again

It seems to me, as a layman – a humanist – that the neurophilosophical evidence in favor of a periperformativist account of reality-creation is quite strong. It seemed that way to Richard Powers in Essay 1, too – but then he is a humanist layman as well. Arrayed against that evidence, of course, is objectivist common sense, backed up by the commonsensical evidence of "the senses": slam your fist into a tree trunk and then ask whether the tree is "really there" or only a performed social construct.

The stutter in this skirmish, I suggest, is that either there is no middle ground between objectivism and social constructivism/periperformativism – an explanatory model that would explain each to the other in mutually satisfactory ways – or such a middle ground exists but is too little known. If reality is a social construct, why does it hurt to slam your fist into a tree? If reality is a collection of stable objects, why do cultural conceptions of it diverge so radically even among normals, and even more radically among sufferers from misidentification disorders?

The cognitive neuroscience of the individual nervous system can explain most of that, along Kantian lines: an "objective" reality exists, but we have no "objective" access to it. All of our experience of that reality is mediated for us by our nervous systems. The pain we feel when we slam a fist into a tree trunk seems pretty immediate – unmediated – but congenital analgesiacs don't feel that pain, or any other pain either. They can run their fingers over the tree trunk with their eyes closed and determine that it *is* a tree; but if they slam their fist into it, they feel no pain. Congenital sensory neuropaths (those with HSAN2/Morvan's disease) are born with the ability to feel pain and sense hot and cold, but lose it in early infancy; their discriminatory touch – the ability to distinguish a rough tree trunk from a smooth one, and both from a telephone pole or a flagpole – is often impaired as well. The "immediate" sensory experience that normals have of objective reality is a neural construct. It is not immediate at all. It only feels that way, thanks to the normal mediatory functioning of our nervous systems.

For a neurological explanation of the social regulatory processes that create discrete cultural regimes and cultural differences, however, we must turn to social neuroscience – or, in my own MH blend of social neuroscience and performance studies, to *icosis*, which incorporates theories of performativity from Austin's speech acts to Derrida's iterability to Sedgwick's periperformativity to Judith Butler's (1990/1999) notion of performative identities. Theatrical performers have known and used the transformative power of mirroring for two-plus millennia; social psychologists began tracking that power in the mid-nineteenth century, a project most notably monumentalized in the so-called Carpenter Effect, named after William Carpenter (1874); the discovery of the mirror-neuron system in the late 1980s not only launched social neuroscience as a powerful new subdiscipline of the neurosciences but gave periperformative theories of truth and identity a shot in the arm. Performance studies are all about embodied interaction, using all five senses, affect, and physical movement to construct, organize, and stage reality – on literal stages, of course, but also in "real life" (though in this periperformativist approach to the world the distinction between performances onstage and performances in the world-as-stage tends to lose its sharp binary teeth). (For MH/cognitive-science approaches to performance, see Shaughnessy 2013, Blair and Cook 2016b, Falletti et al. 2016, and Mermikides and Bouchard 2016. The authors in Mermikides and Bouchard 2016 in particular make much of the medical operating theater as "real-world" stage. I will return to examine theatrical performance more specifically in the Conclusion.)

What this work offers is that important missing link between objectivism and periperformativism: an explanation not only of how individual organisms can be *neuroculturally* transformed so as to conform more fully to shared group norms, but of how that neurocultural transformation can be so successfully naturalized that group members believe it never took place – that they *just are* the way they are, because they're human (isn't everybody this way?), and reality *just is* the way it is, because, well, isn't it obvious? (Slam your fist into that tree trunk.)

As I have been hinting throughout this essay, my icotic model offers a neurocultural explanation of both sides:

- *Essay 2 introduction*. The things that the humanities study, and the orthodox methods they have evolved to study them with, are organized icotically; but the evolution of those methods in each humanistic discipline, subdiscipline, and interdiscipline is also organized icotically. The impression of stability, of stable categories or essences created not just by tradition but by the God of Moses, Socrates, Philo, or Jesus, is icotically managed; but so too is the impression of slow, stately transmutation that emerges when we pay close attention to historical change.
- *Section 2.1*. Freud's reality principle and its repetition-compulsion/death drive is obviously icotic – that is precisely what he means by calling it *das Unbehagen in der Kultur*/ "the malaise in civilization" – but *die Kultur*/ civilization/icosis organizes the pleasure principle just as powerfully. It just doesn't feel as unpleasant as the reality principle. The neat binarization of translationality into "the Translatable" and "the Untranslatable" is also

icotic. That's why there's no real conflict between Apter's description of "the Untranslatable" as "a linguistic form of creative failure with homeopathic uses" and her more essentializing descriptions of Untranslatables as things with "genuine symptoms": the collective homeopathy that organizes certain practices as "creative failure" is the icotic force that reifies the concept as a thing and certain words as its symptoms.

- *Section 2.2.* The dogmatic infallibilization of authoritative source authors (the Seventy, Galen, Jerome, King James's translators, whoever it was who supposedly wrote the Book of Mormon in "Old Egyptian," Dmitri Shostakovich as the "author" of his "memoir") and the restless repeat fallibilization of those and all new authorities are the icoses of competing cultural organizations. This is patently obvious from the simple fact that both Jacobus Sylvius and Andreas Vesalius passionately championed their own radically opposed approaches to Galen as "scientific method" (the traditional name of the icosis governing both sides of that particular debate). Similarly, the pretense that "all this really happened" was arguably the founding icosis of the modern novel – but so too was the antithetical impulse to expose and ridicule that pretense, to have fun with the "impostures" that constitute our sense of reality.
- *Section 2.3.* Objectivism and periperformativism as competing icoses. SIDOLT and translationality as competing icoses.

To be sure, I theorize icosis as specifically grounded in the *continual homeostatic transformation of group response to changing circumstances.* To that extent, icotic theory would appear to take sides: icosis as the guarantor of translationality. But as the group response changes, it always plausibilizes its *current* homeostasis as "reality": icosis as the collective impresario of objective reality, and thus of objectivism.

To sum up my explorations of translationality in this essay, then, everything we do changes as our collective assessment of our environment changes:

1. Our culturally conditioned nervous systems translate the steady stream of sense-data into our current collective (icotic/periperformative) construction of a coherent reality.
2. In order to keep that construction (1) current, they also translate old icoses into new ones, old models of reality into updated adaptive neurocultural models that better manage/fit feedback from changing sense-data.
3. As affective and conative orientations to these changes (1>2) emerge into cognitive awareness, "culture" as group dynamics translates felt neurocultural models into performative constructs like beliefs, values, ideologies, stories, images, melodies, and so on – and beliefs into values, values into ideologies, ideologies into stories, stories into images and melodies, and so on. (This step moves us into the field usually called Adaptation Studies, which Translation Studies scholars like to refer to as "intersemiotic translation," using Roman Jakobson's famous 1959 tripartite model (intralingual, interlingual, and intersemiotic translation).)

4 The adaptation model of textual transformation (3) has also given rise to so-called "translation-chain" experiments shuttling back and forth between poetry and visual images,[17] so that a poem is sent to a visual artist, who transforms the poem into an image or series of images, which is then sent to another poet, who transforms the image(s) into a new poem, which is then sent to another visual artist, and so on; and between poetry and film,[18] shuttling translationality back and forth in similar ways. But "back and forth" is in a sense a misleading description, since there is no generative "going back" to a previous version: the process always moves forward, always transforming each new "source" text in a new "target" direction. It is of course possible to "go back" (and forth) while reading, but the forward movement of the generative process will tend to throw massive obstacles in the way of any attempt to impose a cloning/SIDOLT model on these texts.

5 These intersemiotic translation-chain experiments (4) have also been conducted from poem to poem to poem, of course, based on a serialization of the German notion of *Umdichtung* ("repoeming"): Poem 1 is translated by Poet A from Language 1 into Language 2, making it Poem 2, which is translated by Poet B from Language 2 into Language 3, making it Poem 3, which is translated by Poet C from Language 3 into Language 4, making it Poem 4, and so on. One recent collection of translation-chain experiments would be *Chain 10: translucinación*, edited by Jena Osman and Juliana Spahr (2003), which borrows the Spanish word *translucinación* coined by Andrés Ajens to imply the use of translation to generate trans-lucidity, or, as the editors put it, "how translation is a form of reading and writing that creates new work, new conversations" (iii).[19]

But note what happens when we shift from that mode of text transfer called "adaptation" (3>4) to that mode of text transfer called "translation" (5): suddenly the rules calcify. Suddenly everyone becomes very nervous about translationality as transformationality. Suddenly now things have to *stay the same.* SIDOLT clones become the icotic norm. Translators and translation scholars frequently wring their hands about the impossibility of transferring a text from a source language to a target language perfectly, without loss or change, but the idealized goal remains the perfect transfer of everything: Absolute Equivalence. There are many theories about why this should be so – why translation should be so nervously locked into the requirement of equivalence. There are the obvious pragmatic marketplace theories about target readers needing to know *exactly* what the source text says, for medical or legal or commercial or technical reasons; but see Nord (1991, 23) for the *skopos*/action-oriented/functionalist take on this marketplace context: "Functional equivalence between source and target text is not the 'normal' skopos [purpose] of a translation, but an exceptional case in which the factor 'change of functions' is assigned zero." "Change of functions" in translation(ality), in other words, is the marketplace norm. There are also more "historical" theories about two kings meeting to discuss ending a war or whatnot, and each bringing his own interpreter, because he can't trust the other one's interpreter to reproduce *exactly* what each says to the other – but even that mythic primal scene presumes "change of function," and simply seeks to balance out the likelihood of *functional-change-for-him* with a preemptive provision of *functional-change-for-me.*

Theoretically the requirement of Absolute Equivalence should not be as pressing in literary translation as it is in non-literary translation and political interpreting; but modern concerns for intellectual property rights tend to rigidify thinking about stable translational equivalence there as well. If we translate, say, "Alexander Pushkin" transformatively, creatively – even, *a fortiori,* in a translation chain of creative transformations – in what sense exactly, when we read the series of translations that results, are we reading "Pushkin"? Whose intellectual property is each translated poem? And if, conversely, we translate "him" submissively, worshipfully, in full-on SIDOLT mode, in order to protect the illusion that this is not a new original poem but *Pushkin,* and the resulting "Pushkin" is less brilliant than the Pushkin who wrote in Russian – and SIDOLT means that "he" invariably is, indeed is inferior by default and by definition – how does that protect "his" (reputational rights to that) intellectual property? What recourse does "he" – or some comp lit professor as "his" self-appointed intellectual property lawyer – have if some undergraduate, reading a so-so translation of one of his poems, refuses to believe that Alexander Pushkin is "really" and "truly" a great poet?

Horace's famous warning against "rendering word for word like a faithful translator" *(nec verbum verbo curabit reddere, fidus/Interpres)* – the historical origin of that phrase "word for word" – was of course specifically a clarion call for adaptation, for translationality (though I'm sure he would balk at that usage, because for him translation was the enemy of creativity). What is striking about that call is that he couches it figuratively in terms of transformed or transferred property rights:

> It is a hard task to treat what is common in a way of your own; and you are doing more rightly in breaking the tale of Troy into acts than in giving the world a new story of your own telling. You may acquire private rights in common ground, provided you will neither linger in the one hackneyed and easy round; nor trouble to render word for word with the faithfulness of a translator . . .
>
> (E.C. Wickham's translation; Robinson 1997/2002, 15)

Don't be boring, Horace is saying, like a translator: be *literary.*[20] Both of those rejected courses of action, "linger[ing] in the one hackneyed and easy round" and "render[ing] word for word with the faithfulness of a translator," hunker down timidly in things that stay the same. But we should not conclude therefrom that Horace's imaginary mediocre writer *wants* things to stay the same: s/he just doesn't dare take a risk. S/he is afraid to venture off the beaten path. For this writer, clinging to the hackneyed and the verbatim is not so much an ideal as it is a safe fallback: SIDOLT, the standard inferiorizing definition of literary translation.

Horace's negative exemplar, in other words, is very far from the "scientific" rigidity of either Jacobus Sylvius on Galen or Juliane House on Translation Quality

Assessment. But that is almost certainly because he is envisioning literature as translationality – writing as what Ezra Pound called "making it new." He doesn't feel the competition in the literary field as waged between fiercely dogmatic exponents of destabilization and fiercely dogmatic exponents of stabilization; he sees his opponents as cowards. They stick to the tried and true not because they have a deeply felt commitment to the classics, but because they lack the boldness to respond fully and complexly to changing circumstances. The "fidelity" of the *fidus interpres*/"faithful translator" is for him sheer scribal timidity: fidelity as a self-protective move. (If I'm *stupidly* faithful, at least no one can accuse me of taking liberties. If the Roman *scriba* copied the documents handed to him verbatim, no harm could come to him.[21] Bureaucratic CYA.) His ideal writer is someone like Vesalius or Rabelais, who transforms Galen, or someone like Urquhart, who transforms Rabelais, or someone like Sterne, who transforms Urquhart.

To embrace this model of translationality is to place serial transformation/adaptation at the core not just of the odd poetic experiment[22] but of all literature, indeed all writing: narratives adapting/transforming memoirs and profiles (novels) and memoirs and profiles adapting/transforming novels (creative nonfiction, lifewriting); narratives adapting/transforming critical works (Nabokov's *Pale Fire*), critical works adapting/transforming novels (critical fictions like Lindenberger 1979, Bloom 1980, Steiner 1999), and so on. This perspective, which reimagines literature in terms of its transformative energy, would elevate literary translation to the status not simply of a literary genre in its own right, but of a *prototypical* literary genre. Thus understood, the translation chain may come to be viewed as literature's most characteristic subgenre.

Notes

1 See Derrida (1988) for iterability; for a study of Derrida on translation, see Davis (2001/2014). For traditional Translation Studies arguments in favor of translationality as transformationality, see e.g. Hermans (1985/2014) and Lefevere (1992b).

2 See Emmerich (unpub) for a persuasive critique of Apter's arguments for "the Untranslatable" on another basis – namely, that they are predicated on the normative assumption that there is a stable source text that cannot be adequately represented in any target language. She adds:

> Translation as a mode – like specific translations – will only disappoint if we ask it to do things we already know it can't; translation can only be an "unreliable transmitter" if transmission is what we expect of it. The persistent reliance on the trope of untranslatability in this and other post-poststructuralist writings sets up a kind of conceptual straw man, the false demand that translation provide a "genuine translinguistic encounter with a foreign literature" – a demand translation can never meet.

3 For discussion of Urquhart's involvement in politics and war, see esp. McDowell (2005); Craik (1999, 151–53) and Prescott (2015, 177) also deal in passing with this topic.

4 For additional exuberant celebrations of Urquhart's translation, see Coleman (2003), Doyle (2008), and Prescott (2015).

5 In other versions of this literary history, of course, those "literary monsters" are not novels at all but Menippean satires, or, in the term Northrop Frye preferred, taking Burton's *Anatomy of Melancholy* as his terminological model, "anatomies." Frye distinguishes four main genres of literary prose fiction: novels, romances, confessions, and anatomies. In that classification system, obviously, it is a rather egregious misnomer to call these works early novels.

The category of the Menippean satire, first developed by classical grammarians, was most notably applied to Rabelais by Bakhtin (1940/1984).

6 The phrase *credo quia absurdum*/"I believe because it is absurd" is an established paraphrase of a passage from Tertullian's *De carne Christi* ("On the Flesh of Christ," c. 203–6:

> Crucifixus est Dei Filius, non pudet, quia pudendum est;
> et mortuus est Dei Filius, prorsus credibile est, quia ineptum est;
> et sepultus resurrexit, certum est, quia impossibile.
>
> (*De carne Christi* V, 4)

> The Son of God was crucified: there is no shame, because it is shameful.
> And the Son of God died: it is by all means to be believed, because it is absurd.
> And, buried, He rose again: it is certain, because impossible.

7 This is the beginning of Rabelais's book, from the next-to-last paragraph of the first chapter, as translated by Thomas Urquhart (and edited by Peter le Motteux):

> This Genealogy was found by *John Andrews* in a meadow, which he had near the Pole-arch, under the Olive-tree, as you go to *Marsay:* where, as he was making cast up some ditches, the diggers with their mattocks struck against a great brazen tomb, and unmeasurably long, for they could never find the end thereof, by reason that it entered too farre within the Sluces of *Vienne;* opening this Tomb in a certain place thereof, sealed on the top with the mark of a goblet, about which was written in *Hetrurian* letters HIC BIBITUR; They found nine Flaggons set in such order as they use to rank their kyles in *Gasgonie,* of which that which was placed in the middle, had under it a big, fat, great, gray, pretty, small, mouldy, little pamphlet, smelling stronger, but no better than roses. In that book the said Genealogy was found written all at length, in a Chancery hand, not in paper, not in parchment, nor in wax, but in the bark of an elme-tree, yet so worne with the long tract of time, that hardly could three letters together be there perfectly discerned.
>
> I (though unworthy) was sent for thither, and with much help of those Spectacles, whereby the art of reading dim writings, and letters that do not clearly appear to the sight, is practiced, as *Aristotle* teacheth it, did translate the book as you may see in your *pantagruelising,* that is to say, in drinking stiffly to your own hearts desire; and reading the dreadful and horrifick acts of *Pantagruel:* at the end of the book there was a little Treatise entituled the *Antidoted Fanfreluches,* or a *Galimatia* of extravagant conceits. The rats and mothes or (that I may not lie) other wicked beasts, had nibled off the beginning, the rest I have hereto subjoyned, for the reverence I bear to antiquity.
>
> (1653–93/1994, 26)

8 Thanks to Ivan Delazari for reminding me of Eco's *The Name of the Rose.* Ivan also drew my attention to the authenticity debate over Solomon Volkov's "memoir" of Dmitri Shostakovich, John Fowles's translation of *Eliduc,* and sundry other more minor points.

9 See Emmerich (unpub) for an interesting historical trajectory that brilliantly illustrates what I am calling translationality. First comes Jack Spicer's *After Lorca* (1957/2008), which presents Spicer's translations of twenty-two poems and a

short play by Federico García Lorca interspersed with ten poems and another short play supposedly translated from Lorca, but without source texts – in other words, pseudotranslations – all interspersed with letters to Lorca signed "Love, Jack," which Spicer claims he didn't write (they were "dictated" to him), and prefaced by a letter from Lorca to Spicer. In that introductory letter, Lorca claims that the pseudotranslations are actual translations of poems he sent to Spicer posthumously, but takes his translator to task for "tak[ing] one of my poems and adjoin[ing] to half of it another half of his own, giving rather the effect of an unwilling centaur" (107; quoted in Emmerich). In one of the letters to Lorca, the "author" (narrator? pseudotranslator?) outlines a theory of translationality:

> But things decay, reason argues. Real things become garbage. The piece of lemon you shellac to the canvas begins to develop a mold, the newspaper tells of incredibly ancient events in forgotten slang, the boy becomes a grandfather. Yes, but the garbage of the real still reaches out into the current world making *its* objects, in turn, visible – lemon calls to lemon, newspaper to newspaper, boy to boy. As things decay they bring their equivalents into being.
>
> Things do not connect; they correspond. That is what makes it possible for a poet to translate real objects, to bring them across language as easily as he can bring them across time. That tree you saw in Spain is a tree I could never have seen in California, that lemon has a different smell and a different taste, BUT the answer is this – every place and every time has a real object to *correspond* with your real object – that lemon may become this lemon, or it may even become this piece of seaweed, or this particular color of gray in this ocean. One does not need to imagine that lemon; one needs to discover it.
>
> Even these letters. They *correspond* with something (I don't know what) that you have written (perhaps as unapparently as that lemon corresponds to this piece of seaweed) and, in turn, some future poet will write something which *corresponds* to them. That is how we dead men write to each other.
>
> (133–34)

Spicer would die eight years later, in 1965, at the age of 40, of complications from alcoholism. A gay man, he apparently had no plans of ever becoming a grandfather; but in these lines he is already establishing the equivalence or correspondence between himself as a living man and himself as a dead man, just as the rotting lemon calls out to the fresh one, "the garbage of the real still reach[ing] out into the current world making *its* objects, in turn, visible." Everything decays, and in decaying creates "equivalences" between snapshots along the trajectory of decay, between a freeze-frame boy and a freeze-frame grandfather, between the currency of a newspaper description on the day it is published and the perspective of the reader decades later, "the newspaper tell[ing] of incredibly ancient events in forgotten slang." Things that (supposedly) stay the same are only snapshots of the ever-changing river of time.

The second stage of this trajectory comes at the end of Emmerich's chapter on Spicer, when she pauses to consider a playful pseudotranslation from the Japanese of a fictional poet named Araki Yasunada by Kent Johnson, including a pseudo-back-translation of Yasunada's fictional translation of a Spicer poem, in *Doubled Flowering: From the Notebooks of Araki Yasunada* (1997). This fictional poet was so inspired by Spicer's *After Lorca* that he planned to write a similar work in Japanese, to be called *After Spicer*. When the "authenticity" of Johnson's pseudotranslation began to be challenged (first by Marjorie Perloff), he insisted in interviews that it was a real translation of an actual existing text; but clearly the book had been written to be a playfully *transparent* hoax, and thus, as Brian McHale argued, a "mock-hoax" (237; quoted in Emmerich).

As Emmerich comments:

> My own choice to discuss the translations of a widely influential American poet could likewise be seen as privileging the presumed creative license of the poet-translator over the assumed responsibilities of the translator. My hope, however, is that in focusing on a poet who explicitly rejected ideas about authorial intention, originality, and control over the process and products of writing, this chapter will help deflate rather than exceptionalize the category of poet-translator. Spicer's blurring of the line between writing and translation in *After Lorca* – effected largely through the destabilizing operation of pseudotranslation – can be seen not as an exception to the rule of what translation really is, an exception available only to poets, but rather as a different model for what translation can be, presenting possibilities for all who translate, regardless of what we call them. Particularly in the vacuum left by the fortunate capsizing of paradigms of equivalence, and in an intellectual environment increasingly willing to consider the importance of the visual and material aspects of texts – as well, I hope, as the unstable textual nature of the works our translations seek to further – we are in dire need of good thinking about the nature and limits of translation, how we can translate both differently and with rigor.

Emmerich's citation of Johnson's fictional pseudotranslation *from* the Japanese reminds me also of another intriguing contemporary case *into* Japanese, namely Tawada Yōko's (2007) Japanese novella "Arufabetto-no kizuguchi" (アルファベットの傷口, lit. "Wound in the Alphabet," translated into English by Margret Mitsutani as "St. George and the Translator"). Tawada's story uses the fictionalized process of translating a real story by a real German author – Anne Duden (b. 1942), who is fictionalized but unnamed in the story – as the occasion and setting of her narration. (See Geisel 2001, Esselborn 2007, Gabrakova 2010, and Kaindl 2014. Thanks to Dennitza Gabrakova for bringing this one to my attention.)

10 And that work has been followed up in various venues, such as the special issue of *Linguistica Antverpiensia* titled *Fictionalising Translation and Multilingualism,* coedited by Dirk Delabastita and Rainer Gutman (2005); Christine Lombez's (2005) article in that issue in particular follows up on Toury's approach in the context of French Romantic poetry. That collection would have been an excellent forum for the discussion of the fictional use of translation with which I am concerned here, the found-translation framing device; but it does not broach that subject, focusing instead mostly on the translator as a fictional character.

11 As Hermans (2000, 270) writes:

> Another way of putting this would be to say that the self-reflexive translation makes explicit what remains implicit in more conventional "illusionist" translations (the term is Jiří Levý's). What it makes explicit is the difference between first-order and second-order observation. The self-reflexive translation observes itself observing its original, and in so doing reveals the contingency of its own form, which it makes manifest through the re-entry of the form, i.e. through the demonstration of its contingency. Resistant, recalcitrant or rebarbative translations, whether they are homophonic or abusive, brashly literal or naturalizing or anachronistic, all play havoc with the invitation which the label "translation" carries, an invitation to activate a certain reading attitude, to suspend disbelief, to assume equivalence of one sort or another, to take the re-enactment for the real experience.

Levý's term "illusionistic," unpacked by Hermans as "an invitation . . . to take the re-enactment for the real experience," is what I have been calling the fictional pretense of reality; like metafiction in the novel, metatranslation is explicitly anti-illusionistic. For a brief example of an explicitly self-reflexive (meta)translation of Derrida, see Robinson (1991, 237); for an analysis of a metatranslation of Luther's "Sendbrief vom Dolmetchen" (Robinson 1997/2002, 84–89), see Robinson (1997, 95–96).

12 The convergence between More's defense of the Church and the Messenger's accusations against it was that it was quite true, as More insisted, that the Church was not prohibiting, preventing, and prosecuting *all* vernacular Bible translations, just "heretical" ones – which is to say, Protestant ones – but it was also true, More to the contrary, that the Catholic Church showed no interest in creating their own "orthodox" vernacular translation until late in the century. More makes it sound like the Catholic Church was enthusiastically promoting vernacular Bible translations as long as they were approved, and only prosecuting the unapproved ones; in fact it spent most of the sixteenth century working up the courage to initiate its own vernacular Bible translation, and, since the Protestants were the only ones translating the Bible into the vernacular, cracking down on them hard. The prevailing fear was still derived from the ancient mystery religions: that the Bible, because it was a *mysterious* sacred text – charged with the High Holy Mysteries of Jesus Christ – should not be allowed to fall into the "wrong" (uninitiated) hands. More in fact proposed a system whereby, when (and if) the Catholic Church did actually have the Bible translated into English, the bishop would determine which parishioners were serious and devout enough Christians to be allowed to read it, and would loan those parishioners a copy for twenty-four hours at a time.

13 In the academia.edu workshop on this paper it was suggested – I think tellingly – that it is somehow counterproductive, or perhaps even silly, to borrow a model for the study of literary translation from a theorist who never even mentions translation. Why not call on authorities who know something about literary translation? This is probably what people mean when they call for the consolidation of Translation Studies as a discrete and autonomous discipline: blocking access to neighboring disciplines. As an interdisciplinary scholar I ignore such pressures, preferring instead to cross-pollinate the various disciplines from which I draw – in this case, enhancing literary studies (and perhaps even Genette studies) by smuggling a little TS into it, and enhancing TS by smuggling a little Genette into it.

14 As Deborah Dawkin pointed out in the academia.edu workshop (April 5, 2016), translations of nonfiction (are often taken to) strive for this same fictional illusion – that they are their originals – as well, and are often conditionally assigned "literary" status based on readers' aesthetic response to their style. In other words, the "literary translation" genre that I am suggesting we slot into Genette's empty box consists not of translations-*of*-fiction that are taken to be literary, but translations-*as*-fiction that are taken to be literary – translations that are icotically fictional in the pretense that they are the original and conditionally literary in style.

15 Examples of brilliant translations recategorized as original works would certainly include any translation that deliberately or inadvertently surpasses its source text. As I've mentioned, Chapman's Homer and Urquhart's Rabelais have met with this reception; the translation-chain experiments I mention in the Conclusion offer other examples. More recent works would include Ezra Pound's *Cathay* (the poems in which are often treated as originals because Pound was a brilliant poet in his own right who had no Chinese).

16 Or another Swiftian example: English professors often assign his "Modest Proposal" to undergrads, and love to roll their eyes with colleagues at their students' tendency to take it literally and express their horror that anyone could seriously propose selling Irish babies to the British as food; but in fact such is the brilliance of Swift's satire that it requires advanced literary/interpretive sophistication to pinpoint the textual evidence that he does *not* mean it literally.

17 See e.g. the "Still in Translation" project begun in early 2015 (www.translationgames.net/output/still-in-translation/).

18 See e.g. "Continental Drift: Europe and Translation, Poetry and Film" (www.ingentaconnect.com/contentone/intellect/jafp/2012/00000005/00000001/art00007?crawler=true).

19 For similar projects, see "Translation Chain: Global Literature" (translationchain.deviantart.com/) and "Translation Chain Redux" (tchainredux.deviantart.com/journal/Welcome-to-Translation-Chain-Redux-231250724).

20 It is also significant that translators and translation scholars seeking to assimilate Horace's advice for the *writer* to the task of the *translator* have often read him as saying "Do not worry about rendering word for word, faithful translator, but render sense for sense" (Lefevere 1992a, 15) – an expansive paraphrase that Lefevere presents as an accurate translation of Horace but presumably based not on Horace directly but on Jerome's Horatian extrapolation, "Nec verbo reddere curabit fidus interpres (ait ille) sed sententias, et sensus transferre studebit"/"Nor bother to render the word, faithful translator, but seek to transfer the sentence/sense." Don't translate the pragmatics, or rhetoric, or prosody, or other literary strategies in and around a piece: just give us the meanings of individual sentences without embellishment. In the terms I'm developing here, we might read Horace as saying, "Don't let yourself get sucked down into the SIDOLT prescribed for faithful translators: be original," and Jerome and Lefevere saying more timidly, "To be a faithful translator you must adhere to SIDOLT, but stick to the sense-for-sense kind of SIDOLT." I am arguing that translators too should – and at their best do typically – follow Horace out of the SIDOLT morass.

It is of course telling that Jerome and Lefevere should make the submissive SIDOLT case for sense-for-sense translation by surreptitiously transgressing it – adapting Horace freely, against the source-textual grain, in translating him.

21 When the military force (organized by Brutus after the assassination of Julius Caesar) that had enlisted him as *tribunus militus* (a very high rank for one so young) was crushed by Octavian (later Augustus) and Mark Antony, Horace – now all of 23 years of age – accepted the amnesty proffered by the victors and obtained a sinecure as a *scriba quaestorius*, a high-ranking civil service position at the Treasury that was lucrative and not very demanding, as the officeholder could delegate scribal tasks to the permanent clerks, called *scribae*. Even in his day job, in other words, he was inclined – icotically, I would want to say, through the scribal "community of practice" of the *aerarium*/Treasury – to look down upon the unimaginative work of the *scribae*. It was at this point in his life that he began writing his *Satires* and *Epodes*.

22 See writing.upenn.edu/bernstein/experiments.html for a list of nearly 100 such "odd poetic exercises" based on the radical transformation of existing texts – the first six of them involving translation.

Essay 3 The medical humanities of translation

The social neuroscience of hermeneutics

The study of translation began anecdotally, emerging "organically" out of translators' impulse to explain – sometimes to defend, sometimes to prescribe, quite often to apologize for – their own translation choices, in prefaces or letters. It existed in that desultory form for almost exactly two millennia, from Cicero's 55 BCE comments on his own decision to translate the Greek orations by Demosthenes and others into Latin, by way of training himself to be a better orator in Latin, to the mid-twentieth century, when a few hardy souls (Korney Chukovsky and Andrey Fyodorov in the Soviet Union (1930; see also Chukovsky 1941/2014; Fyodorov 1953; Leighton 1984), Jean-Paul Vinay and Jean Darbelnet in France (1958; Sager and Hamel 1995), Eugene A. Nida in the United States (1964), etc.) began to formulate a more systematic linguistic approach to the study of translation, mainly focused on textual comparisons (equivalence, fidelity, adequacy, etc.; see Pym 2016 for a fuller mid-twentieth-century history). These linguistic approaches tended to dominate the study of translation until the early 1990s, but opposition to the linguistic focus on textual equivalence began to be developed into new methodological paradigms as early as the mid-1970s in Israel and the Low Countries and in the mid-1980s in Germany – and in English began to be called "Translation Studies," or TS:

- The watershed for the movement that would eventually come to be called Descriptive Translation Studies (DTS) was a series of conferences in Europe and Israel: Bratislava in 1968, Leuven in 1976, Tel Aviv in 1978, and Antwerp in 1980. Many of the presenters at those conferences went on to transform the discipline: Itamar Even-Zohar (1979, 1981), Gideon Toury (1980), and others in Israel began to study the shaping influence large sociocultural systems wielded over translation, in an approach that was originally called "polysystem theory"; Theo Hermans (1985), André Lefevere (1992b), and others in the Low Countries began to study translation as "manipulation" around the same time. Toury (1995) – *Descriptive Translation Studies and Beyond* – had the effect of unifying the various strands of the movement under the DTS rubric, originally suggested by James S. Holmes (1975) (Snell-Hornby 1988; Hermans 1999/2014). Susan Bassnett's 1980 introduction titled simply *Translation Studies* was also a summary of this approach.

- Katharina Reiss and Hans Vermeer (1984; Nord 2013), Justa Holz-Mänttäri (1984), and others in Germany began to study the professional networks that commission translations, hire translators, and manage translation projects, in an approach that has been called *skopos* theory, action-oriented translation studies, or functionalist translation studies (Nord 1997).

3.1 Neurocognitive translation studies

Another oppositional methodology that arose in Germany in the mid-1980s, with the publication of Hans Krings's 1986 PhD dissertation *Was in den Köpfen von Übersetzern vorgeht* ("What Transpires in the Heads of Translators"), was explicitly cognitivist. It used Think-Aloud Protocols to track translators' cognitive processes as they translated – and the Think-Aloud Protocol rubric, or TAP, stuck as a cognomen for the approach as a whole, though over the decades since it has also branched out into the use of other empirical research methods as well, such as keylogging (logging an exact history of which keys the translator hits while translating) and eye-tracking (tracking the translator's eye movements across the source text). Obviously combining those two latter methods gives us some very useful clues as to how the translator is processing text: if her eyes jump from the fourth word in line 5 back up to a cluster of words in line 2, then to line 5 again, and then she makes corrections in lines 2, 3, and 5, we can infer that she found a recurring pattern that caused her to rethink the word choices that she had been making for the previous few lines.

Another cognitive approach to the study of multilingual language processing is explicitly neurological: the use of functional brain imaging to study simultaneous interpreting, widely regarded as the most complex communicative act on the planet: "It requires simultaneous encoding of an incoming speech stream in one language, conversion of the content of that stream to a lexically, semantically and syntactically valid form in the target language, production in the target language and ongoing monitoring of the output to ensure message equivalence between source and target languages (Moser 1978; Moser-Mercer et al. 1997)" (Hervais-Adelman et al. 2015, 264). As Hervais-Adelman and his colleagues note, simultaneous interpreting skill begins with linguistic expertise but is built on top of that foundation through "the acquisition of a high degree of control over their language management skills, as well as the development of a non-linguistic cognitive toolkit that ensures mastery of divided attention (attending to speech input and output simultaneously) and efficient use of working memory, in order to enable them to rapidly and dynamically produce an accurate reproduction of the source message in diverse contexts" (264). Considerable neurological research has sought to determine how that control is managed neurally, but without conclusive results; various researchers have found that it works through development of the inferior parietal lobe (Mechelli et al. 2004; Grogan et al. 2012), the left putamen (Abutalebi et al. 2013), the anterior cingulate cortex (Abutalebi et al. 2012), the left inferior frontal gyrus (Stein et al. 2012; Klein et al. 2014), or the left caudate nucleus (Zou et al. 2012). Other cognitive control-related regions identified through functional imaging research include the striatum (e.g., Klein et al. 1994, 1995, 2006; Crinion et al. 2006), the dorsolateral prefrontal cortices, parietal regions, and the inferior frontal gyrus, and parietal regions (Friederici 2006; Hervais-Adelman et al. 2011; Costa and Sebastián-Gallés 2014; these overviews meta-analyzed in Luk et al. 2012).

Other neurocognitive research has sought to establish the benefits of simultaneous interpreting training, which clearly exceed those traditionally attributed to bilingualism alone: improvements of working memory (Darò and Fabbro 1994; Fabbro and Darò 1995; Christoffels et al. 2006; Köpke and Nespoulous 2006; Yudes et al. 2011, 2012; Stavrakaki et al. 2012), for example, and cognitive flexibility (Yudes et al. 2011). Hervais-Adelman and his colleagues (2011, 2014, 2015) have used fMRI scans to study the benefits to "naïve participants"; their research has revealed the "recruitment" of "a broad network of regions, including the pre-supplementary motor area, the dorsal anterior cingulate, the left inferior frontal gyrus, the left posterior temporal areas, the left anterior insula, the left superior and inferior cerebellar lobules as well as the caudate nuclei and the putamen"; in particular, "the caudate nuclei respond to the overall demands of maintaining the lexico-semantic sets of two languages 'live' simultaneously during interpretation, while the right putamen is responsible for the moment-to-moment control of language, ensuring speech production in the appropriate language" (2015, 265). As they summarize their new research:

> In this study, we used fMRI to investigate brain functional plasticity in trainee simultaneous interpreters learning to become professional conference interpreters. We examined cerebral responses during simultaneous interpretation before and after a fifteen-month period of intensive training in a group of 19 trainee interpreters. We compared these to the cerebral responses of 16 multilingual control participants, tested on the same tasks over the same interval. The control participants were students engaged in a course of higher-level study in non-linguistic domains. Our study is the first longitudinal brain imaging study in simultaneous interpreters, and as such, will provide more direct evidence for training-induced brain plasticity than previous cross-sectional investigations. We expect that the acquisition of expertise in simultaneous interpretation training requires the active development and automatization of extreme language control, a skill which overlaps considerably with other domains of executive control. This form of expertise can be expected to be at least partly driven by an increase in automaticity in performing the task, possibly driven by superior management of its multiple component skills.
>
> After training, we expect to observe reductions in the recruitment of regions crucial to SI, due to increased efficiency of these regions during task performance (as proposed by Ericsson et al. 2006; and see also Kelly and Garavan 2005). We are particularly interested in the striatum, since it has been shown to be important in polyglot language control. If changes to striatal recruitment are found as a function of training, this will provide evidence for the importance of the striatum in extreme language control.
>
> (265)

As Hanna Risku (2014, 334) writes of these approaches, they tend to proceed from the assumption that cognitive function does not extend beyond the skull – that it is not *socially* situated – and so does not need to be studied in professional and social contexts. The TAP research draws mostly on the behavioral sciences, especially psychology, and "can be regarded as the mainstream of translation process research"; research design entails "establishing an exact definition of the variables to be studied, hypothesizing a correlation between them, being able to manipulate a particular variable, setting up an experimental and a control sample/group, and analyzing a statistically sufficient amount of data or subjects to verify or falsify the hypotheses." She also notes that TAP research has been subjected to "considerable constructive criticism" (334) related to "fulfilling the requirements set for classic scientific experiments" (335). If TAP research is typically conducted in the lab and follows positivistic protocols, so *a fortiori* is the neurological research.

Since around the turn of the millennium, TS has taken what has been called – especially by Risku's colleague at the University of Graz, Michaela Wolf (2006, 2011; Wolf and Fukari 2007) – a "sociological turn," including ethnographic studies of legal and medical interpreters *in situ,* but also incorporating the sociological and economic theories of translation developed since the late 1980s by Anthony Pym (1990, 1991, 1992, 1995, 2004; Pym et al. 2006), who took a Ph.D. in sociology at the Sorbonne. What Risku does in the article from which I have been quoting is in effect to fold all this newer work, along with the earlier DTS focus on large sociocultural systems and *skopos* work on the professional networking of workflow, into an expanded cognitivist model that includes developments in cognitive science and the philosophy of mind since the mid-1990s:

> However, my main point in this article is that we will also need other methodological paths of inquiry to model the cognitive processes in translation and to establish a deeper understanding of how translations are produced. Present cognitive scientific views of human intelligence, such as the *situated, embodied* and *extended* cognition approaches (see, e.g., Clark and Chalmers 1998; Suchman 2007; Clark 2008), suggest that cognitive processes are context-dependent, i.e., they are dependent on and partly constituted by the social and physical environment in which they are carried out. Cognition is made up of parallel processes like bodily movements and neurological activity, action and perception, externalization and internalization inside and outside the mind (the leaky, situated mind; Clark 1997). Furthermore, these processes are path-dependent processes that do not conform to stable rules but instead depend on the point in time in which the individual cognizers happen to be in the cognitive and environmental dynamics (Clark 1997, 204ff). Cognition itself is heavily dependent on the sequence of prior learning and doing (Elman 1994). Its context- and path-dependency suggests that we will actually also have to study translators in their authentic, personal, historically embedded environments and translation situations if we want to

> be able to describe the cognitive process – i.e., if authentic translation processes are to be included in the research object.
>
> (335)

The resulting research design sounds remarkably like an extended/embedded-cognitivist version of 1980s *skopos* research: "It addresses heterogeneous areas like cooperation with subject matter experts and colleagues, terminology management and contacts with customers" (336).

Other significant moves in the general socio-cognitive research direction mapped here by Risku would include Abdallah (2010, 2012), Abdallah and Koskinen (2007), Ericsson (2010), Martin de León (2013), Muñoz Martín (2010, 2013), and Risku (2009, 2010, 2014). This is very important work; but I propose to chart a different course in this essay. What are the consequences, I want to ask, of approaching the medical humanities of translation hermeneutically rather than positivistically? What is gained and what is lost, in terms of our understanding of "extended translation," in a research design organized [a] positivistically around quantitative variables in laboratory conditions, [b] positivistically around qualitative variables in "authentic" ethnographic contexts, [c] constructivistically/transactionally around qualitative variables in mutually defined ethnographic contexts, or [d] hermeneutically/phenomenologically around consensual or dialogical reconstructions of shared feelings in remembered contexts? (See Lincoln et al. 2011 for discussion of these methodological options.) Risku adopts approach (b), and critiques approach (a) as out of touch with contemporary enactive/embedded/embodied/extended/distributed cognitive science; more radical sociologists of translation, such as Anthony Pym, might lean more strongly toward approach (c), or, with me (see esp. Robinson 2013b for the full defense), toward approach (d).

3.2 The social neuroscience of hermeneutics

What I note about that four-step model in the previous paragraph, however, is the striking split between (a-b) positivistic approaches to the (social/linguistic) "science of translation" and (c-d) "humanistic" approaches to translation as human sociocultural interaction. Those are, of course, effectively C.P. Snow's (1959/2001) "Two Cultures." And one does not cross the DMZ between them. There is no middle ground between the Two Cultures, right?

Or, to put that differently: every conceivable middle ground between them is actually – right? – a disguised version of one or the other. "Interdisciplinary" collaborations between artists/humanists and scientists typically involve artists and humanists remaining artists and humanists and scientists remaining scientists, because the methodological and epistemological differences are just too overwhelmingly necessary to each side. As Matthew Reason and his colleagues (2013, 43) put it:

> In considering these two broad types of relationships between the art[s] and sciences in research, it is worth noting that neither fundamentally challenges the two cultures division at a paradigmatic level. In each relationship there is

> a clear division between object of study and methodological approach, which is seldom blended. It would be possible to argue that arts and humanities/science collaborations are often instrumentalised, with the art "illustrating" the science to the public or science "proving" a disputed thesis. The key epistemological paradigms of what constitute[s] knowledge or expertise or methodology within each discipline remain unchallenged: art remains art and science remains science with neither paradigm fundamentally unchallenged.

Let me confess up front that I have a dog in this race: I have been working in the interstices among neuroscience, cognitive science, and the humanities since the early 1990s, but because the Two Cultures are widely (and hegemonically) understood to be perfectly isolate binaries, my work is typically not understood as exploring that middle ground. Officially – by which I mean "commonsensically," which is to say "intuitively," which is to say normatively – that middle ground doesn't exist. Thus for example when Hanna Risku defines her project as a study of "*extended translation,* i.e., as [a study of] a form of coupled system between human organisms and external entities" (336), she has no obvious reason even to recognize the existence of, let alone to cite and discuss, my late 1990s work on "Cyborg Translation" (2000) and on disaggregated translation agency in Chapter 6 of *Who Translates?* (2001), or, more recently, my exploration of sociality as extended body-becoming-mind in *Feeling Extended* (2013b). True, I don't study translation in that latter book; but I don't reduce the Clark/Chalmers (1998) Extended Mind Thesis to positivistic hypotheses, either, which may be an even more pressing reason for Risku not to cite it. It is a humanistic study of sociality that moves almost exclusively in the realms of cognitive science/philosophy of mind and the neuroscience of empathy. (Is that even possible?) And my theoretical explorations of the middle ground between (a-b) and (c-d) in "Cyborg Translation" and *Who Translates?* are emphatically not (a-b) positivistic, so they must be – *must be* – purely (c-d) humanistic. Right?

Or take another tack: translation has sometimes been studied as a *performance* of the source text in the target language. This metaphor can be exfoliated formalistically – a translation is to its source text as a musical performance is to the score – but when it is channeled through performance studies, as it is in Wechsler (1998), Robinson (2003), Aaltonen (2013), and Bermann (2014), for example, it maps "translation" as situated and embodied social interaction. In January 2014, John Milton and Dennitza Gabrakova and I organized a conference at HKBU on "Performativity and Translation"; in the summer of 2015 we organized a follow-up three-panel session on the same topic at IATIS in Belo Horizonte, Brazil; in Robinson (2016b) I published an omnibus version of the two interwoven talks I gave at those conferences. Performances as situated, embodied, and interactive events involving *doing things to people with verbal and body language* would appear to be very (d), or possibly even [e]: participatory engagements in real time that are socioaffectively powerful but resist reduction to tidy formalistic analyses. In other words, *very* humanistic. And yet Methuen Drama's "Performance and Science" series has been hacking out a groundbreaking middle between (a-b) positivistic neuroscience and (c-d-e) participatory humanistic periperformativity in a series of exploratory essay collections entitled *Affective Performance and Cognitive Science: Body, Brain and Being* (Shaughnessy 2013), *Theatre, Performance and Cognition: Languages, Bodies and Ecologies* (Blair and Cook 2016b), *Theatre and Cognitive Neuroscience* (Falletti et al. 2016), and *Performance and the Medical Body* (Mermikides and Bouchard 2016). I quoted Reason et al. (2013) above – one of the articles in the first of those books – to the effect that the middle sketched out in the series is improbable in the extreme; and yet in article after article we find theater people working closely with cognitive neuroscientists to find a working accommodation between the Two Cultures.

The title of this section is another such (potentially excludable) middle: "The Social Neuroscience of Hermeneutics." What could that possibly entail? Hermeneutics notoriously has about it the reek of the mystical, the touchy-feely, the soft and squishy – the opposite of science. At best it is radically (d-e) humanistic. How could there ever be (a-b) a social neuroscience of it?

One (perhaps contested)[1] history of hermeneutics sets its origin story in the insistence of Johann Gottfried Herder (1744–1803) that understanding requires "feeling yourself into everything":

> *Ganze Natur* der Seele, die durch Alles *herrscht,* die alle übrige Neigungen und Seelenkräfte *nach sich modelt,* noch auch die gleichgültigsten Handlungen *färbet* – um diese mitzufühlen, antworte nicht aus dem Worte, sondern gehe in das Zeitalter, in die Himmelsgegend, die ganze Geschichte, fühle dich in alles hinein – nun allein bist du auf dem Wege, das Wort zu verstehen . . .
>
> (Herder 1774/1967, 37, emphasis in original)

> *The whole nature* of the soul, which *rules* through everything, which *models* all other inclinations and forces of the soul *in accordance with itself,* and in addition *colors* even the most indifferent actions – in order to share in feeling this, do not answer on the basis of the word but go into the age, into the clime, the whole history, feel yourself into everything – only now are you on the way towards understanding the word.
>
> (Forster 2002, 292)

In order "mitzufühlen"/"to share in feeling" the whole nature of an author's soul, you need "dich in alles hineinzufühlen"/to "feel yourself into everything." That sounds very touchy-feely, certainly; but when we remember that, a century after Herder, Robert Vischer (1847–1933) renamed and reframed *das Sich-Hineinfühlen*/"the feeling oneself into" as *die Einfühlung* "empathy," perhaps we will be in less of a hurry to dismiss the social neuroscience of hermeneutics. After all, there *is* a well-established social neuroscience of empathy, which has sprung up since the discovery of the mirror-neuron system in the late 1980s.

But, you may object, the social neuroscience of empathy is the empirical study of responses to facial expressions, gestures, and other body language – empathy in face-to-face encounters – and hermeneutics is the "empathic" study of *texts.*

And as Herderian hermeneutics is reformulated by Friedrich Schleiermacher (1768–1834) – considered by some to be the father of hermeneutics – it does begin again to sound rather mystical:

> Eine Hauptsache beim Interpretiren ist daß man im Stande sein muß aus seiner eignen Gesinnung herauszugehen in die des Schriftstellers.
>
> (Schleiermacher 1959, 32)

> In interpretation it is essential that one step out of one's own frame of mind into that of the author.
>
> (Duke and Forstman 1977, 42 #8)

> Man muß suchen der unmittelbare Leser zu werden um Anspielungen zu verstehen, um die Luft und das besondere Feld der Gleichnisse zu verstehen.
>
> (32)

> The interpreter must try to become the immediate reader of a text in order to understand its allusions, its atmosphere, and its special field of images.
>
> (43 #12)

A hermeneutical approach to a text does not just involve feeling one's way into it; it involves becoming the author, inhabiting the author's mind (note #8), or, more moderately, inhabiting the mind of the "immediate reader" (note #12). Given that all mediated distance between the author and the reader has now disappeared, *of course* one then understands the text: the connection between reader and author has become immediate.

The first corrective to apply to this formulation would be that the "immediacy" in question is not an ontology: it is a *feeling* of unmediated connection, a phenomenology, an experience, a *sense* of becoming the author or the immediate reader. It is not a mystical oneness. Many of the persistent misunderstandings of *Gefühl* and *Einfühlung* in hermeneutical thought arise out of a tenacious – because it is, again, ideologically normative – binarism according to which feeling and empathy are either [1] mystical forces that enable the reader to *merge spiritually* with the author or [Ø] purely private productions of the individual imagination, random subjective and indeed solipsistic projections. Hermeneutical thinkers are commonly taken to be arguing for (1); and, since the exclusion of all fractal middles between (1) and (Ø) is a kind of ideological mandate, the manifest impossibility of (1) seems to dump hermeneutics back into the silly childish solipsism of (Ø). In fact, however, the hermeneutical tradition everywhere insists that *feeling is organized by the community*. More on that as we go along.

The second corrective is that for Herder and Schleiermacher, "feeling one's way into" a textual meaning always had to be supported by extensive linguistic, literary, and historical research – and again, research-based understanding of an author's meaning was only possible because the researcher's reading of inert facts on the page was and is guided by the community, through *collectivized* feeling.

Any reader's feeling-based understanding of an author's meaning is possible because the researcher fills in the cognitive gaps left by the affective vagueness of feeling through research – and is guided to the filling in of those gaps through communally organized feeling.

Still, the fact remains that hermeneutical theorists have not been particularly forthcoming on the social neuroscience behind all this. How exactly – neurally – is feeling organized by the community? How exactly – neurally – is feeling channeled through textuality? How exactly – neurally – does the reader connect empathically with the author? Hans-Georg Gadamer (1960/1990, 188–201; Weinsheimer and Marshall 1989, 184–95) famously critiqued Schleiermacherian hermeneutics on the grounds that Schleiermacher apparently shifted midway through his decades-long process of theorization from a language-based ("grammatical") hermeneutics to a psychological hermeneutics. Of course interpretation has to be channeled either through language or through psyches: all possible middles must be rigorously excluded. According to the commonsensical assumptions on which Gadamer's hermeneutic relies, only the linguistic medium of hermeneutic understanding is evidence-based; as a result, Schleiermacher's supposed binary jump from a verbal to a psychic connection removed the interpreter's evidence for understanding, supposedly leaving behind a channel of interpersonal intuition that seems like (1) "divining" – a mystical connection that, without proper evidence, must collapse in the end into (Ø) guessing – and in any case like bad metaphysics.

But in fact there is no evidence that Schleiermacher made any such leap, or that those are the only two possible channels for hermeneutical understanding, or that a non-linguistic hermeneutic must by definition lack an evidentiary grounding. That is all bad *theory,* based on well-established "intuitions" – hegemonically organized "common sense" – about human interaction. Like the poststructuralist discursivists, Gadamer too seems to have believed that beyond verbal communication there be dragon-myths. If Schleiermacher seems to be imagining other channels of human communication than the verbal, he must have gone off the deep end.

The fact is, if you don't understand how something works, its functioning does tend to seem mystical. And if you don't understand how someone else understands how something works, you tend to accuse that person of mysticism.

Of course a lot more is known about the neurology of communication today than was known when Gadamer was writing *Wahrheit und Methode* in the 1950s; the mirror neurons were not discovered until three decades after the first edition was published. But what Giacomo Rizzolatti and his colleagues discovered was only the brain science behind mirroring-based communication. Sociologists had been studying it for decades; and the psychosocial model was first clearly articulated by William Carpenter in 1874. The nineteenth-century predecessors to today's social neuroscience of empathy were heavily influenced by the German Romantics, going back to Herder. It is easy now, with the mirror-neuron discovery under our belts, to trace that research tradition backwards in time and show that Herder and Schleiermacher were on the right track – and that Gadamer was merely spouting commonsensical prejudice. But of course Gadamer was a philosopher, not a neuroscientist. Even had the mirror neurons been discovered in his day, they wouldn't have been his field. (That seems a bit unfair, perhaps: look how attentively philosophers of mind these days read the cognitive neurosciences. But that too is a relatively recent development.)

But then what about the manifest difference between the empathic reading of body language among speakers physically present to each other and "feeling one's way into" a written text? Surely the mirror-neuron research is irrelevant to readers who are unable to see (and so to mirror) the author's facial expressions, gestures, postures, and so on? Surely Gadamer was right about *textual* hermeneutics?

That is an objectivist protest. It is based on the assumption of objective causality: that the speaker's body does something physical to listeners who are physically present. Teresa Brennan's (2004) theory that empathic response is triggered by pheromones is such an objectivist model: a physical body emits a physical substance, pheromones, which acts as a change agent upon other physical bodies in the same room. Newtonian physics: the cue ball strikes the eight ball, transfers its momentum, and so propels it into the corner pocket. If Brennan is right, it is impossible to respond empathically to people not physically present, because close physical proximity is required for the pheromonal transfer.

But of course we know that we feel empathy over the phone line, and while watching a movie or reading a novel, and even while simply imagining something terrible happening to a loved one. Social neuroscientists have also measured the time lag in empathic response, and found that it is far too rapid – around 300 milliseconds – to be transferred pheromonally (that would take several seconds).

So what is the answer? If we begin not with objectivist theories of causation but at the other end, with Kantian constructivist/periperformativist theories of mimetic projection, it all makes more sense. The empathic connection between author and reader, via the text, is a *projection:* the reader projects it onto the author. It is an empathic construct.

But if it's a projection, then it's a figment of the hermeneut's imagination, right? Nothing *real.* Nothing objective.

Well, no: the empathic connection between two people who are physically present in the same space is also a projection. So is the empathic connection between any one of us and any part of the world outside us. This is how we experience the reality of the world. As the Capgras delusion taught us, we infuse our analytical FFA perception of the world with the somatic "glow" of familiarity. We *perform* the world as real-because-familiar. Our mirror neurons simulate the body states of the people and things around us, inside us, and we feel those body states as our own. We feel them even when we don't see or hear them, but only hear about them in stories, or read about them in books. If we find ourselves unable to simulate those body states, if we feel no trace of the Feeling of the Familiar, the things or people who thus "evade" our empathic projections seem utterly alien to us, and thus not quite real. Hence the terror of the unfamiliar – xenophobia – of which there are so many disturbing horror stories in history, such as the belief that humans who look and dress and act in very different ways from one's own group are not truly human, and can (and perhaps therefore should) be slaughtered or enslaved without moral compunction. Hence the confabulatory paranoia of Capgras sufferers, who through illness or injury stop being able to feel the Feeling of the Familiar in the (visual) presence of their loved ones, including their pets and even their own mirror images, and come to believe that those individuals are trained impostors, or even cleverly programmed robots. In the 1980s a man in Missouri killed his stepfather to prove that he was a robot: he opened up the corpse's neck and was nonplussed to find only human parts.

My theme in this final essay is the medical hermeneutics of translation – translation specifically in the standard interlingual sense of the transfer of textual features from one language to another. If Essay 1 was about medicalized story as a paradigmatic narrativization of the humanities, and Essay 2 was about translationality as a paradigmatic transformationality of medical and narrative literature, Essay 3 is about translational hermeneutics as a paradigmatic social neuroscience of the humanities. As we saw in Essay 1, it is the Capgras sufferer's inability to construct a sustainable sense of reality that teaches us the importance of the glow cast by our emotions over the products of analytical reasoning for the making-real; one of the things we'll be exploring here in Essay 3 is the ways in which the translator's task involves "curing" a kind of Capgras analogue. Foreign cultures where we don't speak the language(s) don't seem quite real to us; the people and places *look* real, but don't *feel* real, because we don't get the emotional glow of reality from them – that glow that is channeled through language but is not fundamentally linguistic in nature. (Yes, Gadamer's critique of Schleiermacher's supposed shift away from a language-based hermeneutics was ignorant – but then, a big part of the problem was that Schleiermacher was just as much in the dark about the reality-creating hermeneutical force.)

My thesis here: we trust translators not only to *represent* those cultures to us by creating cribs to them, but to *realize* those cultures, to make them feel real to us, by recreating foreign texts in ways that we experience as a new affective-becoming-conative channel or conduit of reality.

As we'll see, however, there are many subtle gradations to this translational Feeling of the Real.

3.3 Translation as foreignization, estrangement, and alienation

As we've seen, for Friedrich Schleiermacher the basic situation in hermeneutics is a readerly phenomenology of *immediate connection with the author* – indeed a phenomenology of being inside the author's skin. Strikingly, however, when he comes to theorize translation in his 1813 address to the Royal Academy of the Sciences in Berlin, "Ueber die verschiedenen Methoden des Uebersezens" (1813/2002)/"On the Different Methods of Translating" (Robinson 1997/2002), he takes a very different tack:

> Will nun aber gar die Uebersetzung einen Schauspieldichter reden lassen, als hätte er ursprünglich in ihrer Sprache gedichtet: so kann sie ihn ja vieles gar nicht vorbringen lassen, weil es in diesem Volk nicht einheimisch ist und

> also auch in der Sprache kein Zeichen hat. Der Uebersetzer muß also hier entweder ganz wegschneiden, und so die Kraft und die Form des Ganzen zerstören, oder er muß anderes an die Stelle setzen. Auf diesem Gebiet also führt die Formel vollständig befolgt offenbar auf bloße Nachbildung, oder auf ein noch widerlicher auffallendes und verwirrendes Gemisch von Uebersetzung und Nachbildung, welches den Leser wie einen Ball zwischen seiner und der fremden Welt, zwischen des Verfassers und des Uebersetzers Erfindung und Witz unbarmherzig hin und her wirft, wovon er keinen reinen Genuß haben kann, zulezt aber Schwindel und Ermattung gewiß genug davon trägt.
>
> (90: 19–31)

> Does the translator want to let a playwright speak as if he had originally written in the target language? Then there will be much he will not be able to say, much that is not native to the target culture and thus has no representation in its language. The translator is then faced with the choice between cutting those passages entirely (and thus undoing the power and form of the original whole) and putting something else in their place. Clearly, then, the blanket application of this formula to translations leads either to mere imitation or to an even more strikingly offensive and bewildering hodgepodge of translation and imitation that tosses the reader mercilessly to and fro like a ball, between his world and the foreign one, between the author's and the translator's invention and wit. Nor is there any pure pleasure for him in all that, only exhaustion and a spinning head.
>
> (237)

Here the ideal unmediated hermeneutic between author and reader is ravaged by the translator's mediation: somehow the fact that the translator stands between the source author and the target reader turns the readerly phenomenology of an immediate connection with the author into a nightmare. If Schleiermacher, a German, reads Plato in Greek, his task is to achieve a feeling of hermeneutical oneness with the author; if in translating Plato into German he were to attempt to simulate that feeling of oneness with the author for and in the target reader, he would inevitably "toss[ ] the reader mercilessly to and fro like a ball," creating "only exhaustion and a spinning head."

He doesn't attempt to justify this disturbing imagery, or the apparent divergence it tracks from his hermeneutical model; it would appear not to have occurred to him that anyone might doubt the plausibility of the supposed nightmarish effects of any effort to simulate in the target reader the feeling of hermeneutical oneness with the source author, and thus that he might need to justify it. In Chapter 3 of *Schleiermacher's Icoses* (Robinson 2013c) I speculated on his unstated rationale behind this switch (patriotism, moralism, and mysticism); rather than delving into those reasons again here, let us instead simply register that Schleiermacher is sketching a *hermeneutic of distance,* a strategic hermeneutical disruption of that feeling of oneness with the author that he otherwise posited as the basic enabling condition of interpretation, and explore the medical humanities, the social neuroscience, of that hermeneutic.

Certainly we are aware that a feeling of oneness is not only not possible with everyone we meet – it is not even desirable. Managing social distance hermeneutically is essential for social flexibility and full interactive functionality. Automatic and universal empathy would create an affective cacophony that would be overwhelming in effect. In *Estrangement and the Somatics of Literature* (Robinson 2008) I theorize what I call the "homeostatic regulation of reality" in terms of a homeostatic "titration" of strangeness and familiarity, to explain the odd fact that "both alienation/*otchuzhdenie* and estrangement/*ostranenie* have come to mean opposite things: a passive, pathological isolation from communal feeling and meaning and an active, transformative hypermimesis of that feeling of isolation for the therapeutic purpose of communal reintegration" (97). The artistic purpose of those hypermimetic strategies is specifically "to render things more alien and strange in order to push audiences to break out of their alienated and estranged state" (97) – but that attempt may well backfire, leading to *too much* alienation and estrangement, indeed to depersonalization:

> If your idea is to dealienate audiences by infecting them with a homeopathic or hypermimetic dose of alienation, it is crucial, obviously, to titrate your dosage just right, or you *will* alienate them further; but given the complexity of the somatics of literary response, such precise regulation of estranging dosages is impossible. What is just right for some readers or viewers will alienate others; what is just right for those ideal readers or viewers today may alienate them tomorrow.
>
> (97, emphasis in original)

The medical references there are not metaphors: as medical humanities scholars have long insisted, art can and does serve therapeutic purposes, and those therapies can easily backfire. Like all treatments, art-as-therapy works by trial and error – precisely because people are different, and therapeutic treatments therefore work dialogically, in interaction between therapist and patient.

I conclude:

> What this model points to, in fact, is a kind of somatic homeostatic regulation of our sense of reality. When we feel somatically integrated with the community, when we feel other people's regulatory feelings, we feel connected to reality, grounded in collectively defined reality; but that groundedness can become overfamiliar, anesthetic, numbingly conventionalized, and the resulting depletion of felt connection with collective reality can depersonalize us, flip us over into numb depersonalization. This is the state [Viktor] Shklovsky [1893–1984] seeks to cure by adding strangeness to the mix: if, when life becomes overly conventionalized and we begin to feel numb, a poem can add a little strangeness to the mix, we may be able to reconnect with the sensation of life being lived and resist the pull of depersonalization.

> When on the other hand we feel both somatically integrated with the community and pleasantly different, with an enjoyable sense of the strange, the odd, the dissonant, the off, we feel grounded in a slightly more idiosyncratic but nevertheless collective realty; but that groundedness can become overstrange, nightmarishly surreal, and the resulting depletion of felt connection with individualized collective reality can flip us over into disturbing or disorienting depersonalization.
>
> (99–100)

This theme of estrangement as a channel of artistic revitalization is a very old one; in tracking Viktor Shklovsky's study of estrangement in Leo Tolstoy, Carlo Ginzburg (1996) traces the prehistory of the theme back to Marcus Aurelius (121–180 CE), one of Tolstoy's favorite writers. But estrangement did not become a prominent rallying cry for an entire literary movement until the German and English Romantics in the early nineteenth century; we find it in Coleridge, Wordsworth, and Shelley, in Novalis and Friedrich Schlegel (see Robinson 2008, 79–81, for discussion).

In German Romantic translation theory, by contrast, the focus is not so much on the transformative power of the *strange* as it is on the transformative power of the *foreign* – for obvious reasons, since translators are by definition engaged in the business of domesticating foreign texts, and are therefore professionally exercised by *just how much* to domesticate, how to titrate the dosage of the foreign and the familiar. (Significantly, however, as we'll see, the same German adjective, *fremd,* means "strange," "alien," and "foreign.")

In his Academy address Schleiermacher famously analogizes three titrations of foreignness and familiarity on four different levels: [a] foreign-language learning, [b] reading foreign literary texts, [c] writing original literary texts, and [d] translating literary texts. By "titrations" I mean mixtures between what he calls "das Gefühl des fremden" (which I propose to translate initially here as "the Feeling of the Alien" – the most extreme form of *das fremde*) and what I want to call, building a parallel construction out of his own word "geläufig"/"familiar," in "das Gefühl des geläufigen"/"the Feeling of the Familiar." Something like this (holding off on (d) translation for the nonce):

1 *High Feeling of the Alien, Low Feeling of the Familiar:* the beginning foreign-language learner, who "sich noch mühsam und fast ekelhaft durch das einzelne hindurchstümpert, und deshalb noch nirgend zu einem klaren Ueberschauen des Ganzen, zu einem lebendigen Festhalten des Zusammenhanges gedeiht" (Schleiermacher 1813/2002, 76)/"blunders through the details of a text with great labor and loathing, never succeeding in rising above individual words and phrase to a clear view of the whole, never gaining a vivid sense of its cohesiveness" (Robinson 1997/2002, 230). This type of (1a) foreign-language learner cannot (1b) read foreign literature in the original, and it is so obvious that s/he cannot (1c) write original literary works in the foreign language either that Schleiermacher doesn't even bother to mention it.

2 *Medium Feeling of the Alien, Medium Feeling of the Familiar:* the educated person "dem die fremde Sprache geläufig ist, aber doch immer fremde bleibt, der nicht mehr wie die Schüler sich erst das einzelne wieder in der Muttersprache denken muß, ehe er das Ganze fassen kann, der aber doch auch da wo er am ungestörtesten sich der Schönheiten eines Werkes erfreut, sich immer der Verschiedenheit der Sprache von seiner Muttersprache bewußt bleibt" (78)/"for whom the foreign language is familiar but forever foreign, who needs no longer, like beginning students of the language, translate every word and phrase into his native language before gaining a sense of the whole, but who remains constantly aware, even in its most tranquil enjoyment of its beauties, of its differences from his own native language" (231). This person is actually no longer (2a) a foreign-language *learner,* or at least is not a novice: s/he has learned the foreign language well enough to "run" in it (the root of *geläufig* is *laufen*/"to run"), to get by well enough. S/he (2b) reads literature in the foreign tongue well enough, but never with an experience of immersion – the Feeling of the Alien lingers just insistently enough to maintain a certain detachment – and could never (2c) write original works in it.

3 *Low Feeling of the Alien, High Feeling of the Familiar:* polyglots who learn foreign languages so easily and so fluently that they hardly even notice what language they're speaking, "die solche eigenthümliche Verwandtschaft fühlen zu einem fremden Dasein, daß sie sich in eine fremde Sprache und deren Erzeugnisse ganz hinein leben und denken, und indem sie sich ganz mit einer ausländischen Welt beschäftigen, sich die heimische Welt und heimische Sprache ganz fremd werden lassen" (76)/"who feel so singularly drawn and akin to a foreign culture that they have utterly given themselves over to living and thinking in its language and its texts; and who, at least while caught up body and soul in that foreign world, allow their native language and whole native world to become alien" (230). These "freaks of nature" (as Schleiermacher characterizes them) are no longer (3a) learning the foreign language, except in the sense that we are always learning our native tongues; they (3b) not only read literary texts in the foreign language easily but (3c) may even be able to write original works in it.

Schleiermacher's ideal is (2) – the middle ground – but specifically in the sense that his ideal translation (2d) is one that *mimics* (2b): creates for and in the target reader a mimetic approximation of that medium Feeling of the Alien and medium Feeling of the Familiar felt by educated readers who, no matter how fluently or familiarly they can "run" in the foreign literary text *(wie geläufig sie eine fremde Sprache auch lesen),* in reading it always feel the Feeling of the Foreign *(behalten doch immer dabei das Gefühl des fremden).* The task of the "true" translator, for Schleiermacher, is to "simulate" *(nachzuahmen)* that feeling in, or "transplant" *(fortzupflanzen)* that feeling into, the target reader of the translation – the reader who is reading in his or her native language *as if* it were a foreign one.

The burden of that previous paragraph has been the launching pad for the more recent work of two well-known translation scholars, Antoine Berman (1984; see also Heyvaert 1992) in French and Lawrence Venuti (1995, 1998, etc.) in English. Each adds his own political and ethical spin to Schleiermacher's basic model; that doesn't concern me here.[2] What does concern me is this hermeneutic of distance or disruption that Schleiermacher calls *das Gefühl des fremden:* what it is; where it comes from; how it is maintained; what happens when we translate *das fremde* not as "the Foreign" but as "the Alien" or "the Strange"; how it is differentiated from the Feeling of the Familiar; how those differentiations are fractalized, and so on.

Some basic considerations as a backbone for this essay:

1 A Feeling of the Foreign *(ein Gefühl des fremden)* can often veer suddenly and surprisingly into [a] a Feeling of the Strange *(ein Gefühl des fremden)* or [b] a Feeling of the Alien *(ein Gefühl des fremden)*. The fact that German uses the same adjective – *fremd* – for "foreign," "strange," and "alien" is not surprising, since foreign things are usually (even normatively) experienced as strange and alien; but once one begins familiarizing oneself with the Foreign, it remains endlessly fascinating that a residual Feeling of the Foreign not only can blend and even make common cause with an emergent Feeling of the Familiar (this being the mixture Schleiermacher identified as his ideal) but will sometimes devolve into complete, baffling incomprehension, a feeling of no connection at all (a Feeling of the Alien), or into an intriguing or disturbing feeling of twistedness, oddity (a Feeling of the Strange).
2 A conscious Feeling of the Foreign-and-Alien can be undergirded by an *embodied* Feeling of the Familiar.
3 These feelings are more "social" than "psychological" – more collective than individual. To put that differently, they arise out of our relationships with the people with whom we use the languages more than out of "us ourselves" or the "languages themselves" (whatever either of those might mean). This is the socioaffective aspect of language learning, and of human communication at large. Specifically, this is the *socioaffective ecology* of human communication that I call "icosis," or group plausibilization as becoming-true or becoming-real.
4 The feelings are also often *pressurized* by other people, often for reasons of group loyalty. I call these pressures *affect-becoming-conation*. This is the socioaffective ecology of human communication that I call "ecosis," the becoming-good of the community that is also the becoming-communal of the good (see Robinson 2016a for discussion).

Let's consider those one at a time, dividing (1) into (1a) the Feeling of the Strange and (1b) the Feeling of the Alien – and considering in each case what the consequences might be for the study and act of translation.

3.3.1 The distortion of familiarity: the Feeling of the Strange

As I have noted in other works, there is a striking isomorphism between Romantic theories of foreignization, especially as formulated by Friedrich Schleiermacher and his followers, and Romantic/modernist theories of estrangement, especially as formulated by Viktor Shklovsky (1925/1983) and his followers.

Translation and the Problem of Sway: In Chapter 4 of Robinson (2011), I noted that the Feeling of the Foreign is a phenomenology "that tends to wane with time" (113), and has to be revivified through new estrangements:

> A "foreignized" text may feel foreign at first, but with time it may (and in fact will typically) come to seem more and more familiar, until its "foreignism" or "foreignization," to the extent that it is remembered or noticed at all, comes to feel like a structural *trace* or *vestige* of the original phenomenology of foreignness or strangeness. Any structuralist or poststructuralist attempt to theorize foreignism in stable ways, then, without taking this "phenomenological fade" into account – and I suggest that this is very much the mode in which Venuti discusses foreignism – will tend to focus on those abstract structural traces and bracket the actual historicity of the feeling-foreign.
>
> (114, emphasis in original)

Then, drawing on David Bohm's notion of "the proprioception of the body politic," I explored the possibility that the "foreignness" of a translation is mobilized and managed through a collectivized proprioception, a sociosomatic regulation of the Feeling of the Familiar/Foreign/Strange. From there I moved into a discussion of Viktor Shklovsky's (1925/1983) theorization of «остранение»/"ostranenie"/"estrangement," with special attention to the model he borrowed from Broder Christiansen (1909, 118–19), based on tiny felt deviations from what Christiansen calls the "geltender Kanon"/"canon in force" in a language, which I would here call the Feeling of the Familiar. Those felt deviations, or what Christiansen calls those "Differenzimpressionen"/"differential impressions," summon forth the Feeling of the Strange, which as Shklovsky insists increases the «трудность и долготу восприятия»/"trudnost' i dolgotu vospriyatiya"/"laboriousness and duration of perception," so as to «дать ощущение вещи, как видение, а не как узнавание»/"dat' oshhushheniye veshhi, kak videniye, a ne kak uznavaniye"/"give us the sensation of a thing as seeing rather than as recognizing." This complex he calls the «прием „остранения" вещей»/"priyom 'ostraneniya' veshhey"/"device of the 'estrangement' of things" (Russian text Shklovsky 1925/1983, 12; English translation Robinson 2011, 123). In that sense, I concluded, a foreignizing translation would entail "some sort of strategic deviation from what readers will feel as 'canonical' target-cultural conventions, so that the translation *feels* new and dissonant and strange" (129).

Schleiermacher's Icoses: In Chapter 4 of Robinson (2013c) I explore Schleiermacher's own theory of the Feeling of the Foreign in four steps: (section 4.2) "the power of *conventionalization* to numb our perceptions"; (section 4.3) "the importance of giving the reader a *feeling of an impediment* to perception, so as to goad him or her to shake off the sleep of convention"; (section 4.4) "the importance of reminding the target reader that what s/he is reading is a translation, and so *denaturalizing* the illusion of non-translation"; and (section 4.5) "the possibility that Brecht's estrangement effect on stage might offer a different and more viable way of thinking Schleiermacher on foreignization than the analogical literalism discussed in Chapter 2" (197). My method is to map Shklovsky's argument in «Искусство как прием»/"Iskusstvo kak priyom"/"Art as Device" onto Schleiermacher's argument in "Ueber die verschiedenen Methoden des Uebersezens"/"On the Different Methods of Translating," quoting and discussing the specific passages where Schleiermacher implicitly invokes something like the Romantic theory of estrangement, in order to highlight argumentative possibilities that Schleiermacher himself adumbrated but failed to stress – missed opportunities, in other words. I show, for example, how Schleiermacher fails to "articulate a rationale for leaving the 'Spuren der Mühe'/'traces of labor' in the target text" – what Shklovsky calls the «затруднение»/"zatrudnenie"/"belaboring" (making-laborious) of the perceptual process, which he also identifies as a «заторможение»/"zatormozheniye"/"impeding" of that process.

> The connection between the Traces of Labor [and the "Intuition of an Impediment"] and the Feeling of the Foreign for Schleiermacher is that the translator, like the ideal source reader whose response to the source text he advises the translator to simulate for the target reader, *just is* a foreigner to the source text, and therefore *just does* read it with effort. Schleiermacher doesn't even advise the translator to leave traces of that effort there; he just says that the target text *just is* 'aufgedrückt'/'imprinted' with them. He implies that this is a desirable eventuality, but doesn't even spell that much out, let alone indicating *why* it is desirable.
>
> (214–15, emphasis in original)

Shklovsky, by contrast, has worked it all out; and in his version of Shklovsky's theory for the epic theater, Bertolt Brecht politicizes it, which one might have thought would have been perfect for Venuti's Marxist theorizations.

I conclude:

> In this light, perhaps the most generous (though not necessarily the most Schleiermacherian) way to think the distinction between domesticating and foreignizing translation would be through twentieth-century acting styles: domestication as pretending that the source author originally wrote in the target language as Stanislavskian Method Acting, aimed at convincing the "theatergoer" (target reader) that the action on stage is *really happening in the real world;* foreignization as pretending that the target reader is reading the source text as Brechtian epic theater, aimed at *breaking the theatergoer's illusion of reality* through "estranging" or "distancing" ("quoting" or "third-person") acting styles. To put that differently, Schleiermacher's case in this dramatistic frame would be not that domesticating translation is bad because unrealistic/illusory and that foreignizing translation is equally unrealistic/ illusory but nevertheless good, but that domesticating translation is bad

> because it encourages unthinking *immersion* in the illusion, and foreignizing translation is good because it exposes and denaturalizes the illusion. This is a far subtler distinction than Schleiermacher himself was able to make, because he hadn't lived through the modernist articulation of Romantic aesthetics, and so had no access to Shklovsky or (especially) Brecht.
>
> (233–34, emphasis in original)

Critical Translation Studies: In the first series of Critical Theses in Robinson (2017a) I draw on Sakai's (1997) theory of the regime of homolingual address, "a regime in which each language is ideally isolated from every other, with the speakers of each able to communicate easily and freely, and indeed automatically, with each other, and utterly unable to communicate with the 'foreigners' that have been relegated in advance to other isolated languages" (CT 1.10). That idealized conception of communication – which Sakai builds out of Jean-Luc Nancy's (1986/2004; Connor 1991) Heideggerean ruminations on the mythologization of community as "communion" – at once definitively *forecloses* and *depends* on translation for its proper functioning. Obviously the only way any given homolingual regime could ever communicate with another would be through translation, but the model excludes in advance the very possibility of anyone ever being able to mediate between homolingual regimes. Such mediation relies, Sakai underscores, on what he calls "heterolingual address" – the real-world phenomenology in which we all constantly translate thoughts into words and words into interpretations, in which we are all foreigners to each other and therefore translators of each other's words – but in order to recover that germ of heterolinguality for the regime of homolingual address one must "erase" the translator's mediation from awareness, which is to say, one must instrumentalize and invisibilize the translator. And I conclude:

> The idea remains in the "homolingual" representation of translation that the written or spoken text can be understood by its audience because it is *essentially* homolingual – because the "foreign" author somehow magically wrote or spoke it in the "local" language of its (monolingual) audience. I suggest, in fact, that this is the theoretical critique of "bringing the author to the reader" toward which Friedrich Schleiermacher was so haplessly groping in his 1813 address to the Academy, and that his followers among the foreignizers have so far been unable to formulate more effectively for him: "The assumption that one can make oneself understood without perceptible hindrance, as long as one belongs in the same linguistic community, survives intact here" (ibid.: 10). (See Robinson 2013c: ch. 2 for analysis of the "haplessness."). The difference between domestication and foreignization for Schleiermacher and his many followers should have been – as Sakai would see it – not that the former takes the author to the reader and the latter takes the reader to the author, and not that the former is immoral and unpatriotic and the latter is the only "true" form of translation (as Schleiermacher insists), and not that the former makes the target culture complicit with capitalism

> and the latter makes the target culture dissident (as Venuti insists), but that the former is conditioned by the regime of the homolingual address and the latter is an embrace of the attitude of the heterolingual address.
>
> (11, emphasis in original)

What I notice about all that, however, rereading and summarizing those discussions now, is that in them the Feeling of the Foreign, the Feeling of the Strange, and the Feeling of the Alien all tend to blur together into a single smeary Feeling of the Unfamiliar. But then, as I showed in Robinson (2008), the tradition has tended to blur them as well:

- the precursors to Brecht's *Verfremdung*, namely the *-fremdung* terms that run through the German Idealist/Romantic tradition (and its materialist inversion by Marx), include Novalis's "Befremdung"/"estrangement" and Hegel's and Marx's "Entfremdung"/"alienation";
- Shklovsky and his friends, after Russian Formalism was officially banned in the Soviet Union, began referring not to остранение/*ostranenie*/"estrangement" but to отчуждение/*otchuzhdenie*/"alienation"; and
- Lemon and Reis (1965) first translated Shklovsky's остранение/*ostranenie* as "defamiliarization," and Willett (1964) first translated Brecht's *Verfremdung* as "alienation," neither even hinting at the Feeling of the Strange.

Clearly there is historical warrant for treating foreignization, estrangement, and alienation as wrapped up in the same phenomenology of felt deviation from norms. And as I noted in both *Translation and the Problem of Sway* and *Schleiermacher's Icoses*, it is striking that not one of the three major foreignizers – Schleiermacher, Berman, or Venuti – has ever explored the connections between the Romantic theory of *das Gefühl des fremden*/"the Feeling of the Foreign" and the Romantic theory of *Befremdung/Entfremdung* and its modernist revisions as остранение/*ostranenie*/*Verfremdung*/"estrangement."

But now let us differentiate more thoughtfully among the different Feelings subsumed in German under the blanket term *das Gefühl des fremden*. Yes, there is a high degree of overlap among the Feelings of the Foreign, Alien, and Strange; yes, we like to think that it is "natural" for the foreign to feel alien and strange; yes, as I mentioned above, the convergence of alienation and estrangement with the Feeling of the Foreign is normative, specifically in what Sakai calls the regime of the homolingual address; and yes, even in Sakai's heterolingual address there is a sense in which we are all foreigners to each other, and precisely for that reason aliens and strangers to each other (and ourselves) as well. I think of the time my American high school German class was taking a ferry across Puget Sound to the Olympic Peninsula for a German-only weekend retreat: as we were walking around the ferry speaking German, two crew members sitting drinking coffee audibly cursed us as "goddamn foreigners." That is of course garden-variety heterolinguality heard through a normative homolingual ear, a normative clash between ideological regimes; but I submit that it is a normative clash raised to an absurd power, or to the power of absurdity. It's not just a clash: it's a meta-clash, a self-recursive/self-reflexive clash. Its absurdity derives from its power to engender a sudden disturbing *awareness* of the submerged clash between normative homolinguality (all Americans speak only English, therefore anyone who speaks non-English is a foreigner) and counternormative heterolinguality (we are all foreigners to each other).

A tentative formulation, then: the Feeling of the Foreign is the vague, inchoate sense we have that the regime of the homolingual address is an ideological illusion, that we actually communicate heterolingually; the Feeling of the Strange is the glorious irruption of the absurd in stray moments of *clarity* about that clash.

Or, to shift terms slightly: the reason that the purveyors of "foreignization" from Schleiermacher to Venuti have tended to mystify "the foreign," and have failed to engage with the Romantic/modernist tradition of estrangement, is that estrangement requires a conscious awareness of the slippage between norms and deviations, between conventions and innovations, between the old and the new – and the Feeling of the Foreign, akin as it is to the Feeling of the Strange, can't quite muster that level of self-aware absurdity.

So what consequences do these ruminations have for the study and activity of translation? Take a passage from Aleksis Kivi's brilliant 1870 Finnish novel *Seitsemän veljestä* (*Seven Brothers* – see Robinson 2017c for discussion), where a wolf has fallen into the Jukola brothers' wolf pit, and Timo – the dumbest of the brothers – goes to bang it on the head, but keeps missing, so he runs to get his brothers, forgetting to pull the ladder up out of the pit:

> Siitä, hetken päästä läksivät veljekset, varustettuna seipäillä, köysillä ja kuristimilla, saavuttamaan saalistansa. Mutta tyhjä oli kuoppa heidän ehdittyänsä esiin. Pitkin tikapuita, jotka Timo oli jättänyt jälkeensä kuoppaan, oli heidän sutensa koreasti astunut ylös ja vilkaisnut tiehensä, kiittäen onneansa.
>
> (1870/1984, 134)

Richard Impola (1991, 114) translated that in what Schleiermacher would call the author-to-reader mode, or what Sakai Naoki would call the regime of homolingual address, as if Kivi had originally written the novel in English:

> The brothers soon left the house, equipped with clubs, ropes, and nooses to catch their prey. But when they reached the pit, it was empty. The wolf had climbed neatly up the ladder left behind by Timo and scooted away, thanking its lucky stars.

In the first full published English translation of the novel, Alex Matson (1929/1962, 125) rendered the passage slightly more foreignizingly:

> The brothers soon emerged, furnished with staves, ropes, and nooses, to seize their prey. But when they reached the pit, it was empty. Along the ladder, which Timo had left behind him in the pit, their wolf had climbed to safety and swiftly departed, thanking his lucky stars.

Obviously Impola took a lot of Matson over unchanged; but "along the ladder" is a more literal translation of *pitkin tikapuita* than "up the ladder," and the subordinate clause "which Timo had left behind him in the pit" is an exact syntactic clone of Kivi's *jotka Timo oli jättänyt jälkeensä kuoppaan*. Ironically, Impola's "scooted away" is also a more literal translation of Kivi's *vilkaisnut tiehensä* (lit. "scampered/scurried into his road/path") than Matson's "swiftly departed"; and Matson's "climbed to safety" is a periphrastic unpacking of Kivi's *astunut ylös* (lit. "stepped up").

And we could continue that series, moving in an increasingly foreignizing direction, with a slightly more literal rendition like this:

> From thence, a moment later left the brothers, equipped with poles, ropes and chokers, to apprehend their prey. But empty was the pit when they hove into view. Along the ladder, which Timo had left behind him in the pit, had their wolf prettily stepped up and scurried away, thanking its luck.

That teems with the Feeling of the Foreign, don't you think? It's not quite literal; for example, I can't think of a strictly literal rendition of *ehdittyänsä esiin*, which Matson and Impola render as "reached the pit." *Esiin* is "into view," implying a wolf's-eye perspective on their arrival: the ground above the pit is like a stage on which the brothers make their appearance, like actors entering a scene. But *ehtiä* is "to have time, to arrive in time": *ehdittyänsä esiin* would be literally something like "having had time (to come) into view." The implication is that they're rushing to get to the pit in time to kill the wolf: there is a kind of deadline, which in fact they miss. When they get to the pit the wolf has already decamped. So they don't come in time, which makes the literal translation misleading. The Finnish verb is looser than its literal translation: it can mean just arriving in a rush, even if not in time.

The thing about that foreignizing translation, though, is that it is slightly awkward – deliberately so, of course. It is intended, in accordance with Schleiermacher's proposal to the Royal Academy, to give the target reader the Feeling of the Foreign, the feeling that s/he is reading the Finnish original with mediocre Finnish – with enough of a Feeling of the Familiar to understand the words, but without Impola's kind of easy casual familiarity that might encourage the target reader to gulp the text down without impediment. The subtle awkwardness impedes easy apprehension. For Schleiermacher that impediment serves nationalistic purposes, to remind the target reader that s/he is reading a *foreign* text, not an original local one.

The problem with all that, however, is not just that that sort of nationalism is difficult for us to appreciate these days, nor even just that there are better reasons to advocate for an impediment to easy understanding (denaturalization, etc.) than some kind of nationalistic purity fetish – the problems on which my critique mostly focused in *Schleiermacher's Icoses*. The big problem, it occurs to me now, is that it's not clear *how* the impediment serves the nationalistic purpose – or even, for that matter, the denaturalizing purpose. Precisely how does an awkwardly written text remind the target reader that it is a translation, rather than, say, an awkwardly written original? Why is the awkwardness experienced by a half-competent reader of a foreign text the best denaturalizing feeling for the translator to simulate?

These are questions that Berman and Venuti never ask either, about the Schleiermacherian translation strategy that they espouse. As a result, all three foreignizers mystify the method. All three argue vaguely for a strategy that they themselves don't quite grasp. Hence in fact my suggestion that Schleiermacher's Feeling of the Foreign is the *vague, inchoate* sense we have that the regime of homolingual address is an illusion unconsciously undergirded by heterolingual address, and that it takes the Feeling of the Strange, Novalis's *Befremdung,* Shklovsky's остранение/*ostranenie,* Brecht's *Verfremdung,* to open our eyes and ears to the imposture. We need to be aware of the absurdity – and Schleiermacher's Feeling of the Foreign, I'm suggesting, is powerless to give us that awareness. The semicompetent reader's prevailing experience of a foreign text – the experience that Schleiermacher's foreignizing translator is to simulate in the target language – is one of groping and grasping for *some* vague sense of the text. The most Schleiermacher expects such a reader to bring back from his or her encounter with the foreign text is that nagging discomfort that he calls the Feeling of the Foreign. It requires a far subtler sensitivity to the turbulences in the textual current to come back with a Feeling of the Strange.

Two things that the reader with only minimally competent Finnish might miss in Kivi's novel are his archaism and his playfulness – and especially the playfulness of his archaisms, the fact that he doesn't just use archaic Finnish but uses it for humorous effect. The result does often feel strange – so strange, in fact, that the most significant critical response to the novel early on was a series of vituperous attacks on it (two in Swedish while it was still in production, a third in Finnish after it had been released to a hundred-plus subscribers) by August Ahlqvist (1826–1889) for its indecency, its utter lack of realism, its "bad Finnish," and so on. Ahlqvist was not just the only professor of Finnish in what was then an autonomous Grand Duchy of Russia; he was also the acknowledged bastard son of the most powerful man in the Grand Duchy, Baron Johan Mauritz Nordenstam (1802–1882). Understandably, then, the committee behind its publication at the Finnish Literature Society, panicking at the intensity of this attack from such a powerful figure, withheld the novel from publication, pending further study – and Kivi, who had devoted ten years of his life to writing it, and knew that it was great, went crazy and died (in 1872, at the age of 38) before its eventual release to bookstores in 1873. Within a decade of his death Kivi was recognized as a great Finnish writer, but fear of Ahlqvist's retaliation checked public expressions of admiration for his novel until after Ahlqvist had died in 1889; support for it grew apace around the turn of the century, and by 1915 it had been canonized as the greatest work of Finnish literature – a status that it not only retains today, but, according to Finnish literature mavens, is unlikely ever to lose.

The novel, in short, gives off a Feeling of the Strange – but a playful, brilliant, disturbingly wonderful Feeling of the Strange. It was for Finns an acquired taste – one that has now been acquired and assimilated and canonized by the culture as a whole, but still has to be acquired by each new reader of the novel. As Finland's greatest novel it is regularly assigned to Finnish schoolchildren to read, and many of them hate it, because it's strange, and difficult to read (all those unfamiliar words!), and because to appreciate its humor you probably need to be an adult – indeed an adult with a certain twisted sense of humor, a love of the absurd, the grotesque, and the carnivalistic.

And so to translate that, you're going to simulate the response of someone who can't read the Finnish very well, and so squints at it through Coke-bottle lenses, making out only the blurriest outlines? This is an *intelligent* approach to a brilliantly difficult novel?

Here is what I do with that passage:

> In a trice birr'd the boys to the pit, arm'd to the teeth with their stangs and their ropes and their noose wands, to seize their spoils. But whenas they 'd hove into view of the pit, la, 'twas empty. Featly 'd debouch'd de loop up de stee delaps'd by de man in de pit and dash'd to freedom, thanking his loopy luck.
>
> (Robinson 2017d, 157)

The archaisms there are Shakespearean: to birr is to run fast, a stang is a pole, featly means nimbly or neatly, and a stee is a ladder. Kivi loved Shakespeare, read him (in Swedish translation) obsessively, and had memorized several whole plays – and, as one might expect, frequently used Shakespearean phrases and allusions in his own writing. This archaism in my translation is more intense than Kivi's own: my translation is in fact stranger than Kivi's original. (Is it a character flaw that I consider that a good thing?)

What I'm happiest about in that translation, though, is the running gag built around "de": "debouch'd de loop up de stee delaps'd by de man in de pit." Inspired by the Frenchy archaism "debouch'd" and the roller-coaster loop-de-loop, the series picks up on the French for wolf *(loup)*, which is then reprised in "loopy luck," and also along the way gestures gently toward Paul de Man. There is a punny Latinate line that I loved as a child, too, which probably worked on me as well: "Defeat of deduct went over defense before detail." The (uncomfortable?) fact, of course, is that there is no *textual* warrant for this gag in the Finnish line it renders. I made it up myself. I would like to claim that it was inspired not just by "debouch'd" and "loop-de-loop" and "defeat of deduct" but by Kivi's love of such running gags, but that may just be my projection. The inescapable fact is that it was inspired by the delight *I* take in the Feeling of the Strange I get while reading the novel in Finnish. (This is a big part of what I call translationality.)

But then what is the impact of my estranging translation on the target reader? That is not for me to say, of course; but I designed it to feel strange, humorously strange, and to channel that Feeling of the Strange into epistemological interrogations of homolinguality. It's not just the French loopiness or the Latinate deductivity that comes a-creepin' into that passage; it's also the slave dialect of Negro Spirituals:

Place one foot upon de dry land
Fare you well, fare you well
Place de other on de sea
Fare you well, fare you well
Den you'll see de coffin bustin'
Fare you well, fare you well
See de dry bones come a-creepin'
Fare you well, fare you well

Like the wolf, the enslaved African-Americans in the antebellum South imagine themselves "climbin' Jacob's ladder" – "every round goes higher and higher" – and escaping into freedom. But *what are those black slaves doing in a Finnish novel?* And *why are they playing with the French word for "wolf"?* It makes no sense at all. Yes, the novel is set in the 1840s, the time also of American slavery; and yes, Kivi's seven brothers are illiterate farmers whose social status is not much higher than slaves. But they are free – Finland never had any form of slavery or serfdom – and even if they weren't, there is a significant cultural gap and difference between 1840s conditions in the American South and the Finnish South. Even "the South" means very different things in the two lands – though August Ahlqvist, who came from Eastern Finland, sneered of the southern dialect stylized in the novel that Kivi "oli syntynyt milt'ei huonoimpaan murteeseen, mitä Suomen kielen alalla on" (176)/"was born into what must be nearly the worst dialect in the entire scope of the Finnish language," an attitude that many New England Brahmins would also have held even about Southern white aristocratic English in those days, and *a fortiori* about slave dialect.

In other words, the clash of cultures in my translation is designed not to reveal some deeper objective *truth* about Finns or Americans, peasants or slaves, but simply or complexly to perform/elicit the Feeling of the Strange. Why? Because I take that to be Kivi's project in the novel: not just to portray Finnish peasants of his parents' generation with some kind of ethnographic realism, but to *estrange* that ethnographic scene, and to estrange it playfully. There was a concerted attempt, especially as realism took hold in Finnish literature in the waning decades of the nineteenth century, to defend the realism of Kivi's novel against Ahlqvist's attacks; I would suggest that one way of understanding Kivi's realism is that it is an *estranging heterolingual* realism, a realism that estranges in part by building heterolinguality into the emerging national literature of Finland, and so, to paraphrase Deleuze and Guattari (1975; Polan 1986) on Kafka, to minoritize its future majority.

3.3.3 The loss of familiarity: the Feeling of the Alien

Schleiermacher's Feeling of the Foreign, you'll recall, is basically a medium titration of the Feeling of the Familiar and the Feeling of the Alien; but what happens when the Feeling of the Familiar is suddenly vaporized out of the dosage? This is not a possibility Schleiermacher ponders: the Feeling of the Alien for him (though that is not his phrase for it) is experienced only by schoolboys who are forced to learn a foreign language and hate every moment of it, because nothing makes sense to them. What happens when the phenomenological sedimentation of many years of experience and training in a language seems to dissipate into the air, leaving nothing behind? What happens when one expects the Feeling of the Familiar, or even the Feeling of the Foreign, and gets instead the Feeling of the Alien?

I think for example of the times in my life when non-Finns, hearing that I speak Finnish, ask me to "say something in Finnish" – and I go blank. Nothing comes. What I have felt in those moments is panic: where did it go, that proficiency in Finnish that has stood me in such good stead since I first began to feel at home in Finnish, at age 17? That experience reminds me of the opening of Otto Friedrich's book *Going Crazy,* where he remembers walking to work through Times Square in the early seventies, when he was working at *Time* magazine, and "going crazy":

> Then, as I was about to cross 45th Street, the strange thing happened: I couldn't figure out how to cross the street. I stood there at the curb in a state of bewilderment, unable at first even to realize what it was that I couldn't figure out. I carefully told myself that it would be all right to cross the street whenever the traffic stopped, but as I watched the trucks and taxis flowing south along Broadway, I couldn't determine which part of the traffic was supposed to stop, or which street I was trying to cross. Then I thought, as one always does at moments of crisis, "This can't be happening." Then I felt a touch, just a touch, of fear – panic. Even while I kept reassuring myself that this couldn't be happening, I also saw myself standing utterly helpless in the middle of Times Square – intellectually incapable of finding out how to cross the street, but repeatedly warning myself that if I made a mistake, the oncoming traffic would kill me.
>
> (3–4)

What I have typically done whenever that Feeling of the (Finnish) Alien has come over me is to ask my interlocutor to say something in English for me to translate into Finnish. That always works. Then some translation automatism kicks in, and the Feeling of the Familiar spurts forth into an easy Finnish equivalent. Like Friedrich in this next passage, I then realize that the problem is one of context: it's not that I can't speak Finnish, but that I have nothing to say, and no speech context to say it in. If I have to satisfy an abstract request like "say something in Finnish" – Friedrich's counterpart might be something like "explain what it means to cross a street" – I need a prompt, a kick-start. As Friedrich continues:

> The scene lasted no more than ten seconds, perhaps only five, perhaps only one or a fraction of one. Then something clicked, some gear shifted, and I realized what had happened. It was my custom, daydreaming, only half awake, to walk to the office as though on automatic pilot. That is, I didn't really pay much attention to where I was going but somnambulistically

> crossed streets whenever some half-functioning message system told me that the light was green. What had happened on 45th Street was that the traffic light had broken, so my automatic system didn't work, and it took me a moment or two to realize it.
>
> (4)

When I'm in conversation with Finns, especially in Finland, my "automatic system" generates plenty of things to "say in Finnish"; when the context that activates that automatic system is absent or fractured in some way, it takes me too "a moment or two to realize it," and correct for it, by asking for a source text that I can translate.

What's interesting about Friedrich's example, though, is that he spins it as "going crazy" – as the opening anecdote for his book by that title:

> During that moment or two, I think, I was standing on the border of what we call insanity. The main symptoms were all there: a breakdown in the machinery of perception, or a breakdown in the rational mind's ability to receive and combine perceptions and to make judgments from them. And a sense of helplessness, together with a perfectly clear vision of one's own helplessness. And panic. It was, in retrospect, like experiencing some sort of time warp, like catching a glimpse of another century or another civilization. Yet that world where the mad live is not so remote. Most of us come near it at one time or another, sometimes only for a moment, sometimes for days or even for months. "In all of us," Herman Melville once wrote, "lodges the same fuel to light the same fire. And he who has never felt, momentarily, what madness is, has but a mouthful of brains." We have felt it, if nowhere else, in the chaotic world that we inhabit in our dreams, that world of half-forgotten messages and half-remembered images. There, night after night, we all go mad.
>
> (4)

Okay, fine: but now, again, what practical or theoretical significance does any of this have for translation? Theoretically it seems to me useful to have a phenomenological boundary or limit for the Feeling of the Familiar that we would normally take to be a *sine qua non* for the very possibility of translation. If there is nothing familiar about a text, how can it possibly be translated? But obviously "*nothing* familiar" is an extreme binary pole that gives us little sense of the excluded middle. So let us ask instead: *how much* unfamiliarity can we tolerate and still manage to translate a text? To someone accustomed to translating texts written clearly and coherently in ordinary language, the threshold to untranslatability may be quite low; someone accustomed to translating modern or postmodern poetry may have far more tolerance for disruptions in the flow of conventionalized meaning-making. But is there a *theoretical* limit to that tolerance?

Viktor Shklovsky took most of his examples of literary estrangement from Tolstoy, but it has often been noted in the literature that the Russian writers closest to him, who indeed had a far greater impact on his thinking than Tolstoy, were the Russian Futurists, like Велимир Хлебников (Velimir Khlebnikov, 1885–1922) and Алексей Елисеевич Крученых (Aleksey Eliseyevich Kruchyonykh,[3] 1886–1968), whose transrational заумь/*zaum'*/"beyond reason" poetry deliberately pushed on the furthermost boundaries of meaning. Here, for example, is an early (and famous) poem by Kruchyonykh from 1913, quoted in Harte (2009, 80):

Дыр бул щыл
Убешщур

скум
вы со бу
р л эз

Or, romanized:

Dyr bul shhyl
Ubeshshhur

skum
vy so bu
r l ez

This is what is commonly known as "nonsense" poetry – here reframed as "transrational" poetry. As Tim Harte comments:

> Transrational poetry, "Dyr bul shchyl" suggests, constituted a bold statement of contemporaneity, despite all its primordial, grunt like sounds. As Kruchenykh explained in "New Ways of the Word (the language of the future, death to Symbolism)" ("Novye puti slova [iazyk budushchego smert' simvolizmu]"), one of the major theoretical discussions of *zaum'*, "We loosened up grammar and syntax; we recognised that in order to depict our dizzy contemporary life and the even more impetuous future, we must combine words in a new way, and the more disorder we introduce into the sentence structure the better." Non-grammatical word constructions and their indeterminacy of meaning indeed fostered a lexical simulation of modernity's "dizzying contemporary life" and its alteration of visual reality. *Zaum'*, it could therefore be argued, introduced linguistic "disorder" into poetry in a manner comparable to the way speed distorts our surroundings to the point of non objectivity. In fact, Kruchenykh went on to explain in "New Ways of the Word" how "the irregular structuring of a sentence (in terms of logic and word formation) generates *movement and a new perception of the world* and conversely, that movement and psychological variation generate strange 'nonsensical' combinations of words and letters." For Kruchenykh, movement, a new abstract "perception of the world," and "nonsensical" transrational word creations had merged, as his irregular verse gave rise to an abstract impression of speed, and vice versa. Constituting a non-representational

> form of verse, *zaum'* altered phenomenal reality and anticipated, in Kruchenykh's words, the "impetuous future."
>
> (Harte 2009, 81, emphasis in original)

One slight clarification there: when Harte writes that "transrational poetry, 'Dyr bul shchyl' suggests, constituted a bold statement of contemporaneity, despite all its primordial, grunt like sounds," that "despite" would appear to be predicated on his association of the poem's "grunt like sounds" with primordiality, which is to say the distant past. Despite the poem's aural evocation of prehistoric experience, it is a commentary on contemporaneity. That seems to me a problematic temporal prejudice: the narrow-minded assumption that "grunting" is something only our distant ancestors, perhaps even our prehuman ancestors did, and we don't do. As I read Harte's account, however, that prejudice is actually not his: he is anticipating and tacitly correcting *readers'* prejudices, in order to second Kruchyonykh's insistence on this version of contemporaneity, in which our Enlightenment ideal of the imposition of rational order on reality is increasingly fatally disrupted.

We should not, I suggest, have far to look for the practical implications of the disruptive irruption of the Feeling of the Alien in the midst of expected familiarity: I would argue that both the "domesticators" and the "foreignizers" would consider Kruchyonykh's poem untranslatable – or, perhaps, more moderately, *not in need* of translation. It doesn't have enough coherent rational "meaning" to lend itself to domesticated translation, and it doesn't generate a sufficient Feeling of the Familiar to make foreignization – the simulation of a Feeling of the Foreign – possible. And in any case if it was written as nonsense in Russian, it is equally nonsensical in English, so all we need to do is romanize it.

But the poem is not just "nonsense *in* Russian"; it is Russian nonsense. It is nonsense that, to the extent that it gives the impression of hovering just beyond the reach of rational sense, hovers beyond the reach of *Russian* rational sense. The Feeling of the Alien that it invokes, in other words, stands in a transgressive relation to a culturally specific Feeling of the Familiar. The rational sense that it seeks to transgress is not universal. It invokes a Feeling of the *Russian* Alien: a Feeling of the Almost-Familiar to Russians; a Feeling of the Slightly-Less-Familiar/Slightly-More-Alien to non-Russians like me with some knowledge of Russian.

Дыр/*Dyr*, for example, is almost but not quite a дыра/дырка//*dyra/dyrka*//"hole." Бул/*bul* is almost but not quite a булка/*bulka*/"bun" or "small white loaf of bread." Щыл/*shhyl* is almost but not quite a щи/*shhi*/"cabbage soup" that has been oddly inflected with the verbal past tense ending -л/-l. Убешщур/*Ubeshshhur* seems to be stitched together from убежать/*ubezhat'*/"to run away," бешенный/*beshennyi*/"rabid," and щуриться/*shhurit'sya*/"squint": a rabid dog that ran away squinting? Скум/*skum* looks more like English scum than any Russian word, but would be pronounced *skoom*. С/*s* is "with" and кум/*kum* is "godfather," so that с кумом/*s kumom* would be "with godfather"; and a mackerel is скумбрия/*skumbriya* (also called scomber in English). Вы/*vy* is actually an existing Russian word, the polite/plural form of "you." Со/*so* looks in Cyrillic script like roman "co," and is actually used the same way, as a sight-borrowing from Latin: a соавтор/*soavtor* is a coauthor. Бу/*bu* is the beginning of several hundred Russian words, including quite a few borrowed from the same foreign terms as their English equivalents (and some even from English), such as бубон/*bubon*/"bubo" and бубонный/*bubonnyi*/"bubonic," буддизм/*buddizm*/"Buddhism," будка/*budka*/"booth," будуар/*buduar*/"boudoir," буёк/*buyok*/"buoy," буза/*buza*/"bouza," буйвол/*buyvol*/"buffalo," бук/*buk*/"beech," бука/*buka*/"boogeyman," букет/*buket*/"bouquet," буколика/*bukolika*/"bucolic literature," булла/*bulla*/"Papal bull," булинь/*bulin'*/"bowline," бульвар/*bul'var*/"boulevard," бульдог/*bul'dog*/"bulldog," бульдозер/*bul'dozer*/"bulldozer," бульон/*bul'on*/"bouillon," бум/*bum*/"boom," бумеранг/*bumerang*/"boomerang," бункер/*bunker*/"bunker," бур/*bur*/"Boer," бура/*bura*/"borax," буравить/*buravit'*/"to bore/drill," бургомистр/*burgomistr*/"burgomaster," бургундское/*burgundskoe*/"burgundy," буржуа/*burzhua*/"bourgeois," бутил/*butyl*/"butyl," бутоньерка/*buton'erka*/"boutonnière," бутылка/*butylka*/"bottle," буфер/*buffer*/"buffer," буфет/*buffet*/"buffet," буфф/*buff*/"buffo," and буффон/*buffon*/"buffoon."

That partial list of Russian бу-words alone contains thirty-five shared loanwords; is that enough to make "bu" a good nonsense translation of бу? Well, no, because *boo* means things in English (what a ghost or girlfriend says) that no бу-word in Russian even hints at; and the shared loanwords make up only a small portion of the бу-words in Russian, most of which are Slavic in origin. In fact in Russian бу!/*bu*! on its own is a colloquial interjection indicating unhappiness with what's going on. ("Не бубукай!"/"ne bubukay"/"don't bu," as my wife might say, in the sense of "stop whining." Бубунить/*bubunit'* is a similar verb, meaning to drone on and on in a monotonous mumble, the implication being that mumbling on and on about boring things is like saying бу, бу, бу/bu, bu, bu – or hearing that in someone else's mumbling.) But perhaps running "vy so bu" on a line between "skum" and "r l ez" vitiates those objections? Perhaps. But perhaps even then "skum/vy so bu" also looks in English as if it could be read as "(you) scum, why so boo?" in a Russian accent.

That impulse to *make* nonsense make sense reminds us that "nonsense" is not a thing in itself, not a stable absence of sense: it is an audience effect, a phenomenology. Or, to put it in the terms I'm adapting from Schleiermacher, it's not an alienness or an alienation but a *Feeling* of the Alien. When I feel I can't say anything in Finnish or Otto Friedrich feels he can't cross 45th Street at Broadway, that emphatically does not mean that we lack the ability to do those things; it means rather that we feel temporarily *alienated* from that ability. And just as for Schleiermacher foreignizing translation involves simulating the *Feeling* of the Foreign felt by an educated reader reading a foreign text in a language s/he doesn't know particularly well, so too, I suggest, might "alienating translation" involve simulating the Feeling of the Alien felt by a competent speaker/reader of the source language who suddenly, mysteriously, loses that expected Feeling of the Familiar.

So what might an alienating translation of "Дыр бул щыл"/"Dyr bul shhyl" look like? The simplest and most conventional way to create one, it seems to me, would be to apply a Modified Nida (dive down from source-textual surface structure to deep structure, then resurface in the target language):

Hol bre sou
Erabruns

mack
ye so bu
r l ez

There "hol" is the beginning of "hole," "bre" is the beginning of "bread," "sou" is the beginning of "soup," "Erabruns" runs an Updikean "rabid run" together and tacks on a Latin "e-" prefix to signify "out or away" and an "-s" suffix to hint at "squint," "mack" is the beginning of mackerel, "ye" is the archaic plural "you," and "so" on (boo). But that's not only kind of boring; it seems to me to tame the process out of the realm of the Feeling of the Alien. No, that's not quite right: the Feeling of the Alien is not a realm, doesn't have boundaries, doesn't have an inside and an outside. What I suppose I mean is actually that I don't just want the *product* of my translational work to have an alienating effect on the target reader; I want the translation *process* to feel alienating, to give me, as the translator, the Feeling of the Alien. And that Modified Nida just doesn't do it for me.

So let's take a different tack, and try a Modified Zukovsky (play with the sounds, as in the famous Catullus translation from 1969):

Drr bool shll
Oobshhhsoor

mux
boosovyy
r l □z

That's better, isn't it? At least it feels more alienating to me, as I drop vowels, add extra letters to "Oobshhhsoor" and "boosovyy," and reverse the order of "skum" to make "muks">"mux" and "vyy so boo" to make "boosovyy." The repetition of "oo" in three lines seems to promise order, too, and thus meaning, and even an echoic do-wah-diddy scat – but then reneges on its promise.

Or, as that эmpty box suggests, we could play a little more with typography:

D♪r b♫l sh♮hl
□□βšš□□ρ

kc□□m
Vy s□ 6y
¶ √ εξ

I like that one a lot – so much, in fact, that I grow suspicious. Isn't that sort of play clichéd by now, in our postmodern era?

For that matter, is it even possible to simulate the Feeling of the Alien in a translation of this poem, more than a century after the source text was first published? Isn't the "contemporaneity" of this sort of alienating translation always already old hat?

(In fact what occurs to me there is that the Zukovskys' homophonic Catullus is itself an alienating translation. That is an entirely apt characterization of their project. If this section has no other practical value, it has at least given us a name for one of the most famous weird translations of the twentieth century. And of course its "weirdness" strikes us today, a half century later, as rather tame and quaint. For other homophonic translations, see van Rooten 1967; Melnick 1983.)

3.3.4 Embodied familiarity: the (Feeling of the) Alien Hand

On a train in Europe once when I was 17, traveling around on an Interrail card, I found myself sharing a couchette (a six-seater compartment convertible to beds at night) with a young Spanish man with whom I shared not a single language. I had had Spanish in primary school, and thought I knew some, but the two of us quickly established that we couldn't communicate, and more or less gave up. But then at one point he said to me "¿Qué hora es?" I said in English "I don't understand" and then suddenly realized that my body did: I had lifted and twisted my left arm around to look at my watch. Spanish no longer felt familiar, as it had in childhood, but in that moment I got a Feeling of the Alien-but-Familiar from it. Later, in my thirties, I began to regret having forgotten my Spanish, and took some classes to "get it back." It turned out I'd never had much, and basically had to learn the language from scratch; but the Feeling of the Familiar survived from my childhood.

I liken that moment to alien hand syndrome for continuity's sake, though as I mentioned in the Preface the "alien hand" or "devil hand" or "imp" is actually far more disruptive than my left hand was; all it wanted to do was to remind me that at some deep level I understood the Spanish question. If the Feeling of the Foreign deviates just slightly from the "automated" regime of homolingual address, the Feeling of the Strange deviates more strikingly (but still makes "sense" that can be assimilated to homolinguality), and the Feeling of the Alien deviates most strikingly of all (but still deliberately), the (Feeling of the) Alien Hand is no longer a deliberate distortion of homolingual sense-making. It is out of our control.

A much more germane neurological parallel with that incident on the train might be the experiments Michael Gazzaniga began performing on split-brain patients in the early 1960s, as Roger Sperry's Ph.D. student at Caltech (see Gazzaniga et al. 1962, 1965; Gazzaniga 2015): in one experiment, the subject would sit staring at a screen with a finger on a telegraph key beneath the table, with the instruction to tap the key *and* provide verbal confirmation every time s/he saw an image. The images were flashed to the far right or the far left of the screen, to test the effects of split hemisphericity on recognition. When an image appeared on the far right edge, a right-handed split-brain subject would process perception in his or her left brain and both tap the key and state that s/he had seen one. But when an image appeared on the far left edge of the screen, the subject would tap the key, but say nothing, and have no idea that s/he had seen the image. The subject's left *hand* knew that an image had appeared, but his or her left *brain* was clueless. (Actually, of course, the subject's right brain knew that the image had appeared, and activated the left hand, but, due to the corpus callosotomy, had no access to the language centers in the left brain.)

Now, my corpus callosum is intact: I am not a split-brain patient. But there does seem to be a suggestive similarity between the split-brain patient's left hand "seeing" the image and left brain not seeing it, on the one hand (so to speak), and my left hand understanding the Spanish question and left brain not understanding it, on the other. There is, clearly, a channel of foreign-language familiarity that is embodied in kinesthetic response even when conscious memory is not activated.

Not only that: what happened in that train couchette when I noticed that I had raised my arm and glanced down at my watch was that conscious memory suddenly *was* activated – after the fact, as it were. I suddenly "heard" the Spanish phrase, *¿qué hora es?* and suddenly realized that I did understand it. As we would normally narrativize that event, I should [1] hear the question, *¿qué hora es?*, [2] recognize it as Spanish, [3] analyze the syntax and semantics ("what hour is?"), [4] translate it into idiomatic English ("what time is it?"), and *then* [5] raise my arm and look at my watch. Instead, I (5) raised my arm and looked at my watch, (4) realized (seemingly out of nowhere, but most likely from the watch-checking gesture) that the man was asking the time, (2) recognized that it was in Spanish, (1) very belatedly (retroactively) heard the actual words in the question, and then (3) realized that I had a vague memory of what the individual words meant and how they worked together in that common phrase.

Cognitive neuroscience research over the past two or three decades has begun to explain events like this through the close neural links between gesture and speech. Iverson and Thelen (1999), for example, drawing on McNeill (1992), track the ways in which "gesture and speech form a single system of communication based on a common underlying thought process. Gesture and speech are tightly connected to one another, and there are links between gesture and speech throughout the process of speech production, occurring at the levels of discourse, syntax, semantics, and prosody" (21). More specifically, they note,

> four lines of research from neurophysiology and neuropsychology provide converging evidence of links between language and movement at the neural level. These studies have revealed that: a) some language and motor functions share underlying brain mechanisms; b) brain regions typically associated with motor functions (e.g., motor cortex, premotor area, cerebellum) are involved in language tasks; c) classical "language areas" (e.g. Broca's

area) are activated during motor tasks; and d) patterns of breakdown and recovery in certain language and motor functions appear to be closely linked in some patient populations.[4]

Tapping into this research, along with Dynamic Systems Theory, John Lutterbie (2013, 107–10) has explored the meaning-making impact of gestures in onstage and on-the-street communication, noting that the complex affiliations between the language and motor functions in the brain often cause gestures to prime, and even to preempt, verbal communication. My (5) unconscious gesture of raising my arm and looking at my watch, for example, *primed* my ability to react: first (4) primed the "holistic" (right-brain?) realization that the man was asking the time, then (2>1) cross-cued the language-processing circuits in my left brain, which helped me identify first the language, then the actual words, and finally (3) activated the memory-retrieval circuits from somewhere/somewhen deep in my primary-school experiences that helped me "translate" the words as "What time is it?"

I put scare quotes around "translate" there to highlight the striking fact that the *only* part of that performative event that would have interested both the linguists who began to formulate a "science" of translation in the mid-twentieth century – Fyodorov, Vinay and Darbelnet, Nida, etc. – and the hermeneutical thinkers from Hans-Georg Gadamer to the poststructuralist discursivists would have been (3) the interlingual processing of *¿qué hora es?* as "What time is it?" For those two strains in the emerging history of translation studies, it was only to the extent that mutually understandable language was exchanged that translation could be said to be occurring as an analyzable event, and only the linguistic part of the exchange was analytically relevant. Everything else – everything that cognitive scientists are now calling the situated, embodied, enactive, extended parts of the communicative event – not only could be but had to be suppressed (indeed was not even noticed).

This for me was the interesting takeaway of that train incident in the light of my reading in brain science in the early 1990s: that kinesthetic response can trigger or prime foreign-language memory. This realization became the genesis of my thinking for my 1997 textbook, *Becoming a Translator*. Sometime in the summer of 1994 I was sitting in my study in Peoria, Illinois, translating a chainsaw manual from English into Finnish, and I started noticing what I would do whenever I came across a lexical item I couldn't remember: I would remember the times I used a chainsaw in Finland, showing a movie in my head and participating kinetically in the movie with body movements rather than voiced words. The text would mention the importance of clearing debris off a log before cutting into it, for example, and I would lift my right hand off the keyboard and run it down an imaginary log. In my mind, sitting there in the summer heat, I would be in a snowy forest with my brother-in-law or a good friend, picking up a log from a snow-covered pile and running my gloved hand down it, removing the majority of the snow and frozen leaves to expose the surface of the log. Or I would come across the warning that the chainsaw might buck, and ask myself how you say "buck" in Finnish. What happened next inspired the textbook: I noticed that I *lifted my right shoulder*, as you do when using a chainsaw, and the Finnish word popped into my head: *potkia*/"to kick." I moved my body in a kind of partial simulation of actually sawing with a chainsaw, and the word I was looking for came to me. That kinesthetic prompt was accompanied by the movie in my head, of course – mentally, imaginatively, I was in that snowy Finnish forest, cutting firewood – but it was the *body movement* that triggered the verbal memory. That realization melded with my memory of the incident in the train from 1972, more than two decades before, and generated what I took to be an exciting and *useful* approach to translator training.

That same summer, based on *The Translator's Turn* (Robinson 1991), I received an invitation to come to Tlaxcala, Mexico, to give a weeklong workshop on translation the following November. I was thrilled: I've loved Mexico ever since those weekend trips my elementary school class made with Señor Guevara, and the workshop would be an excellent opportunity to develop and try out my ideas for the textbook's chapters and exercises. On the second day of the workshop, I was at breakfast with Eileen Sullivan, who had invited me, and I was looking through the menu, trying to decide what to order, and came across a word I didn't know: what kind of chicken is *pollo desfilado*? I asked Eileen what *desfilado* meant, and she made a preparatory chicken-shredding motion with the fingers on both hands, and *then* remembered and voiced the English word: "shredded." So that day in the workshop I told that story; and then, at lunch, I was sitting around a table with two or three of the local teachers, including Eileen, and another speaker, a top-flight interpreter from Cuba, who was doing a parallel workshop with the same students and teachers in the afternoons. This woman had traveled all over the world, interpreting for top Cuban political leaders; at one point she stopped to try and remember an Arabic word she had learned in the Middle East. It just wouldn't come to her. Eileen said to her with a little laugh, "Doug needs to give you a hand gesture." I smiled and said, "No, no need for a hand gesture," and picked up a napkin and held it in front of the woman's face. Suddenly the Arabic word exploded out of her mouth; her eyes went wide and she clapped both hands over her mouth, as if to prevent more verbal escapees. Again, bodily movement had triggered her memory.

As I worked on the textbook, and did my own world traveling to trial my ideas for it, more examples of this principle kept coming to me, both from my own experience and from the experience of the people attending my lectures and workshops. I remembered, for example, the many times I couldn't think of a word, and reached for the dictionary, opened it, and started paging through it, looking for the entry that would give me the word I needed – and that word would come to me before I actually reached the right page. Somehow the kinesthetics of flipping through the pages of the dictionary would trigger my memory.

One of the points I was making was that translating is a *job* – you do it to make money – and the faster you translate, the more money you make (at least as a freelancer, but there are some in-house jobs that bill by the word or character count as well). Every time you stop to look up a word in a dictionary, or do more elaborate research, you aren't producing text, which means you're earning less money. Back in the early 1990s I was hired to translate a legal deposition from a nurse in a specific hospital in Finland, and contacted a Finnish doctor friend of mine to ask about some unfamiliar words; she told me that that was local slang, probably used only in that hospital. So I called that hospital (from the U.S.) and found a nurse that was willing to help me out by explaining their slang. That was interesting and exciting – but I was not only not translating during those two transatlantic phone calls; I was paying for them out of pocket. Obviously in sheer economic terms, the faster your memory works on the words and phrases in transit from the source text to the target language, the more money you make.

Of course sheer speed isn't enough: if you translate so fast that you make egregious mistakes, you will damage your professional credibility, and you will lose clients. One of the things I sought to develop in *Becoming a Translator* was a series of exercises that would train what I called "pretranslation skills" – exercises that would put translators in the right frame of mind to enhance speed *and* accuracy of recall, as well as enjoyment. And, coming out of my realizations about what I myself did to enhance speech and accuracy of recall, those exercises all used visualization and dramatization. They were designed to activate embodied triggers for memory that didn't necessarily go through conscious propositional processes. The situated and embodied neuroscience of hermeneutics.

3.4 Chinese philosophy

In *The Dao of Translation: An East-West Dialogue* (Robinson 2015a) I returned to the model I had developed in *Becoming a Translator* in response to an interesting challenge to it from Ritva Hartama-Heinonen (2008, 256), who, citing my approach and a few others, exclaimed in disapproving mock-astonishment:

> What is surprising about these descriptions and what also characterizes the various theoretical orientations to professional translating in general, is that action and secondness somehow become highlighted. Instead of translators being "in as passive and receptive a state" (*CP* 7.45) as possible, they adopt the role of active searchers and, in this agency, seem to forget Peirce's own experience "that those things . . . done spontaneously were the best done" (*CP* 7.45; cf. Peirce's view in fn11, above). Abduction is, nevertheless, action without effort, and requires *letting* the sign address the mind (*CP* 2.228), or as earlier stated concerning the translator's part of the contrast, *not* intervening (Gorlée 1994, 222). Abductive thought therefore entails "a surrender to the Insistence of an Idea" (*CP* 4.581), in translating, an "unconditional surrender" to the sign (Gorlée 1994, 194). Characteristic of the descriptions above is also the aspect of finding single solutions to problems. But abduction is an attitude that covers all action and every step, and it is inseparable: a feeling that integrates and permeates, and flows into a habit, that of abductive thought. In this light, translating is not about my thinking and finding and solving; it is about letting thoughts I have create wider alliances.

As I argued in Robinson (2015a), this sounds very Daoist – though specifically "Daoist" in the mystical sense, with Laozi's concept of 無爲/*wuwei* (lit. "without acting" or "non-action") interpreted mystically as involving no action at all. Mengzi (or Mencius) too, the greatest Confucian thinker after Confucius, has his own version of 無爲/*wuwei*, namely 勿助長/*wu zhu zhang* "don't help grow": rather than trying to stretch plants to help them grow, the gardener should just get out of their way and *let* them grow. The Daoists and Confucians were supposedly great opposites and opponents in Warring States China, and certainly they did take different paths politically, the Confucians advising emperors and the Daoists refusing political appointments; but on many philosophical points they shared a foundational belief in the ecological emergence of everything out of everything. Hartama-Heinonen never ties her theory of "abductive translation" specifically to Daoist or more generally to early Chinese thinking, but it does seem to be quite close to this assumption about action: the translator does not need to *translate* the text, because the text knows how to translate itself. The translator's task is to get out of the text's way, not intervene in the text's self-translation process.

This is extreme, obviously; and as I show in Robinson (2015a, ch. 4), late in her book Hartama-Heinonen backs off the extremism that informs the rest of her argument. But note three things about that extremism while it lasts:

- *Thing 1.* While she attacks my Peircean model in *Becoming a Translator* as a habit-based "straitjacket" (245) – "Robinson is, in other words, interested most in the actual process of hardening habits – habit-forming through experience in translation" (246) – I take the focus on habits from Peirce, to whom she too declares fealty. I show in Robinson (2015a, 30–34) that Hartama-Heinonen actually deviates quite strikingly from Peirce, ending up with a "Peircean" theory of translation that is surprisingly anti-Peircean; but at least in principle she and I are on the same page in our admiration for the semeiotic of Charles Sanders Peirce.
- *Thing 2.* In their "philosophical translation" of Laozi, Roger T. Ames and David L. Hall (2003) argue persuasively that Laozi's 無為/*wuwei* is not about *not* acting: it's about *habitualized* acting. Because right action has become so habitualized that it has come to feel like second nature, the Daoist sage acts without bending himself to a purpose: action flows out of him, without conscious deliberation or determination. Translated to Hartama-Heinonen's "abductive" semiosis of translation, this would mean that it's not that the "Daoist" translator refuses to translate, but that s/he is such a consummate professional that s/he is able to rely on habitual or subliminal processes to accomplish most of the work – and, in so doing, is freed from much of the drudgery that plagues novice translators.
- *Thing 3.* Hartama-Heinonen invented the part about me insisting on the "hardening" of habits: for both Peirce and me, as for Viktor Shklovsky, habits are an automatization of action that *can* harden, which is why it is so important to have access to cognitive strategies that will keep loosening

> them up. For Hartama-Heinonen what is dangerous about my model is that it not only recognizes the existence of habits but allows that habits may even sometimes be useful.

In fact, note that "automaticity" – specifically the homeostatic management of automaticity – has become something of a scarlet thread running through this essay. On the one hand, as we saw Hervais-Adelman et al. (2015) noting, "We expect that the acquisition of expertise in simultaneous interpretation training requires the active development and automatization of extreme language control, a skill which overlaps considerably with other domains of executive control. This form of expertise can be expected to be at least partly driven by an increase in automaticity in performing the task, possibly driven by superior management of its multiple component skills" (265). This habitualization or automatization of language control certainly makes simultaneous interpreting possible; without intensive training and the resulting automatization, most bilinguals find simultaneous interpreting too difficult even to imagine. My argument in *Becoming a Translator* is that the same "increase in automaticity in performing the task, possibly driven by superior management of its multiple component skills," makes it faster and more enjoyable to translate written texts accurately as well. And indeed we saw that an unexpected hitch in that "translation automatism," like the unexpected failure of Otto Friedrich's "automatic pilot" on his walk to work, can create those disturbing Feelings of the Alien, and shut us down completely for a few moments.

On the other hand, however, too much automatization can be numbing. Viktor Shklovsky, quoting a passage from Leo Tolstoy's journal, where the Count is wiping dust off the furniture in his room at the home of his friends the Olsuf'evs and can't remember whether he wiped one chair, notes that habit can devour our whole lives, so that it seems to us that we aren't living at all. It is precisely to counteract that numbing that Shklovsky theorizes estrangement, the Feeling of the Strange that shakes us awake, rouses us from our numbed, habitualized stupor, and makes us feel completely alive again – "makes the stone stony," in his memorable phrase. There is, I would argue, a strong kinship between Shklovsky's theory of остранение/*ostranenie* – the Feeling of the Strange – and Hartama-Heinonen's theory of abductive translation: both bubble up out of the pleasure principle/life drive, laying waste to deathly repetition. Unlike Hartama-Heinonen, however, who explicitly chastises translation scholars who even *admit the existence* of habitualized drudgery in the translator's professional work, because she prefers to believe that "abduction captures the essence of translational activity, involving novelty, creativity, and playfulness" (273) – that there is *nothing but* novelty, creativity, and playfulness – Peirce, Shklovsky, and I all theorize a shuttle movement back and forth between habitualization and dehabitualization. Habit is a useful shortcut past the boring stuff, but would quickly pall if life were nothing else. Abduction is exciting, but would also quickly pall if life were nothing else.

Compare also my description in Robinson (2017a) of Sakai's theory of the regime of homolingual address, which is "a regime in which each language is ideally isolated from every other, with the speakers of each able to communicate easily and freely, and indeed automatically, with each other, and utterly unable to communicate with the 'foreigners' that have been relegated in advance to other isolated languages" (CT 1.10). Sakai theorizes this as an *illusory* automatization of communication – actually people who speak our language are more foreign to us than we like to think, and our own speech often thwarts our automatized intentions – but it is certainly true that conversing in our first language with other native speakers of that language tends to *feel* automatic, precisely because, as Peirce would insist, it has become habitualized through lifelong repetition. That automatization can come to feel numbing – endless small talk without surprise or other intensity – and what Peirce calls abduction, what Shklovsky calls estrangement, and what Sakai calls heterolinguality would all be welcome disruptions of that numbness.

The interesting question to ask about Hartama-Heinonen's "Daoist" theory of translation, though, is: how can it possibly be Daoist, if she gives no indication of drawing explicitly on Daoist thought, indeed no sign that she even knows anything about it? She identifies her approach as Peircean, and, like Peirce himself, situates herself sympathetically in the history of Romanticism and Idealism as well – so where do such transparently Daoist notions as "abduction is, nevertheless, action without effort" (256) come from?

In the two sections that follow, I offer two answers to that question. In the first (3.4.1) I show not only that the Romantics and Idealists in early nineteenth-century Germany, England, and America were avid readers of the Chinese philosophical classics, but also that the Romantic/Idealist opposition to mainstream Enlightenment thinking was itself preconditioned by two centuries of European translations of the Daoist and Confucian classics and the powerful influence those translations had on esoteric thought. In the second (3.4.2) I explore the congruences between Romantic/Idealist/hermeneutic thought about *Gefühl*/"feeling" and Daoist/Confucian thought about 心/*xin*/"feeling."

3.4.1 *The influence of Chinese thought on the peripheralized (anti-)West*

The story of the impact ancient Chinese thought had on Western esoterics beginning in around the beginning of the seventeenth century is not widely known. The story begins with the Jesuit mission to China in the late 1570s and early 1580s, especially with Michele Ruggieri (1543–1607), sent to Macao from Portuguese India in 1579, and Matteo Ricci (1552–1610), who joined Ruggieri in Macao three years later, in 1582. Ruggieri and Ricci tried their hands at translating Laozi and the Confucian "four books" early on, but did not manage to produce publishable texts; part of the trouble was that Ruggieri embraced Daoism and Ricci embraced Confucianism, each man believing that his preference was closer to Christianity. Over the twenty-seven years Ricci was working in China, until his death in 1610, he kept detailed journals in Italian, often reflecting in them on what later came to be known as his "accommodationist" theology: his belief that, because Confucianism was compatible with Christianity, the aim of the mission should be not to quell the former and replace it with the latter, but to find and expand the convergences. When after his death those journals were found by his colleagues in his Beijing office, the China Mission's Superior, Niccolo Longobardi (1559–1654), assigned the job of editing, expanding, and translating them into Latin to Nicholas Trigault (1577–1628). This labor Trigault undertook on his way back to Europe from China in 1613–1614; the resulting Latin work was published as *De Christiana Expeditione apud Sinas Suscepta ab Societate Jesu* ("About Christian Expeditions to China Undertaken by the Society of Jesus") in 1615. A later German Jesuit Sinologist named Athanasius Kircher (c. 1601–1680) published *China monumentis, qua sacris qua profanis, nec non variis naturae and artis spectaculis, aliarumque rerum memorabilium argumentis illustrata* (usually known simply as *China Illustrata,* 1667). The Confucian classic "four books" were first published in Latin translation in 1687, under the title *Confucius Sinarum Philosophus* ("Kongzi, Philosopher of the Chinese"), translated by Jesuit Fathers Philippe Couplet (1623–1693), Prospero Intorcetta (1626–1696), and others.

The story of the influence of Chinese thought on *oppositional* Western thought begins to get interesting around the turn of the eighteenth century, when G.W. Leibniz (1646–1716) began synthesizing all that was then known in the West about the Daoist and Confucian classics. Leibniz was an advocate of Agostino Steuco's (1497–1548) theory of a "perennial philosophy" (see Schmitt 1966), the supposed universal source from which all religious traditions draw; what he was ultimately looking for in Chinese thought was confirmation of his mystical assumptions. To that end he read everything published about China in Europe and all existing European translations of Chinese works, and also corresponded extensively with the Jesuit missionary Joachim Bouvet (1656–1730), an eminent mathematician and member of the Paris Academy of Science who had traveled to China to undertake his mission in 1687 – one of six Jesuits sent to China on the first French mission. Bouvet's version of the *philosophia perennis* was the then quite widespread notion that the Hebrew Bible was the universal source of all religions and all knowledge. Leibniz's late Idealist metaphysical treatise *La Monadologie* (1714) in particular reflects this mystical view: the monads are eternal and indecomposable centers of force, each of which mirrors the entire harmonious panpsychic universe in a ceaseless unfolding. As Perkins (2004, 108) writes:

> Leibniz showed an interest in China and other cultures from an early age, and, of Europeans who never left Europe, he became one of the most knowledgeable about China, particularly in the breadth of his knowledge. His interpretation of Confucian thought has serious flaws, but stands well above those of his contemporaries, and even some of the missionaries. From his research into Leibniz's sources, David Mungello [1982] concluded that Leibniz had probably read or was familiar with every significant book that had been written on China. Leibniz mentions almost all of them at some point in his correspondence.

In his study of *Leibniz and Confucianism*, Mungello (1977) reports that his research met with considerable surprise among colleagues; Perkins (2004, 9) reports the same more than a quarter century later. Somehow it seems counterintuitive that Leibniz could have been so respectfully attentive to the Chinese philosophical classics. Surely such an influential European thinker should have been primarily influenced by *European* thought – and his own genius? What Leibniz was doing was in fact *channeling* the European esoteric work he was reading – by the Neoplatonists (Plotinus, Porphyry, Iamblichus, etc.), by "Hermes Trismegistus" as translated by Marsilio Ficino (1433–1499) and Giovanni Pico della Mirandola (1463–1494), by the Christian theosophists and early seventeenth-century Rosicrucians, by the Huguenot philosopher Phillippe du Plessis-Mornay (1549–1623) – into and through his reading in ancient Chinese thought, and transmitting it into the oppositional eighteenth century and beyond. (For studies of Leibniz and Chinese philosophy, see also Lach 1957; Zempliner 1970, 1971; Mungello 1982; Ahn 1990; Ching and Oxtoby 1992; and Lai 1998.)

Another influential protagonist in this story is Emanuel Swedenborg (1688–1772), who drew heavily in his esoteric work both on ancient philosophical texts from China and on the reports of Moravian missionaries. It would be difficult to overemphasize Swedenborg's influence on nineteenth-century thought: Catherine the Great, Kant, Goethe, Lavater, Coleridge, Carlyle, Balzac, Baudelaire, and many other influential thinkers and writers were reading Swedenborg carefully. In *Kant's Critical Religion*, Stephen R. Palmquist (2000, chs. II and X) argues persuasively that Kant developed his "Copernican Hypothesis" – his realization that space and time are a subjective projection, not stable properties of an objective world – while reading and responding to Swedenborg. If Palmquist is right, the driving philosophical force behind all influential Idealisms and most (post-)Romanticisms over the past two-plus centuries is indebted to Kant's critical reading of Swedenborgian mysticism, which was steeped in Freemasonry, Rosicrucianism, the Kabbalah, and ancient Chinese thought. Henry James Sr. (1811–1882), father to William (the psychologist and philosopher) and Henry (the novelist), was a devoted Swedenborgian. Indeed all of the Transcendentalists, including Emerson, Thoreau, and Bronson Alcott, read Swedenborg avidly (and Emerson wrote a chapter of *Representative Men* on him), as did Transcendentalist-influenced writers like Whitman and Melville.

Emerson (1803–1882) and Thoreau (1817–1862) were in fact strongly drawn to Daoism and Confucianism through direct translations into French and English (see Christy 1963; Cheng 2000, 219n1): when Thoreau first stayed in Emerson's house in 1841, he found French translations of the Daoist classics by the French Orientalist Guillaume Pauthier (1801–1873), *The Works of Confucius* (1809) by the Baptist missionary to Calcutta Joshua Marshman (1768–1837), and *The Chinese Classical Work Commonly Called the Four Books* (1828) by David Collie (d. 1828), the third headmaster of the Ying Wa College (英華書院), the world's first Anglo-Chinese college. Both men pored over these books avidly, and discussed them frequently; Emerson published a selection (translated by Thoreau from Pauthier's French) of "Sayings of Confucius" in the 1843 *Dial*, and Thoreau quoted extensively from Mengzi in *Walden*. (Charles Sanders Peirce, by the way, was born in 1839 in Cambridge, Massachusetts; his father was a preeminent Harvard professor of mathematics and a close friend of Emerson, and Emerson's thought was profoundly influential for Peirce's later philosophical development.)

By the early nineteenth century, in other words, various forms of ancient Chinese and Western esoteric thought were circulating through the intellectual bloodstream of Europe, especially the Romantic and Idealist dissidents and utopians of the age. The German Romantics and Idealists at first looked upon Chinese thought with disdain, possibly in reaction against the superficiality of Enlightenment chinoiserie. Over the first two or three decades of the nineteenth century, however, all of the major German Romantics, including Johann Gottfried von Herder (1744–1803) and Friedrich von Schlegel (1772–1829), and all of the major Idealists, including G.W.F. Hegel (1770–1831) and Wilhelm von Humboldt (1767–1835), seem to have undergone a gradual "conversion" vis-à-vis the value of Chinese writing: Chinese philosophy and literature, they began to realize, were not after all "mummified, reactionary, and unimaginative" (Linder 2003, 254) but a sinuous and tenacious ally against the forces of conservatism that surrounded them. Arguably the German Romantics and Idealists found in the Chinese thinkers kindred spirits because they had been prepared for that kinship by two centuries of "peripheral" Western thinkers incorporating Chinese thought into the esoteric tradition. As they read and responded to Leibniz and Swedenborg and the others, in other words, they were at some level responding to lingering traces and echoes of Chinese thought already stockpiled into the counterhegemonic power source from which they drew. As Yan (n.d.) argues, German post-Romantics and post-Idealists like Richard Wagner (1813–1883), Friedrich Nietzsche (1844–1900), Hermann Hesse (1877–1962), Alfred Döblin (1878–1957), and Bertolt Brecht (1898–1956) continued to draw heavily on Chinese thought either directly or indirectly for their transformative engagements with the mainstream Western thought of their eras.

3.4.2 The 心 of the foreign

My title for this section is a bilingual translation of Schleiermacher's catchphrase "das Gefühl des fremden"/"the Feeling of the Foreign": if 心/*xin* is the Chinese character for the heart, and is used to mean the verb "to feel" and the noun "feeling," the counterhegemonic influence of Chinese thought on the Romantics (and their esoteric precursors and pragmatic and phenomenological successors) suggests that Schleiermacher's definitive insight into the different methods of translating might yield to a superimposition of Daoist/Confucian 心/*xin* on Romantic/hermeneutic *Gefühl*/"feeling." Let us consider, then, the consequences for *-fremdung* approaches to translation of three ancient Chinese ways of thinking about 心/*xin*: (section 3.4.2.1) Mengzi's insistence that the heart thinks, (section 3.4.2.2) the use of feeling as an energy in the dispositional training of the body, and (section 3.4.2.3) the notion of a group heart-becoming-mind or feeling-becoming-thinking as a utopian model of society.

3.4.2.1 Feeling-becoming-thinking

心/*xin* is a pictographic representation of the cardiac muscle, but Chinese people also use it to refer to something like "mind," and some Sinologists have taken to translating it "heart-mind." Indeed Mengzi famously writes that the organs of the eyes and ears cannot think, and so are easily deceived, but 心之官則思, 思則得之, 不思則不得/*xin zhi guan ze si, si ze de zhi, bu si ze bu de* (6A15), literally "the heart's office/function is to think, thinks and engages, doesn't think doesn't engage." Shun (1997, 150) notes that in contemporary (Warring States) Confucian texts, 思/*si* means not thinking in general, and certainly not logical, propositional thought, but rather something like "directing the attention to," especially to something one feels *inclined* to do. If 心/*xin* is feeling or affect, then, and affect channels inclinations (conations) into guidance for thinking (cognition), the character might be translated expansively as affect-becoming-conation-becoming-cognition. 官/*guan* originally meant a government office, later a government officer, someone in charge of making decisions; in that etymological light, we might think of 心之官則思/*xin zhi guan ze si*/"the heart's office is to think" as something like "the heart is the officer that manages thought." The affective directing/guiding/managing/commanding of thought/attention/perception/focus in effect *saturates* cognitive/conscious apperception of the world with managerial or "officious" (conative) affect. This is in fact almost exactly Damasio's (1994) somatic-marker hypothesis. So far from being some strange "Eastern" conception of the heart at a thinking organ, in other words, 心/*xin* is very close to Western understandings of affect and conation as *guides* to cognition – as in common English phrases like "the heart knows better than the head," which we take to imply that the cold cognitive logic that we trope as "the head" is weak and ultimately powerless without the guiding force of the affects and conations that we trope as "the heart."

If accordingly we modify the emerging "heart-mind" translation of 心/*xin* as "heart-becoming-mind" or "feeling-becoming-thinking," then, the 心/*xin des fremden* might be the Feeling-becoming-Thinking of the Foreign, the Feeling-becoming-Thinking of the Strange, or the Feeling-becoming-Thinking of the Alien. What effect does this slight shift have on our explorations of the foreignization, alienation, and estrangement of translation in section 3.3 above?

Our answer to that question would depend, obviously, on who is doing the Feeling-becoming-Thinking about those things: (1) the translator, (2) the target reader, or (3) the stereoscopic reader (comparing the translation with the original) who becomes the translation scholar. Let us consider each of those in turn.

1. *The translator.* As Schleiermacher sets up his model, of course, the translator is not expected to *feel* the foreignness of the current source text: s/he is supposed to *simulate* the Feeling of the Foreign felt by an imaginary person, a source reader who is neither a native nor a particularly fluent reader of the source language, *for* the target reader. For the purposes of that simulation it is, obviously, advantageous for the translator to retain a strong embodied

memory of the Feeling of the Foreign, either in an earlier stage of his or her engagement with the source language or in her or his current engagement with some other language. There is, to be sure, no need for that Feeling to become Thinking in the full-on propositional sense – the translator does not need to think consciously, logically, coherently about the Feeling of the Foreign – but if we follow Shun Kwong-Loi in reading 思/*si* as *guidance* for thought rather than conscious propositional thought in its own right, that's not really a problem: the main thing for Schleiermacher is that the translator be able to channel a remembered Feeling of the Foreign into guidance for the translating process, so that the target reader will feel the Feeling of the Foreign while reading the translation. From the translator's point of view, nothing in that model changes significantly when we move from the Feeling-becoming-Thinking of the Foreign to the Feeling-becoming-Thinking of the Strange or the Feeling-becoming-Thinking of the Alien: each specific channeling of that Feeling-becoming-Thinking is a translation *strategy*. It is a way of guiding translatorial choices. The examples I gave of translating Aleksis Kivi estrangingly in section 3.3.1 and заумь/*zaum'* alienatingly in section 3.3.2 fit this model exactly.

2. *The target reader*. Things become more complicated, and therefore considerably more interesting, when we move to what the target reader Feels-becoming-Thinks in reading the translation. The complication stems, as I began to suggest in section 3.3, from my sense that the target reader reading an awkward translation is highly unlikely to convert that awkwardness into a Feeling-becoming-*Thinking of the Foreign*. Certainly, if the foreignizing translator has done her or his job well enough, the target reader will feel some sort of Feeling of the Awkward; but what aspect of an awkward text will guide the target reader to convert the Feeling of the Awkward into a Feeling-becoming-Thinking of the *Foreign*? In order to experience the Feeling-Becoming-Thinking of the Foreign, to be sure, the target reader does not have to Think, consciously, words like "this is a foreign text"; s/he only has to have an inchoate affective certainty of the text's foreignness. But there does, it seems to me, have to be some kind of Felt-becoming-Thought difference between domestic awkwardness and foreign awkwardness. There are, after all, so many different subgenres of domestic awkwardness – bureaucratese, legalese, textbookese, freshman-compese, and so on, produced through a shifting collection of convergences between weak writing and genre restraints – and it is so much likelier that target readers will have extensive experience with those domestic forms of awkwardness than with foreign awkwardness, that it will almost certainly require an extra push to get target readers to Feel-becoming-Think the Foreignness of the awkward.

And then, one step further: the target reader is also likely to have some experience with *unintentionally* awkward foreign texts: lists of ingredients on foreign-made food products, instruction manuals translated by non-native speakers of the various target languages, and so on. This is the subgenre of foreign awkwardness called "translationese," which is, obviously, the default label slapped onto a Schleiermacherian foreignized translation by the unwary. The target reader properly primed to dismiss that default label as inappropriate would obviously need to Feel (and perhaps even to Think) a heightening of the difference between translationese and (stylized)/foreignized translation, so that the latter is at *least* feelingly distinguished from the former. (And of course "distinguishing" is a becoming-Thinking kind of Feeling.)

Those complications become even more interesting when we move to the Feeling-becoming-Thinking of the Strange or the Feeling-becoming-Thinking of the Alien. The first question concerns whether the Feeling-becoming-Thinking of the Strange and the Feeling-becoming-Thinking of the Alien must *also* be Feelings-etc. of the Foreign. How we answer that question will depend on what we take the purpose of titrating Feelings-etc. of the Familiar and the Unfamiliar to be:

- *Purpose 1: nationalism.* If, following Schleiermacher, the purpose of this congeries of approaches is the patriotic one of reminding the target reader that s/he is *not* reading a work originally written in the target language – that there is a qualitative difference between "local" writing and "foreign" writing – then our answer must be *yes: das Gefühl des fremden* must be at least in part a Feeling-becoming-Thinking of the Foreign, Feelingly guiding the target reader to a Thinking of national pride, domestic prowess. P1 would thus tend to reinforce what Sakai Naoki calls the regime of homolingual address: if original domestic literature creates in the reader a *high* dosage of the Feeling(-becoming-Thinking) of the Familiar and a *low* dosage of the Feeling (-becoming-Thinking) of the Unfamiliar, it may become possible to suppress all Thinking of the latter, and even eventually the Feeling of the latter, and thus to idealize the Feeling-becoming-Thinking of the Familiar as "automatic" communication among native speakers, or what Sakai calls homolinguality. Presumably P1 would be served equally well by the Feeling of the Strange or the Alien – anything that makes the target reader shake his or her head at "them weird (goddamned) foreigners" – except that in each case the Feeling of the Weird would need to become a *Thinking* of the Foreign alone. Nationalism is not served by a generalized Feeling of the Weird that does not culminate in a conscious tracking of that Feeling to the Foreign.
- *Purpose 2: denaturalization.* If, following Berman and Venuti, the purpose of these approaches is the anti-illusionistic one of reminding the target reader that s/he is reading a translation, and thus also, by extension, of disrupting the (P1) "homolingualization" or automatization of the local culture, then the answer must again be *yes: das Gefühl des fremden* must be at least in part a Feeling-becoming-Thinking of the Foreign, Feelingly guiding the target reader to a transformative Thinking of what Sakai calls heterolinguality, the attitude that we are all foreigners to each other, and even to ourselves, and therefore that we are always translating, that all communication is translation.

- *Purpose 3: ostranenie/estrangement.* If, following Shklovsky, the purpose of these approaches is the estranging/defamiliarizing one of shaking the target reader out of a habitualized numbness to embodied experience, the answer is *not necessarily: das Gefühl des fremden* could be a Feeling-becoming-Thinking of the Foreign, but all it really has to be is a Feeling-becoming-Thinking of the Strange or a Feeling-becoming-Thinking of the Alien. Reading a translation produced using one of those latter two strategies would only need to make the target reader feel more alive.
- *Purpose 4: Verfremdung/estrangement.* If, following Brecht, the purpose of these approaches is the *politicized estranging* one of shaking the target reader out of a habitualized numbness to oppression, to the ways s/he is being both exploited and numbed to that exploitation, then the answer is again *not necessarily:* the important thing would be guiding the Feeling of the Foreign/Alien/Strange into the Thinking of political resistance to power. Ideally, of course, for Brecht that would mean a Marxist Thinking, but Brecht never explicitly theorizes how *Verfremdung* channels the Feeling of the Strange into a Thinking (and ultimately an activist Pursuing) of Marxist revolution. One should also note that this ethos is also very close to the Marxist Thinking promoted by Lawrence Venuti, who, however, never invokes Brecht or Brechtian *Verfremdung,* never raises the possibility of a Feeling-becoming-Thinking of the Strange that does not involve a Feeling-becoming-Thinking of the Foreign. (Not that he ever thematizes foreignization as involving Feeling anyway, let alone Feeling-becoming-Thinking.)

3. *The stereoscopic reader as critic/scholar/theorist.* Factually, the stereoscopic reader – who reads both the original and the translation and compares them with each other – is also a target reader, and as such is covered in (2); historically, the stereoscopic reader who becomes a translation critic, a translation scholar, or a translation theorist has almost always been a translator as well, and so is also covered in (1). The stereoscopic activity of comparing the translation with the original, however, transforms both (1) and (2); and the professional activity of *writing about translation* by default also intensifies the *becoming-Thinking* part of 心/*xin* – to the point even, especially in the West, of driving some scholars to deny the entire relevance of Feeling to Thinking. I began writing out "Feeling-becoming-Thinking" at some point in the 1990s in reaction against a fairly widespread simplistic reading of *The Translator's Turn* that took me to be saying something like "the translator doesn't need to think, s/he can just translate any way s/he feels." Any talk of Feeling, in this binary oversimplification, cancels out Thinking. I also began grounding talk of Feeling-becoming-Thinking in the neo-Jamesian neurological tradition, and specifically in Damasio's somatic-marker hypothesis, because in Damasio's neo-Jamesian approach to neuroscience emotion is a mapping of body states, feeling is a mapping of emotion, and thinking is a mapping of feeling: each emerges out of the lower bodily level by mapping it as emergent mind. But also the great liberation I felt living in Greater China for most of the second decade of the new

millennium stemmed in part from the fact that Chinese people *never* binarize Feeling and Thinking in this way, because 心/*xin* in Chinese covers the entire range of heart-becoming-mind.

It also seems to me, however, that simply grounding the emergence of Thinking out of Feeling does not exhaust the complexity of the 心/*xin des fremdes.* I have already hinted at the additional complications in noting that in theorizing the foreignization of translation Schleiermacher, Berman, and Venuti do not *Think* the emergence of the Thinking of the Foreign out of the Feeling of the Foreign in any of the three potential constituencies: (1) translators, (2) target readers, and (3) stereoscopic readers like themselves. They all tend to mystify that whole process, leading me to suspect a break in the flow of Feeling into the Thinking of the Foreign not just in their Underthinking (under-theorizing or non-theorizing) but in the social organization of the reading of translations. It seems likely to me that target readers are "taught" or "conditioned" icotically to read textual awkwardness and the Feeling of the Awkward it provokes in them primarily as domestic rather than foreign subgenres of textual awkwardness, like bureaucratese and textbookese, and, secondarily, to the extent that they recognize the text they're reading as a translation, as translationese rather than as foreignization. Foreignized translation, therefore, would seem to me extremely unlikely to have any of the desired effects projected onto it by Schleiermacher, Berman, and Venuti. I infer therefrom that the only reason that they are able to promote it so enthusiastically is that they are not asking the important theoretical questions about it – they are, in other words, massively Underthinking it, and so rendering it incapable of performing or facilitating any worthwhile scholarly work. (Which is not to say, of course, that it is incapable of facilitating any scholarly work at all: witness the hundreds of MA theses that have been written around the world showing that Translation X is domesticated and Translation Y is foreignized. While one could argue that such scholarly work is "worthwhile" in the sense that it allows otherwise unpromising MA students to obtain their degree, I'm not convinced that is a particularly convincing argument.)

The relative extremism of the Feeling-becoming-Thinking of the Strange and the Feeling-becoming-Thinking of the Alien, by contrast, combined with the relative clarity and coherence of the Romantic/modernist Thinking of estrangement devices and alienation effects in literature, combined further with the freedom to incite and explore *Verfremdungseffekten* without a mandatory Feeling-becoming-Thinking of the *Foreign,* would seem conducive to a more productive medical humanities of translation – and other kinds of literary production.

3.4.2.2 *The dispositional training of the body*

As I mentioned earlier, Ames and Hall (2003) argue that the Daoist 無為/*wuwei* "without-acting" is actually not at all an instruction not to act, as it seems to be in Ritva Hartama-Heinonen's putatively "Daoist" theory of abductive translation, but a kind of *noncoercive* action emerging "naturally" (unconsciously) out of habitualized dispositions. Ames and Hall identify several other constructions in Laozi based on the 無/*wu*/"without" character as well: 無知/*wuzhi*/"without knowing," 無欲/*wuyu*/"without desiring," and 無心/*wuxin*/"without feeling." These constructions, which they call the *wu*-forms, become the basis for their reading of Laozi as promoting the dispositional development of good habits:

> What the *Daodejing* has to offer, on the other hand, is much simpler. It encourages the cultivation of a disposition that is captured in what we have chosen to call its *wu*-forms. The *wu*-forms free up the energy required to sustain the abstract cognitive and moral sensibilities of technical philosophy, allowing this energy, now unmediated by concepts, theories, and contrived moral precepts, to be expressed as those concrete feelings that inspire the ordinary business of the day. It is through these concrete feelings that one is able to know the world and to optimize the human experience.
>
> (36)

Thus for example 無為/*wuwei* becomes "noncoercive actions in accordance with the *de* ('particular focus') of things"; 無知/*wuzhi* becomes "a sort of knowing without resort to rules or principles"; and 無欲/*wuyu* becomes "desiring which does not seek to possess or control its 'object' " (38). Their sensible understanding of how Daoists are to cultivate these "withouts" – these apparent renunciations of acting, knowing, and desiring – is that the way to the withouts leads through habitualization:

> The developed customs and habits of mind of the Daoist are a resource that conditions, influences, and attempts to optimize the range of creative possibilities without in fact causally determining the crafting of novel experiences. Such aggregated habits are irreducibly social, and are the unannounced social propensity out of which individual hearts-and-minds express themselves as overt actions.
>
> For example, the insistent particularity associated with the uniqueness of a particular person must be understood both relationally and as a dynamic process within the context of a given natural, social, and cultural world. Particular character is an interpenetration of habits that has organized and made meaningful the more primary but not more important natural impulses. Considered synchronically, persons are irreducibly relational, entailing what they do for this specific community as well as the personal enrichment they derive from participating in its communal life-forms and culture. Viewed diachronically, each particular personality must also be understood as an ongoing and unrelenting awareness that attends every gesture and thought, and that is expressed as a refined disposition in all of its activities.
>
> (48–49)

The notion that this dispositional habitualization works through the training of the body, however, comes from Mengzi:

> 中天下而立，定四海之民，君子樂之，所性不存焉。君子所性，雖大行不加焉，雖窮居不損焉，分定故也。君子所性，仁義禮智根於心，其生色也，睟然見於面，盎於背，施於四體，四體不言而喻。
>
> (7A21)
>
> *zhong tianxia er li, zi hai zhi min, junzi le zhi, suo xing bu cun yan. junzi suo xing, sui da xing bu jia yan, sui qiong ju bu sun yan, fen ding gu ye. junzi suo xing, ren yi li zhi gen yu xin, qi sheng se ye, sui ran xian yu mian, ang yu bei, shi yu siti, siti buyan eryu.*
>
> To stand in the center of the Empire, to bring an orderly life to the people within the four seas: this gives the exemplary person pleasure, but s/he does not embody that pleasure as a propensity toward virtue. The exemplary person embodies virtue so robustly that, no matter how great or straitened the conditions in which s/he lives, s/he is not buffeted by external circumstance. S/he embodies fellow-feeling, rightness, ritual propriety, and wisdom by rooting them deeply in feeling-becoming-thinking, so that they put out new growth as a clarity in the face and a fullness in the back and shoulders, and on into the four limbs, so that they communicate clearly even though they cannot speak.
>
> (translation Robinson 2015a, 57–60)

Shun (1997, 159) notes that Chinese commentators have tended to take the four limbs there as signifying *conduct,* but surely what Mengzi is referring to here is not conduct in general but specifically *posture* as a corporeal (and so 不言/*buyan*/"unspeaking") display of the virtue or vice that has shaped or trained it.

One less obviously embodied disposition resulting from this sort of training would be the "language control" that makes simultaneous interpreting possible – less obvious because the embodiment of language control is neural, and so not visible to the naked eye. Such "dispositions" are only detectable through functional and other brain-imaging research; but they can certainly be Felt (and even Thought) by simultaneous interpreters, who settle into their embodied dispositions as they set up in the booth. A more obviously embodied disposition resulting from professional training or long professional experience would be the professional translator's Feeling – which also occasionally becomes a Thinking, and in my case generated *Becoming a Translator* – that translating is mostly performed by the body: kinesthetic reenactments of past experiences do the remembering; the fingers do the translating; and man, look at those fingers go! The fact that "the fingers" can only do the translating as long as no problems arise – no unfamiliar words or phrases requiring research, no garbled syntax or bad spellings – serves as a reminder that translation is *also* an intelligent activity; and Thinking the Feeling that the body does the translating, Thinking that Feeling as the product of the automatization of long training or experience, serves as a reminder further that translation is *always* an intelligent activity. *Pace* Hartama-Heinonen, it just doesn't always seem that way.

3.4.2.3 The utopian group heart-becoming-mind

In the previous section I mentioned what Ames and Hall called the *wu*-forms, and listed 無心/*wuxin*/"without heart" as one of them – but then did not give Ames and Hall's (re)definition of that form. Let us now look at an interesting example of that form, in Chapter 49 of the *Laozi:*

> 聖人恆無心，以百姓心為心。
>
> *shengren heng wuxin, yi baixing xin wei xin.*
>
> Sage constant without heart/feeling, takes hundred surnames' heart as heart.
> (literal translation DR)

> The sage has no invariable mind of his own; he makes the mind of the people his mind.
> (Legge)

The sage lacks a heart? The sage feels nothing? The heart that the sage has is not the constant heart – or as Legge has it, "invariable mind" – but the people's heart? What is going on there?

Ames and Hall give us:

> Sages really think and feel immediately.
> They take the thoughts and feelings of the common people as their own.
> (153)

The significant retranslation there is their rendering of 無/*wu*/"without" as "immediate(ly)" – the implication being that the negation in 無/*wu* is a negation not of heart/feeling but of mediation. The sage feels what the "hundred surnames" (a common euphemism for "the masses") feel without a protective "membrane" that filters out whatever might be unpleasant. In a modern Western rationalist/individualist purview, 無心/*wuxin* might be translated negatively as "codependency"; to get back to the social neurology of hermeneutics, another translation might be German *Einfühlung* or English "empathy." A Herderian translation might go:

> Die Weisen fühlen sich in alles hinein.
> Sie nehmen die Gefühle und die Gedanken der Massen als ihre eigenen an.
>
> Sages feel their way into everything.
> They take the feelings and the thoughts of the masses as their own.

I have elsewhere called this transmission of feeling through bodies "transfeeling": we "transfeel" other people's feelings in the sense that we not only receive them but transmit them onward to yet others. Feelings circulate through a group: what I call the somatic exchange. Every member of a group of friends present at a conversational event transfeels the affective orientations of every other present member. Another term often used for it is "identification," but it is not simply a matter of mapping of our identities cognitively onto someone else's, or theirs onto ours; it is an empathic projection, or what Ickes (1997; Ickes and Aronson 2003) calls "mind-reading." I would call it an affective, or affective-becoming-cognitive, projection; and, since affect is generally taken to be more fully embodied than cognition, and is typically displayed in "legible" form on the stage of the body, it might more accurately be called not mind reading but "body-becoming-mind-reading." We *feel* other people's body states, from inside our own bodies. This is what makes the socioaffective phenomenon we call "face" possible: it is a *collective* evaluation of any given participant's contribution to the conversation, and the various individual members of the group participate in that collective evaluation affectively, without necessarily becoming aware of doing so.

If 無心/*wuxin* is an "empathic projection," then, would we be justified in translating it as "the Golden Rule" – the rule that you should feel your way into another person's being? Given that Ames and Hall translates 無知/*wuzhi* as "a sort of knowing without resort to rules or principles" (38), perhaps we should add that 無心/*wuxin* would be the Golden Rule-without-Rule, the *habitualized* Golden Rule, or perhaps the Golden Disposition?

Interestingly, when Kongzi (Confucius) wanted to formulate that Rule, he borrowed the ancient Chinese concept of 仁/*ren,* which up to that point had meant something like "benevolence"; and "benevolence" was the translation chosen for the character in the Confucian *Four Books* by David Collie in 1828 and James Legge in 1861. And, while a countertradition began to emerge in the middle of the twentieth century, with Chan (1963), Dobson (1963), Hinton (1998), Bloom (2009), and others translating it "humanity" or "humaneness," it continues to be rendered "benevolence" by many English translators and Sinologists even today (most recently by Bryan W. Van Norden in 2008).[5]

Mengzi, however, a century after Kongzi, added a new twist to the concept, renaming the *outward* projection of transfeeling (what Kongzi means by 仁/*ren*) 恕/*shu,* and transforming 仁/*ren* either into its opposite, an *inward* transfeeling, an introjection of other people's feelings, or, more likely, into a larger umbrella concept that includes both the outward projection and the inward introjection of transfeeling, and thus the circulation of feeling through the members of a group.

In other words, 仁/*ren* is neither "benevolence" nor "humanness." As I argued at some length in Robinson (2015a, 71–75, and 2016a, 67–76, 91–102), what Mengzi means by the expanded Kongzian concept is specifically an interactive phenomenology of shared feeling, a socioaffective ecology. This construction of 仁/*ren* obviously brings us remarkably close to Laozi's 無心/*wuxin* and 心為心/*xin wei xin:* if as I suggested above the negation in 無/*wu*/"without" signals the removal of the regulatory membrane through which most people *transfeel a little* (not too much to be unsettling) of other people's feelings, the sage's goal is not only to let the common people's feelings circulate through him or her, but to let 無心/*wuxin* become a "sedimented habit of engagement" (Ames and Hall 2003, 153). For it is only when 無心/*wuxin* is "second nature" – not something one constantly strives to attain but what feels like the most natural thing in the world – that the sage becomes what Mengzi calls 仁人/*ren ren,* a fellow-feeling fellow, someone who allows other people's feelings, the feelings of the whole group, to flow through his or her actions, thoughts, words, and relationships.

But this all seems very vague: "one big happy family"–type thinking. "One is all and all are one." How exactly does the circulation of people's feelings through a group work in translation?

Consider the kinds of texts nonliterary freelance translators translate: technical, legal, commercial, medical, governmental. In any given week a translator may translate an instruction manual for a diesel engine, a series of depositions for a court case, an advertisement and two pharmaceutical inserts (one intended for doctors, the other for patients) of a new drug, and a toxic-waste environmental-impact statement for a proposed new pulp mill. These documents are not just words and phrases that can be translated as "pure language" (whatever that might be): they are human communications created for specific purposes, charged with agency, designed to bring about change in the world. They are interpersonal exchanges – not usually one-to-one exchanges, but exchanges nonetheless. In them people are trying to do things to other people with words. And all of the people involved are very different – people who have been shaped by their jobs in very different ways. They not only talk about their experience of the world differently; they actually Feel and Think about it differently. In an important sense they live in different worlds: their Feeling-becoming-Thinking "worlds" different "realities" forth.

The instruction manual may have been written by a technical writer with input from an engineer, or a technician, or a whole team of technicians, who may not all have agreed on specific points; the tech writer may not have internalized the input as fully or complexly as the technicians might have hoped. Or it may have been written by a technician who understood the diesel engine extremely well but had no idea how to write about it, who even hated writing, and was assigned the job by a supervisor who knew nothing about writing either, and didn't really care. Some members of the team who contributed to the creation of the instruction manual probably cared a great deal about the engine – more even, perhaps, than about his or her coworkers. Others might have cared more about the words than the machine; others still more about the money, or the boss's praise. In principle they should all care most about the end user, the reader, and his or her interactions with the diesel engine – but to expect the whole team to assign top priority to that reader would be utopian.

The depositions would be word-for-word transcripts of oral testimony by a series of witnesses, conducted out of court by a lawyer or a group of lawyers and transcribed by a court reporter, either from a recording or through shorthand. The transcripts would reflect not only a variety of personalities – the lawyers, the witnesses – but the complexities of human conversation (misunderstandings, imprecise memories, sloppy descriptions, etc.) as refracted across the gap between legal experts and laypeople. Again, the work of taking and transcribing these depositions should ideally be organized toward the end of making a case in court; but people's motivations vary.

The advertisement and the two pharmaceutical inserts would provide roughly the same information about the new drug, but for different purposes and to different target audiences – mainly doctors and patients, obviously. The advertising copy would be designed to sell the drug; the inserts, how and when to prescribe it (doctors) or take it (patients). Pharmaceutical companies spend huge amounts of money developing new drugs, and obviously want to sell as many units as they can, to recuperate their investment; but the people who create the ad copy and pharmaceutical inserts may not care at all about the company's investment, which the texts they write are intended to protect.

The toxic-waste environmental-impact statement for the new pulp mill is a governmental document, required before the new mill can open; one would think such things would be routine, purely and indeed facelessly factual, without the kind of "agency" (or spin) that we expect from, say, advertising texts. But of course there's always room for spin; and even if the mill truly does meet all governmental requirements, there is the chance that environmentalists will use the document to protest the laxity of governmental standards.

In each job, in other words, all within the space of a single hypothetical week, this one translator must feel his or her way into a dozen or more *different* hermeneutical encounters, each of which is organized verbally and cognitively, obviously, but also affectively, and conatively, around real or imagined human relationships. In Mengzi's terms, each is its own separate 仁/*ren*/"fellow-feeling" or regulatory group 心/*xin*/"Feeling-becoming-Thinking." S/he must, like the Daoist sage as imagined by Laozi, take that 心為心/*xin wei xin*/"group heart as heart" – must be enough of a 仁人/*ren ren*/"fellow-feeling fellow" to be 無心/*wuxin*, which is to say, not to insist on retaining the personal agency of a separate individualistic Feeling-becoming-Thinking.

This means not only identifying with the various social actors involved in each group interaction – commissioners, supervisors, project managers, researchers, writers, speakers, readers, users – but entering imaginatively into the interaction itself, feeling one's way into the transaction. How does one do that? How is that even possible? This is not a mystical model of human communication; one does not "divine" these things. Rather, one guesses, imagines, projects – but does so in an "educated" way, through educated guesses that are affectively guided by research. Without that ability to enter into the regulatory affect of a group, it is in fact impossible to write to or for that group. Most adult humans have been sufficiently socialized to be 仁者/*ren zhe*/"fellow-feelingists" (Mengzi 4A8, 7A24, 7B1) in face-to-face encounters. It is quite common, however, for people to hate to write: why? We might use Mengzi's "social neuroscience of hermeneutics" model to suggest that across the spatiotemporal gaps that open between writers and readers, they are 不仁者/*buren zhe*/"non-fellow-feelingists": they don't feel the guidance of the group when they read, and so are unable to feel or wield that guidance when they write. Written texts thus become abstractions to them, strings of words that they cannot Feel as group guidance, and so cannot use to channel Feeling-becoming-Thinking back through the group either.

3.5 The icosis/ecosis of hermeneutics

In the Preface I posed the core MH question of this book as follows: "Sense-data move through our sensory apparatus to our central nervous systems, and there are translated not only into a coherent picture of reality but a coherent picture of reality *shared by other members of our culture*. How does that happen? How does a culture shape the neural translation of sense-data into a coherent picture of reality in all or most of its member individuals?"

The answer toward which I have been moving throughout the book involves what I have called "the neurocultural regulation of human social life," or "the regulatory social neurology of hermeneutics," or, more briefly, "icosis" and "ecosis." Icosis, as I've mentioned along the way, is my coinage from Aristotle's *eikos*/"plausible" and *ta eikota*/"the plausibilities," and means the sociosomatic ecology of plausibilization; ecosis is my coinage from Attic Greek *oikos*/"household, community," and means the sociosomatic ecology of communal normativization, or what I call either the becoming-good of the community or the becoming-communal of norms of goodness. Icosis is all about "truth," "reality," and "identity" – making the group opinions that structure those ideals *feel real* – and thus my main medical-humanities concern in this book. Ecosis is all about "right and wrong," "good and evil," "good citizenship," "morality," "ethics" – making the group opinions that structure *those* ideals feel real – and thus also extremely important to the medical humanities, just not the central concern of this book.

Both icosis and ecosis involve the circulation of evaluative affect – approval and disapproval, praise and blame, pride and shame, honor and dishonor – through the group as conation (motivation), which is effectively pressure to conform to group norms. This repurposing of shared evaluative affect as conation may also become conscious awareness in its participants, or what I call affect-becoming-conation-becoming-cognition; but it often works without emerging into consciousness. The key movement is affect-becoming-conation, feeling-becoming-pressure – the affects of approval and disapproval shading over into the pressure to conform to group norms – but that movement as organized "ecotically" as the becoming-good of the community, and "icotically" as the becoming-true or becoming-real of group opinion.

Icosis and ecosis are socioecological versions of post-Kantian social constructivism/periperformativism, based on Kant's "Copernican Hypothesis" that we do not simply "register" the objects around us but actively (if unconsciously) *construct/periperform reality*. As I noted in the Preface, this post-Kantian thought was modeled for one influential twentieth-century school of neuroscience by William James; the neurological team whose work has most powerfully influenced mine has been the one in the neo-Jamesian lab of Antonio R. Damasio.

I also noted in the Preface that, while social constructivism/periperformativism is the phenomenological/hermeneutical ground on which "critical theory" stands – "the best thinking in the humanities," I called it there – there seems to be virtually no recognition among humanistic critical thinkers of the parallel work being done in the social neuroscience of empathy. And I would suggest that it is as an indirect result of this neglect that social constructivism/periperformativism is dismissed as "only a theory" by many humanist thinkers – only one theory among many, including the preposterous theory of simulacra offered by Jean Baudrillard. Because the fact is that without confirmation from neuroscience, social constructivism/periperformativism seems unable to explain the most fundamental, and problematic, aspect of its own model: the fact that social constructs/performances *feel real.*

Take one of the bones of contention between the cultures of liberalism and conservatism, for example: whether state support for the poor is a good thing (liberals) or a bad thing (conservatives). If you are a liberal, it seems not only *humane* but a simple indelible fact – a reality – that the poor are trapped in poverty by a hundred social, political, and economic restraints, and therefore that they *need* state support; and therefore that the only possible explanation for conservative attacks on social welfare must be that conservatives are selfish beasts who don't want to share their income with those worse off than themselves. If you are a conservative, it seems equally *real* that human beings are motivated by need to strive for a better life, and that by diminishing need, social welfare actually *hurts* the poor, indeed traps them in poverty; and therefore that the only possible explanation for liberal defenses of social welfare for the poor is that liberals benefit in some nefarious way from a bloated state welfare apparatus. Each side takes its own view to be grounded in *reality* – after all, it *feels real* – and the other side to be motivated by mere superficial (and indefensible) self-interest. After all, the views of a culture not your own typically feel like cloud castles.

The widespread dismissal of social constructivism/periperformativism by many humanists may have something to do with the fact that social constructivism/periperformativism tends to be philosophically congruent with liberalism, so that to conservatives it too seems like cloud castles – mere empty theorizing without any basis in (what they take to be) reality. But I suggest that it is also more than that. Not all liberals, after all, are social constructivists/periperformativists. Liberalism and social constructivism/periperformativism are isomorphic but not coterminous. It is not only possible to be a liberal objectivist; objectivism is the *dominant* metaphysics in the West. It is, therefore, "normal" or "natural" (read: ideologically normative) for everyone, liberals and conservatives alike, to believe that what they take to be reality *is* objectively real. Philosophical orientations that challenge the normativity of that hegemonic view are therefore "obviously" (normatively) not true, and anyone who claims to believe such drivel is "obviously" either seriously deluded or horribly perverted.

Nor is that all. The version of post-Kantian social constructivism/periperformativism that has reigned in the non-medical humanities for roughly the past century has notably lacked an explanation of what *makes* this or that social construct/performance feel real. Without that kind of explanation, one's own views feel real but one's opponents' views do not – and because one is philosophically unable to explain how "their" views might *be* socially constructed/periperformed but *feel* like objective reality, one is also philosophically unable to convince "them" that one's own periperformativist account of reality is the most realistic explanatory model we have.

The attraction of the research on the Capgras delusion for me is that it offers a powerful neuroscience explanation of that "feeling of reality": the analytical work done by the fusiform face area (FFA) is roughly similar to the abstract humanistic model of social construction *without* an explanation of what makes such "constructions" as face recognition feel real, and the emotional "glow" of familiarity – the Feeling of the Familiar – that is disrupted by Capgras syndrome offers a useful neurological differentiation between things that feel real and things that don't.

In order to explain the phenomenon of *shared/performed* reality-construction, however, it is not enough to study the neural functioning of individuals: one needs social neuroscience. As Insel (2010, 768) writes:

> Social neuroscience has come a long way in a short time. Two decades ago, a gap existed between behavioral neuroscience, systems neuroscience, behavioral ecology, and social psychology. Today, the field of social neuroscience fills this gap with abundance: social neuroscience now has its own journals, textbooks, societies, and, according to PubMed, nearly 3000 research papers (as of February 22, 2010). Much of this stunning growth has been driven by human neuroimaging studies seeking the neural correlates of psychological processes, from face perception to social preferences.

The Damasio team has been involved in this effort right from the start; indeed their first published proposal of the somatic-marker hypothesis, one year before that term first appeared in a title ("Somatic Markers and the Guidance of Behavior: Theory and Preliminary Testing," Damasio et al. 1991), came in an article titled "Individuals with Sociopathic Behavior Caused by Frontal Damage Fail to Respond Autonomically to Social Stimuli" (Damasio et al. 1990a), published exactly two decades before Insel's 2010 remark about "two decades ago," and it was explicitly social in its orientation. This is the article's abstract:

> Following damage to ventromedial frontal cortices, adults with previously normal personalities develop defects in decision-making and planning that are especially revealed in an abnormal social conduct. The defect repeatedly leads to negative personal consequences. The physiopathology of this disorder is an enigma. We propose that the defect is due to an inability to activate somatic states linked to punishment and reward, that were previously experienced in association with specific social situations, and that must be reactivated in connection with anticipated outcomes of response options. During the processing that follows the perception of a social event, the experience of certain anticipated outcomes of response options would be marked

> by the reactivation of an appropriate somatic state. Failure to reactivate pertinent somatic markers would deprive the individual of an automatic device to signal ultimately deleterious consequences relative to responses that might nevertheless bring immediate reward (or, alternatively, signal ultimately advantageous outcomes relative to responses that might bring immediate pain). As an example, activation of somatic markers would (1) force attention to future negative consequences, permitting conscious suppression of the responses leading to them and deliberate selection of biologically advantageous responses, and (2) trigger non-conscious inhibition of response states by engagement of subcortical neurotransmitter systems linked to appetitive behaviors. An investigation of this theory in patients with frontal damage reveals that their autonomic responses to socially meaningful stimuli are indeed abnormal, suggesting that such stimuli fail to activate somatic states at the most basic level. On the contrary, elementary unconditioned stimuli (e.g. a loud noise) produce normal autonomic responses.

Note there the explanatory gap toward which Insel points: "The physiopathology of this disorder is an enigma." Damasio and his colleagues "*propose* that the defect is due to an inability to activate somatic states linked to punishment and reward" – that would be the somatic-marker *hypothesis* – but of course that is still just a proposal, just a hypothesis. Above all, they still lack an explanation for the dissemination of somatic states through a population – for how else would those "somatic states [be] *linked* to punishment and reward"? What would "link" them, if not some sort of mimetic dissemination/circulation system?

It is not until the late 1990s that the Damasio group begins to integrate the mirror-neuron research coming out of Italy (Di Pellegrino et al. 1992; Gallese et al. 1996; Rizzolatti et al. 1996) into their studies of the ventromedial frontal cortices, and thereby to suggest ways in which "somatic states" are linked socially to group values regulating what I call the "ecotic" morality of approved vs. disapproved behaviors, and thus "the experience of certain anticipated outcomes of response options," including "punishment and reward." The Rizzolatti team's discovery of the mirror neurons in the late 1980s was the turning point in the move from behavioral to social neuroscience: now, finally, it became possible to track the mimetic *sharing* of somatic markers throughout a group. As I have noted in earlier essays, my reformulation of these developments for the medical humanities works on four levels:

1. *Somatic markers* are the autonomic nervous system's reminders of lessons learned through experience, stored in the ventromedial frontal cortices and represented in pleasurable or painful somatic responses. Because they are stored and activated in more or less stable ways – stabilized by experience – they also tend to stabilize the values and value-driven inclinations they signal in each individual.
2. *Somatic mimesis* is the simulation of somatic markers (and other somatic states) from body to body through the mirror-neuron system, based on

visual, auditory, or narrated evidence. Because the somatic markers that are thus shared have a stabilizing effect on each individual's perception of true and false and right and wrong, that stabilizing effect is also shared throughout the group.

3 The *somatic exchange* is the almost instantaneous circulation of regulatory somatic mimeses through an entire group. This is the "neurocultural" stabilization of group norms.

4 An *icosis* or *ecosis* is a socioaffective ecology of value (good and bad, honor and dishonor, glory and shame, approval and disapproval) that turns the somatic exchange into a collective engine of reality-construction/-periperformance (icosis) and morality-construction/-periperformance (ecosis).

How then might we apply that four-tier model to the reformulation of hermeneutics – say, Herder's principle that you must "feel yourself into everything" – as a social ecology, something that might be studied through social neuroscience? Perhaps something like this:

1 *Somatic markers.* The feelings you have about texts/people/events in the world are not random turbulences in your rational assessment of reality: they are socialized responses coded neurally to "mark" your orientation to this or that behavioral option positively or negatively, based on past experience. Social feelings, in other words, are such useful channels of interpretation because as somatic markers they guide the way we think.

2 *Somatic mimesis.* Your ability to "feel your way into" a text may feel like divination – mystical or nonmystical guessing – but it is actually conditioned by our hardwired tendency to simulate other people's body states. Normals do this "automatically" (unconsciously) with people they either know well or see and hear physically; transferring that mirroring ability to the reading of a written text requires considerable practice. Somatic markers are not by nature private experiences: they are by default shared with other people mimetically, in the sense that your body simulates their somatic markers and other somatic states, and their bodies simulate yours. This means that you can to a very high degree "read their minds," as Ickes (1997; Ickes and Aronson 2003) claims. This is the social neuroscience of empathy. But it also means that your ability to read (bodies-becoming-)minds is itself conditioned somatomimetically: you learn how to read other people by simulating not just their body states but the group's somatic markers guiding the reading of body states. Just as it is possible to block other people's "default" ability to read your mind, by developing a "poker face" (or what we might want to call a "poker body": gestural and postural blank pages), or by performing a misleading verbal/bodily edifice (lying, misdirecting, spinning, etc.), and just as such bodily defenses are fragile and vulnerable to collapse, so too is it possible for a writer to conceal his or her intentions in a written text – but it is very difficult to conceal them completely. A good deal of literary criticism and philosophical/theoretical deconstruction is devoted to reading past obfuscations to what the critic or theorist *feels* is the author's true meaning.

3 *Somatic exchange.* In face-to-face encounters, the somatic exchange involves the internalization/simulation of other people's body language as your own body states and the externalization/display of your body states as body language for other people to "read" and simulate. In textual hermeneutics this internalization/externalization cycle becomes the internalization of prosody and other stylistic features as feeling and the externalization of feeling as interpretation. When Herder and Schleiermacher and other early hermeneutical theorists insist that "feeling" must always be accompanied by "research," too, the idea is that "feeling your way" into a single author's text is actually a collective enterprise: you are reading not just that one author but a whole textual conversation, a whole collection of interlocutions as feelings-becoming-texts-becoming-feelings-becoming-interpretations-becoming-texts.

4 *Icosis/ecosis.* Somatic exchanges do not consist of whatever evaluative affects specific groups happen to be circulating at any given moment: somatic exchanges strive to *organize* evaluative somatic mimeses normatively, which is to say, strive to get all of their members to feel the same way about things. Hermeneutics, in other words, is not just a feeling-based channel of interpretation; it is a group *regulation* of interpretation. Hermeneusis-as-icosis is a normative plausibilization of felt values, circulated as "truths" or "realities" through a group. Hermeneusis-as-ecosis is a normative communalization of felt values, circulated as "morals" or "ethics" through a group.

But note that this is all *normal* hermeneusis – and as Sakai Naoki would insist, that hermeneutical normativity will tend to congeal into the regime of homolingual address, in which we are taught to "plausibilize" or icotize the supposed "reality" that we all converse easily and automatically with other native speakers of our first language and cannot communicate at all with foreigners. The regime of homolingual address is specifically an icotic regime. It is icotically regimented, in the sense that its members come to take its ideological norms to be a "natural" "human" reality, and to ignore – not-see, not-hear, not-think – any evidence that would tend to undermine the regime.

The bulk of the essay, however, was devoted to a discussion of potentially counternormative ("heterolingual") Feelings-becoming-Thinkings, or feeling-based hermeneutics. The Feeling(-becoming-Thinking) of the Foreign, emerging out of Schleiermacher's 1813 Academy address on the different methods of translating, was the first cautious foray into the counternormative realm of heterolinguality: it is not only possible, Schleiermacher was arguing, but *desirable* to simulate the Feeling of the Foreign in the translation of foreign texts into the local language, thus signaling the difference between locally and nonlocally sourced texts. The other Feelings-becoming-Thinkings in the essay, of the Strange, the Alien, and the Alien Hand, constituted a series of progressively more counternormative/heterolingual hermeneusis – but note that the gradated scale of "progressively" implies not only a shifting middle ground between extremes (homo-/heterolingual, normative/counternormative) but the regulatory impulse to *manage* the shifting of that middle ground. And certainly the Feelings of the Foreign and the Strange seek precisely a managed middleness that heterolingualizes but still *makes sense;*

and it is not until the Feeling of the Alien that we encounter a deliberate attempt to relinquish sense-making, and the (Feeling of the) Alien Hand is an irruption of senselessness out of the ruins of homolingual automatization.

Notes

1 Arguably the first "hermeneutical" study was Aristotle's *On Interpretation,* the second text from his *Organon* – in Greek, *peri hermeneias.* Modern hermeneutics arises out of, and in part responds to, the long patristic and scholastic tradition of biblical exegesis; its "founder" is variously identified as Johann Gottfried Herder, Friedrich Schleiermacher, and Wilhelm Dilthey.

2 Three other things that don't concern me here, because I have dealt with them elsewhere: (1: Robinson 2013c, 148–65) the nationalism of Schleiermacher's basic preference for (2d), and (2: Robinson 1996, 176–81) the scary moralism and (3: Robinson 2013c, ch. 2) appalling logic that he mobilizes in support of his nationalistic agenda. The first is the fact that for Schleiermacher, German readers should always feel the foreignness of the translated works they read, so that they never fail to notice and respect the superiority of works originally written in German; the second is his sick "joke" that trying to write well in a foreign language would be "eine frevelhafte und magische Kunst. . ., wie das Doppeltgehen, womit der Mensch nicht nur der Geseze der Natur zu spotten, sondern auch andere zu verwirren gedächte“ (88)/"a wicked and magical art akin to going doubled, an attempt at once to flout the laws of nature and to perplex others" (236); and the third is the mind-boggling absurdity of his claim that because no one can *write* well in a foreign language, and therefore also that no one can *translate* well into a foreign language, it is also impossible to simulate in the target reader the feeling that s/he is *reading* well in a foreign language (~~3a~~>~~3b~~>~~3c~~>3d).

3 In the discussion that follows, my romanization differs slightly from the American Library Association/Library of Congress romanization Harte uses. In ALA/LC, ё is romanized "e" and щ is romanized "shch": thus Крученых is Kruchenykh, щыл is "shchyl," and Убешщур is "Ubeshshchur." In Russian ё is pronounced not [e] but [jo:] and щ is pronounced not as a voiceless palato-alveolar sibilant fricative [ʃ]/sh followed by a voiceless palato-alveolar sibilant affricate [tʃ]/ch but as a voiceless alveolo-palatal fricative [ɕ]/shh. As a result of the ALA/LC romanizations, English speakers pronounce the surname of the Soviet Premier from 1958 to 1964, Хрущёв, as CROOSH-chev; in Russian his name is pronounced hru-SHOAF. To avoid that kind of mispronunciation, I prefer to use the GOST 7.79 (2002) romanization system, which renders ё as "yo" and щ as "shh." Thus Крученых is Kruchyonykh, щыл is "shhyl," and Убешщур is "Ubeshshhur." The extended fricative in that last should be pronounced like the sound of the air being let out of a tire, with a deep mouth-pursed sh gradually modulating into a high mouth-wide sh.

4 Lutterbie (2013, 109) "quotes" this exact passage, verbatim, without quotation marks, as if he had written it himself. He does change Iverson and Thelen's letters (a, b, c, d) to lowercase Roman numerals (i, ii, iiii, iv).

5 Of course, the philosophical transformation of 仁/*ren* by Kongzi into something like the Golden Rule – the expansion of self to encompass the other, or at least to prefeel the other powerfully enough to anticipate the other's preferences and feel inclined to honor them – does not exactly render the "benevolence" translation tradition incorrect or obsolete: a person who is inclined to do unto others as s/he would have others do unto her or him is likely to behave in benevolent ways. But it does tend to render the core "niceness" sense of benevolence in English a secondary byproduct of transfeeling projected outwards.

Conclusion: The humanities of translational medicine

The performative phenomenology of (self-)care

For health-care professionals, translational medicine (TM) covers the translation of medical research into clinical trials, and clinically trialed devices and drugs into patient care. The goal is healing the sick and injured in the most effective way possible. A medical humanities approach to translational medicine (TM+MH=TMH) would want to add that its goal is healing the sick and the injured in the most *humane* way possible – but of course humane patient care does not trump effective medical treatment. It's not a zero-sum game: effectiveness vs. humaneness. If humane care can be superadded to effective care, that's a win-win. If to achieve effectiveness a certain modicum of humaneness has to be sacrificed, that isn't ideal, but it still beats ineffective care.

As I mentioned in the Preface, I am not a health-care professional, and so tend to come at the TMH dynamic from a different angle – namely, the patient's. From the patient's point of view, patient care is the *whole* medical experience. And it makes a significant difference whether care at the hands of the medical profession is effective, of course – it is important to get well – but of equal importance is how *humane* that care feels. A suffering person seeks medical care in a state of extreme vulnerability, often existential dread. Important as a cure is in that state, human love and support may be even more important. Certainly a cure is never guaranteed, and in the end of every life medical care ultimately fails – and that inevitability of failure makes the precarious but all-important success of human love and support that much more important.

In section 2.2.7 I paused toward the end of the literary history of translationality I was tracking to argue that Manuel Portela's Portuguese translation of Sterne's *Tristram Shandy* was a similar kind of TMH: Sterne first translates the experience of dying into a performative phenomenology for his reader to experience in English; Portela then translates that primary translation into a performative phenomenology for his target reader to experience in Portuguese. "Like a medical clinician," I wrote there, "Portela must do more than diagnose: he must devise a strategy by which the 'patient' might be helped to adapt to and so enter and engage and embody a transformed future."

Now let us begin to draw the various threads of this series of essays together by considering a humanistic approach to TM more carefully. Specifically, I want to explore the experiential translations that humans who are not health-care professionals make in order to help build humane support systems for (coping with) care – and especially self-care, since, as medical humanists know, only self-care is sustainable. Patient care that seeks to repair a meat-machine that lacks all agency, lacks subjectivity, lacks affect, lacks fears and hopes and plans and hope and despair, may repair the machine temporarily, but will not heal it sustainably. Patients who take care of themselves, who care for their physical bodies through diet and exercise and their affective bodies through communal support, are more likely to survive longer than patients who take no responsibility at all for their own mental, emotional, and physical health – who only trust the doctors passively. What series of humanistic medical "translations" can get us to that sort of sustainability?

The most powerful MH study I've ever seen does not mention MH at all. It appears in Nicola Shaughnessy's 2013 edited essay collection *Affective Performance and Cognitive Science: Body, Brain and Being* – which of course makes it a better fit with my prevailing concerns in this book than studies more specifically targeting future health-care professionals. The article is "Between Faulty Intellects and Failing Bodies: An Economy of Reciprocity in *Wit* and *33 Variations*" by Naomi Rokotnitz, a lecturer in the Department of Theatre Arts at Tel-Aviv University; it deals with theatrical performances of two plays with similar medical themes, Margaret Edson's *Wit* (1993) and Moises Kaufman's *33 Variations* (2008). Rokotnitz (2013, 118) summarizes the similarities between the two plays:

> Both dramatise the last few weeks in the life of a successful academic who is dying of an incurable disease. Edson's protagonist, Vivian Bearing, professor of literature, and Kaufman's protagonist, Katherine Brandt, professor of musicology, are both world-renowned authorities in their respective fields of study; their intellectual prowess is unequivocal. However, both are brisk, disciplined and demanding, having dedicated their lives to the study of art, and yet restricted their engagement with it to critical analysis. Both women remained dispassionate for most of their lives, having deliberately shunned emotional ties and intimacy with others. The advent of her illness propels each stridently independent woman into a state of dependency upon others. In addition to contending with ever-increasing pain, physical disintegration, invasive clinical examinations, and fear of death, each woman is also forced to reflect upon her professional and her personal life choices, and upon the dynamics of intra- and inter-corporeality. Biology, psychology, technology and art are intertwined in both the subject matter of each play and its dramatic presentation, creating a productive economy of reciprocity.

In other words, both plays are trained dramatically on a scene from TM, the translation of clinical trials into patient care – but specifically a *humanistic* version of TM, with primary attention to the phenomenology of patient care, which is to say, *how it feels to the patient* to be ill or injured and dependent on others, and, in these two cases, dying.

And indeed Rokotnitz's statement of her approach is a cognitive-science account of this humanistic/hermeneutic phenomenology: "My interest here," she writes, "is primarily the ano[e]tic, pre-reflective, embodied dimensions of affect, and the crucial role these play in determining and changing both somatic identity and philosophical (autonoetic) conceptions" (118). In other words, her model is very close to what I have since Robinson (1991) been calling somatic theory, but with one key element missing – more on that in a moment. For now, note that her nominalizations – "the . . . dimensions of affect" that determine and change "somatic identity and philosophical (autonoetic) conceptions" – would appear to imply that those determinations channel a depersonalized force ("dimensions") without human agency. I find that phrasing problematic, because it seems suspiciously complicit with the dehumanizing tendencies of both traditional TM and the two academic protagonists in the plays she is studying. Rokotnitz seems to be hinting that she is not interested in *how it feels to be living in a diseased and dying body,* let alone *how dealing kinesthetically and emotionally with illness and the approach of death changes your sense of who you are* (repersonalized paraphrases of those abstract nominalizations above). She *is* interested in those more personalized experiences, of course; specifically, she is interested in how drama situates us vicariously as viewers (and even as readers) in the embodied phenomenology of those changes. It's just that academic writing, especially when it draws on the natural sciences, seems to require this kind of rhetorical depersonalization. Might I humbly submit that scholars pushing this particular interdisciplinary envelope might want to rethink their rhetorical strategies as well?

She goes on: "Filtering my analysis of the plays through current research into embodied receptiveness, empathetic 'motor equivalence', and physiotherapy, I explore how dramatic performance may demonstrate the value of bodily forms of apprehension and communication" (118) – though her actual analysis exceeds this rather cautious statement of intent in interesting and significant ways. She doesn't just explore "how dramatic performance may *demonstrate* the value of bodily forms of apprehension and communication"; she is mainly interested in how dramatic performance *embodies* the "forms of apprehension and communication" she tracks, how through "empathetic 'motor equivalence'" we actually *experience* the phenomenological hermeneusis of end-of-life embodiment acted out onstage by the two leading actors.

The trajectory Rokotnitz follows from *Wit* to *33 Variations* is in fact a very MH one, moving us strategically from a cautionary "before" to a more hopeful "after": the patient-unfriendly patient care dramatized in *Wit* is precisely the kind of horror story adduced by MH scholar-teachers by way of warning future health-care professionals of the *need* for a humanistic/humanizing approach to medicine; the patient-friendly patient care dramatized in *33 Variations* might well work as a kind of MH poster child. This trajectory makes Rokotnitz's article an exemplary MH text. For my TM purposes here in the Conclusion, however, I only really need her remarks on *Wit,* and will limit my commentary to that section of her piece.

Most of the dramatic action in *Wit* consists of dialogues between Vivian, the patient, and the oncologist's "ambitious research fellow, Jason" (119), for whom getting to know patients as people is a "colossal waste of time for researchers"

(Edson 1993/2012, 35; quoted in Rokotnitz 2013, 119). Jason is a former student of Vivian's, and a significant part of Edson's dramatic strategy in the play is to have Jason's aloof coldness mirror Vivian's:

> Over-empathising with patients may present doctors from maintaining the distance necessary to treat them, and a certain dulling of emotions is sometimes necessary for decisive actions. Nonetheless, through experiencing Jason's professional competence and his empathetic incompetence, Vivian recognizes her own deficiencies: while she was a rigorous scholar, she was deaf to her students' personal pleas, remaining entirely unmoved by their individual or collective troubles, just as she brushed aside Donne's. Her strictly logical view of justice therefore determines that, to her mind, she cannot justifiably expect kindness now that she is in need.
>
> (120)

The leading edge of what interests Rokotnitz about this dramatic presentation is that Edson doesn't spell out for her audiences that this unemotional/detached approach to the world is ultimately destructive: she lets them figure it out for themselves. And, Rokotnitz insists, she apparently *trusts* them to figure it out for themselves: "This sophisticated dramaturgy-of-affect allows the playwright to remain – as her title suggests – in the realm of wit, while simultaneously undermining her characters, demonstrating instead the benefits of embodied communication" (121). The pressing question for Rokotnitz, however, is *how* she manages this: how it is possible for a playwright not only to get audiences to figure out her "message" or "point" in the play, but to trust them to do so. It is a truism of playwriting that too much explicit guidance – writing "on the nose," as the jargon has it, without much subtext – is a bad thing, a hallmark of bad playwriting; but how exactly, in cognitive neuroscience terms, does "good playwriting" work? How do what Grice would call the "implicatures" of subtle playwriting get through, come across, make contact, hit home?

Rokotnitz's answer to that invokes the mirror-neuron system:

> Of particular importance to this present study is research into our inborn inclination to imitate, indeed simulate, actions we observe others perform. This capacity for "motor equivalence" [Thompson 2007, 119] allows us to utilize our shared motor schemata to interpret the actions of others – in life and on stage. The meanings of a dramatic performance arise from its embodied effects just as much as its discursive registers, and performative communication depends upon empathetic resonance. . . . I adhere to the definition of empathy as "a complex experience of another person through cognitive, evaluative and affective processes" [Gregg and Siegworth 2002, 5–6] allowing us to resonate with another agent through body-based simulation which provides "experiential insights into other minds" [Massumi 1980, xvi] as well as "pain, touch, or tickling" [Gregg and Siegworth 2002, 6].

> Mapping the neural correlates of this resonance corresponds in interesting ways with mirror-neuron studies and provides evidence that empathy is an innate capacity, hardwired into our cognitive architecture.
>
> (121–22)

Edson does not have to *write* (explicitate) the implicatures of Vivian's and Jason's inability to connect on a human level, "on the nose": the audience picks those implicatures up from the actors' body language, through that innate "motor equivalence," which resonates empathically, through what Antonio Damasio (1999, 80) calls the "as-if body loop," or through what William Ickes calls "accurate mind-reading" (Ickes 1997; Ickes and Aronson 2003) but might more accurately be called "body-becoming-mind reading" (see also Tomasello 2008, 321 and 335–37, for "recursive mindreading"). The social neuroscience of empathy is rife with evidence-based debates over whether what the audience feels while simulating the actors' pain-based body states onstage is only "affective pain" (Singer et al. 2004) or affective *and* sensory pain (Loggia et al. 2008); but they do, social neuroscientists agree, "feel the pain." Rokotnitz also notes that "emotional correlation does not equal emotional contagion. Although humans have 'the tendency to automatically mimic or synchronize facial expressions, vocalizations, postures and movements with those of another person' [Gregg and Siegworth 2002, 7–8], empathy does not by any means guarantee sympathy, as the history of torture attests" (122): not all audience members will respond with the same quality or quality of empathy to the bodies onstage. "Personal dispositions to empathy vary," she admits; but she then quickly goes on to assure us that "Edson can trust that, despite Vivian and Jason's emotional inhibitions, audience members will respond – through our mirror-resonance systems – to the physical cues of the performance" (122).

But this is too simple. There are actually at least four "translations" – in the TM sense of that word, in this case phenomenological translations of pain and suffering – involved in this theatrical mirroring process, and Rokotnitz only addresses the fourth, [4] from actors' pain to audience's pain, and only very vaguely hints at the full range of potential turbulence in that translation alone (the critical debates over Aristotle's theory of catharsis would contain an introductory sampling of that turbulence). The third is [3] from cancer patients' pain to actors' pain – or, for Megan Cole playing Vivian Bearing in the 1995 production of *Wit* at the South Coast Repertory Theater in Costa Mesa, California, what would have been known as "getting into character." This is a considerably more fraught translational process than Rokotnitz indicates in her article, and fraught in at least five different ways:

a Translating (3) "naturally arising" body states in "real people" into simulated body states onstage requires what is known as "good acting"; and "bad acting" tends to generate another kind of (4) actor-to-audience pain-translation, from weak imitation to strong irritation, or perhaps at best carefully suppressed embarrassment for the actors (another kind of empathic response).

b (3a) is complicated by the fact that there are theoretical and directorial differences in preferred acting styles. The two most commonly known are Stanislavskian "Method Acting," which implicitly undergirds the thinking behind (3a), and the Brechtian epic-theatrical "Verfremdungseffekt"/estrangement effect, which explicitly *rejects and proscribes* the theory and practice of (3a). Like the (Schleiermacherian/Shklovskian) translational stylization of the Feeling of the Foreign/Strange/Alien in Essay 3, which can easily be mistaken for "bad translation," so too can the (Shklovskian/Brechtian) translational stylization of the Feeling of the Foreign/Strange/Alien onstage be easily mistaken for "bad acting."

c The (3) "natural"-to-simulated translation of body states never produces an exact one-to-one correspondence. In the terms I developed in Essay 2, "motor equivalence" is never objective equivalence (cloning). It is always transformational, or what we might call "performational" – steeped in translationality and (peri)performativity. Acting always *stylizes* body states. This is a big part of what we call "theatricality."

d Following out of (3c), in the *Rhetoric* (2.8.12–13, 1386a19–24) Aristotle notes that it is typically easier for (4) an audience to respond empathically to emotions in an oration (or, by extension, onstage) than it is for "real people" to respond to the real-life emotions simulated by orators (or actors), because the performance (*hupokrisis*/"acting, delivery") tends to purify real-life complexities out of relationships. (When it's your own mother dying you have a lifetime of relationship complexities clogging or churning up your empathic response; when it's an imaginary mother dying onstage you are more fully and simply able to simulate the vicarious sufferer's body states.)

e Another complication attendant on (3cd) is that we tend to stylize the body states we imitate in "real life" too. This is more or less the problematic that Jacques Derrida (1977/1988) addresses in his deconstruction of Austin on the performative: that it is only because we can reperform or reiterate performatives, and *change* them slightly in so doing, that we can communicate at all. Iterability as the repeat performability/stylizability of performatives is endemic to all human social interaction. We are all actors and audience members. We all reperform other people's body states. We are all onstage when we are in the audience, and audience members when we are onstage. We all try to be (3a) "good" actors, but our efforts in that direction are (3b) often hit or miss, trial and error, directed at a variety of purposes that are often not clear to us as we act, and (3cd) we always iterate past performances in new ways.

The second translation in the humanistic/hermeneutic/phenomenological/performative TMH scene that I am outlining here is [2] from the playwright through the director to the actors. Actors don't just (3) imitate/simulate "real-life" body states, with all the complexities outlined in (3abcde): they build their characters out of the words written by the playwright, and they are guided in that character-building by the director, often with the playwright in attendance at rehearsals. The director translates the playwright's words for the actors; the playwright, explicitly if s/he is present at rehearsals but implicitly even if s/he is not, translates the words on the page for the director.

To underscore the importance of this (2) translation from playwright to director to actors, note that *Wit* won a Pulitzer Prize for its powerful dramatization of the human pathos of dying – but the "pathos" of that dramatization was not "in" the script. It was a product of (2) the translation of the words on the page into acted body states onstage. And those words could have been translated/dramatized differently. They could have been played as farce – as slapstick, say, with pratfalls, or what the *commedia dell'arte* called *lazzi,* in the style of a Dario Fo play or a *Monty Python's Flying Circus* sketch, or as a comedy of manners, in the style of *Much Ado About Nothing* (Shakespeare, c. 1599), or *The Way of the World* (Congreve, 1700), or *She Stoops to Conquer* (Goldsmith, 1773), or *The Importance of Being Earnest* (Wilde 1895), or any of the contemporary sitcoms that follow those models. I quoted the "colossal waste of time for a researcher" remark Jason makes, above; imagine that scene played by the Marx Brothers:

JASON: **(playing an up-tempo ragtime piece on a golden grand piano, leaning over the keyboard in a standing position in tails and a top hat, with a short unlit cigar gripped between bared teeth)**. I'm simplifying for you.

VIVIAN: **(draped languidly over the piano top in her Hello Kitty hospital gown, her blank smile matching the cartoon's on her gown)**. Thank you. (**She bats her lashes and honks a Harpo horn**.)

JASON: **(jumping with feet splayed up onto the piano bench, without missing a note)**. We're supposed to.

VIVIAN: **(to the tune of the music he's playing, belting the four syllables out to the back rows)**. Bedside manner.

JASON: Yeah **(arching his back to spit the cigar high in the air)**, there's a whole course on it in med school. It's required. Colossal **(plays a dramatic suspended chord)** waste **(plays another suspended chord)** of time **(plays a third suspended chord)** for researchers. (*He* **plays a showy arpeggio, blows the audience a kiss, gives a sly wink and then an exaggerated moue of surprise, doffs his top hat and bows deeply, revealing a bald spot on top of his head with BOO! written on it in red felt-tip pen, and** *turns to go.*) (Edson 1993/2012, 35; bolded text added by DR)

"Translated" (staged) that way, I think it's fair to say, it would not have won the Pulitzer.

This line of thinking seems to demean Edson's powerful one-act, perhaps – even to profane it. There is something sacred, taboo, about dying. We are not supposed to joke about it. The idea of introducing *lazzi* and anarchistically "witty" Marx Brothers gags into *Wit* seems shocking. But of course the impulse to protect the sacredness of a specific dramatic/theatrical tradition of "translating" (staging) a given play is what generates the "deadly theater"

Peter Brook (1968/2008) describes: Chekhov, say, performed exactly the same way for a century and more, for people who need things to stay the same, because things that change are so terrifying. Staging *Hamlet* with one-for-one gender reversals, or an all-dwarf cast, or all actors playing naked, or the like is the kind of radical "revival" translation of a classic play that seeks to bring deadly theater back to (new) life.[1]

What possible translation is left to go at the top of the flowchart, then? I suggest that it is [1] the socio-regulatory effect of icosis/ecosis – the translation of icotic/ecotic impulses by and for and as our inclinations to act in certain ways. This is in fact the element that I hinted early on was missing from Rokotnitz's model: when she writes about the "ano[e]tic, pre-reflective, embodied dimensions of affect, and the crucial role these play in determining and changing both somatic identity and philosophical (autonoetic) conceptions" (118), I think she means something like the icotic "determinations" of reality and identity that I have theorized – but she has no provision in her model for a socio-regulatory role for those "embodied dimensions" to play in determining such things. This makes those determinations seem somewhat random – as if our "somatic identity and philosophical (autonoetic) conceptions" were shaped and changed by whatever "embodied dimensions of affect" happened to be coming down the pike at any given moment. She can't possibly mean for that "crucial role" to be as random as it appears here; but she fails to account for any kind of social ("neurocultural") guiding force.

Other terms for what I'm setting at the top of the hierarchy would include the internalization of mastery (Nietzsche), *das Man* (Heidegger), structures of feeling (Williams), the political unconscious (Jameson), and so on. I envision it as *any* kind of internalized cultural normativity – not just Gramscian hegemony, for example, at the very top, and not necessarily a single normativity unifying an entire national or macrospatial culture, or even one dividing a large-scale culture in half (liberalism vs. conservatism). It could be the deep-seated and overlapping prejudices of a racial culture (racism), class culture (classism), sex/gender culture (sexism, homophobia), etc. It could be dominant orientations toward altruism and self-sacrifice. It could be the ethos of a family, a small workplace, or the regulars at a bar or café.

Just how much is at stake in this top-level "translation" can be demonstrated by a look at the complaint lodged by Martin Welton (2013), drawing on Ruth Leys (2011), against affect theorists who want to "reduce" affect to "autonomic responses that are held to occur below the threshold of consciousness and cognition and to be rooted in the body" (Leys 437; quoted in Welton 160). Welton says that he shares with Leys "a sense of unease in the reductive move by which affect becomes shorn of intentional content in its reduction to pre-cognitive bodily states" (160) – bodily states, in Leys's words, that are "independent of consciousness and the mind's control" (443; quoted in Welton 160).

Leys calls this set of assumptions "the Basic Emotions paradigm" (439); she attributes its ascendancy to the pioneering work of Silvan S. Tomkins (1962–1992) and his student Paul Ekman (1985), but insists that Joseph E. LeDoux

(1984, 1996) and Antonio R. Damasio (1994, 1999, 2003, 2010) are also proponents of the approach, and indeed argues that, despite a smattering of voices raised against it, "the Basic Emotions paradigm continues to dominate the research field" (440). Key to her critique is the fact that affective neuroscientists like Damasio and LeDoux (she could have included Jaak Panksepp 1998 in her indictment) tend to focus on "emotions as comprising six or seven or eight or nine 'affect programs' located subcortically in the brain and defined in evolutionary terms as universal or pancultural categories or 'natural kinds'" (438); while these "basic emotions" do "minimally include the emotions of fear, anger, disgust, joy, sadness, and surprise," she charges, they "are viewed as genetically hard-wired, reflexlike responses, each of which manifests itself in distinct physiological-autonomic and behavioral patterns of response, especially in characteristic facial expressions" (438). And indeed one could easily cite textual corroboration for her charges; in Damasio (2010, 35), for example, we find descriptions of "affect" in single-celled organisms like amoebae and paramecia as a hardwired *desire* for survival:

> Deprived of conscious knowledge, deprived of access to the byzantine devices of deliberation available in our brains, the single cell seems to have an attitude: it wants to live out its prescribed genetic allowance. Strange as it may seem, the want, and all that is necessary to implement it, *precedes* explicit knowledge and deliberation regarding life conditions, since the cell clearly has neither. The nucleus and the cytoplasm interact and carry out complex computations aimed at keeping the cell alive. They deal with the moment-to-moment problems posed by the living conditions and adapt the cell to the situation in a survivable manner. Depending on the environmental conditions, they rearrange the position and distribution of molecules in their interior, and they change the shape of subcomponents, such as microtubules, in an astounding display of precision. They respond under duress and under nice treatment, too.

But basing a global assessment of Damasio's approach to the emotions on passages like this would be extremely selective citing. As a neo-Jamesian neuroscientist, Damasio is interested not just in these "basic emotions" (which he calls "primary emotions": happiness, sadness, fear, anger, surprise, disgust, etc.) but in an even lower level of emotional response, which he calls "background emotions" (well-being or unease), and, more to the point, a higher level of emotional response as well, namely "secondary emotions," which he also characterizes as "social emotions": embarrassment, shame, and guilt, contempt and indignation, sympathy and compassion, awe, wonder, gratitude, and pride, jealousy and envy. And these social emotions only become possible through what William James (1890/1950) teaches Damasio to call a feeling-emotion loop: affects-as-feelings mapping affects-as-emotions and other body states. What a feeling will generate specifically, Damasio's team has found in the lab, is both a series of mental representations or mappings of body states and a style and speed by which those mappings are brought into consciousness. The former aspect (representation) pushes toward the "mental," toward "thoughts" and "ideas," while the latter (style and speed) charges the thoughts so generated with what still seems like the submental or bodily "experience" that we typically associate with feelings.

The emotion-inducing event may be feeling-laden thoughts or images of your own humiliation (generating embarrassment), a competitor's humiliation (generating contempt), your own triumph (generating pride), your unfair treatment at the hands of another (generating indignation), loss of a love object to a competitor (generating jealousy), the harm you have caused someone else (generating guilt or shame), someone else's suffering as if it were your own (generating sympathy or compassion), or someone else's good fortune which you wish were your own (generating envy). (See Damasio 1994, 131–39; 1999, 281–89; 2003, 44–49. This model is also, of course, very close to Aristotle's account of the emotions in Book II of the *Rhetoric;* see Robinson 2016a, 126–41, for discussion.)

Not only that: what Damasio (2010, ch. 5) finds emerging out of feelings mapping lower body states, especially the appetites (I feel hungry, I feel thirsty) and emotions (I feel angry, I feel sad), is *a conscious sense of the self that feels these things.* This is Damasio's affective-becoming-cognitive model of the origins of consciousness. Indeed feelings map thoughts as well: I feel certain that I'm right; I feel there's something missing in my argumentation here; I feel this draft is now ready to send off. Damasio's somatic-marker hypothesis arises out of precisely this intertwining of affect and cognition in all human (and indeed mammalian) decision-making and intentionality.

Now compare this model with Leys's caricature: "On this view, whose origins are frequently traced back to the work of Charles Darwin and William James, the affects can and do combine with the cognitive processing systems of the brain, but they are essentially separate from those" (437). It is difficult to believe, reading an assessment like this, that Leys has actually read Damasio. Where exactly in Damasio's contributions to neuroscience is the "essential separation" she imagines? Where for that matter is it in LeDoux, or his Ph.D. supervisor Gazzaniga?[2] If "on this view . . . the affects can and do combine with the cognitive processing systems of the brain," could the "essentially" in "essentially separate from those" possibly be Leys's essentializing/stabilizing attempt to binarize what these affect theorists in fact find complexly and shiftingly *blending* in affective-becoming-cognitive neuroscience? Could the "separation" she attacks be an artifact of her own binary reading?

Icotic/ecotic theory takes Damasio's line of thought several steps further, suggesting, as we've seen, that somatic states are not only mirrored and simulated, as Rokotnitz agrees they are (what I call the somatic transfer, or somatic mimesis), and not only circulated mimetically and almost simultaneously through a group, as Rokotnitz does not say they are (what I call the somatic exchange), but *organized normatively.* This would be affective intentionality wielded becoming-cognitively by the group. As a result of the icotic "plausibilization" of reality and identity, for example, we *know* – though it might take us a minute to work through our icotic inclinations to an articulation of what we know – that a slapstick staging of Edson's *Wit* would be dramatistically wrong or "off": not true to "the play," or to "the reality" that the play depicts. As a result of the ecotic "moralization" of communal values, we know – though again our knowing may hover just shy of propositional articulation, unless we are pressed to verbalize it – that a slapstick staging of Edson's play would be unworthy, base, demeaning, not only of the play but of our neurocultural understanding of the experience of death and dying. As I said earlier, we know that we are not supposed to joke about death. We do it, sometimes – but we do it only in situations when we *feel* that it would be somehow socially acceptable, even perhaps that it would meet some inchoate communal need.

Something tells directors of Edson's play, in other words, that the play needs to be staged as a serious drama – not as slapstick. Edson herself may tell them that; but even in productions where she has not been present at rehearsals, or discussed it with the directors, *something* tells directors not to play it for giggles. The directors, I suggest – and perhaps even Edson herself – know how to play the piece because they are (1) translating icotic/ecotic norms into guidance for the production. Communal affective intentionality.

This (1) top-level act of translation offers a new perspective on Rokotnitz's claim, quoted earlier, that "this sophisticated dramaturgy-of-affect allows the playwright to remain – as her title suggests – in the realm of wit, while simultaneously undermining her characters, demonstrating instead the benefits of embodied communication" (121). Yes, of course Edson manages to "remain . . . in the realm of wit" on the verbal surface while subtextually "undermining her characters"; yes, working the affective dramaturgy on those two levels simultaneously is sophisticated (although on a level of sophistication that is pretty much standard among produced playwrights). What makes it work, however, is not just Edson's skill with words: it is her ability to translate complexly intertwined icotic/ecotic pressures from "the culture" *through* those words into guidance for (1) directors, (2–3) actors, and (4) audiences.

That this skill seems to Edson's admirers among theater people to be mainly verbal is only to be expected, because it channels regulatory neurocultural intentionality through (1–4) the neurophenomenology of the performative collective at a precognitive affective level of which most of us are not aware.

When the collection of humanistic texts in question is medically themed, then – as Richard Powers's *The Echo Maker* novel was in Essay 1, as Robert Burton's *Anatomy of Melancholy,* François Rabelais's *Gargantua and Pantagruel,* and Laurence Sterne's *Life and Opinions of Tristram Shandy, Gentleman* were in Essay 2, and as *Wit* and *33 Variations* are here in the Conclusion – it is tempting to map overlapping schemata of TM: [TM1] health-care professionals translating medical research into clinical trials and clinically trialed drugs and devices into patient care, and [TM2] writers, directors, actors, and audiences translating neurocultural norms into imaginative texts, texts into performances, performances into "patient care" (coping strategies) for audiences. As one might expect, given the fragility of human life, and the super-value we place on wellness and well-being, both TM schemata culminate in patient care. They take very different pathways to that destination, of course, TM1 prioritizing the medical efficacy of care, TM2 prioritizing the communal efficacy of self-care. But they are also strikingly similar. Both, after all, are top-down, moving from normativized culture down through top-flight professionals (researchers, writers, directors) through front-line practitioners (clinicians, actors) to suffering people in need of care. Both are organized by an overriding concern for the efficacy of care. They simply bring different professionalized affects to bear on the notion of efficacy.

Perhaps we can tie together my various combinatory vectors here by rethinking Roman Jakobson's (1959) famous tripartite distinction among *intralingual, interlingual,* and *intersemiotic translation.* I suggested in passing that Richard Powers's "neurological novel," *The Echo Maker,* is a kind of intersemiotic translation, in the sense that Powers reframes the narratives in one written genre (or semiotic world), popular or "narrative" neuroscience, as a narrative in a different written genre (or semiotic world), the novel. But what kind of translation is at work in translational medicine (TM)? It is similar to what medieval thinkers called the *translatio studii,* the translation of learning, also known as the transfer or transmission of knowledge – which is never a "cloning" of knowledge, of course, but always involves what I'm calling translationality: adaptation, transformation.

Thinking about that, we might want to expand Jakobson's framework by naming the sort of translation at work in TM *interepistemic translation:* translation from one "epistemic system" (George A. Miller, quoted in Gazzaniga 2015, 376) to another. But then, wouldn't the translation from cognitive neuroscience to the novel in Powers's creation of *The Echo Maker* also be an interepistemic translation? And, more radically: when Gazzaniga and his colleagues study the split-brain patients – the basic medical research that in TM is then "translated" interepistemically into clinical trials, and then on into patient care – aren't they also working to translate from the split-brain subjects' epistemic systems into the epistemic system of neuroscience? And when Gazzaniga (2015) recalls that half-century history of basic neurological research in his memoir of "a life in neuroscience," isn't he essaying a secondary interepistemic translation, from the *experience* of doing the research (lots of drudgery and social interaction punctuated by brilliant flashes of insight and discovery, backed by funding and other forms of institutional support, and networked through friends and colleagues) into a single coherent narrative that is novelistic in its form and tone?

To generalize: is the big picture of TM not in fact something like the series of interepistemic translations diagrammed in Figure 4.1?

- *ES2a to ES3a to ES4a* would be the standard trajectory for TM. Implicit in that trajectory, I'm guessing, is also a concern for the patient's *experience* of patient care *(ES4a to ES1)* – but only implicit. The insistence on taking that phenomenological extension of TM into consideration is a signal contribution of MH to TM.
- *ES1 to ES2a to ES3b* would be the series of interepistemic translations made by practicing neuroscientists (like Sacks, Ramachandran, Gazzaniga, Damasio, and Powers's Weber) who also write popular narrative neurology.
- *ES3b to ES4b* would be the translational trajectory followed by Richard Powers in creating *The Echo Maker.*

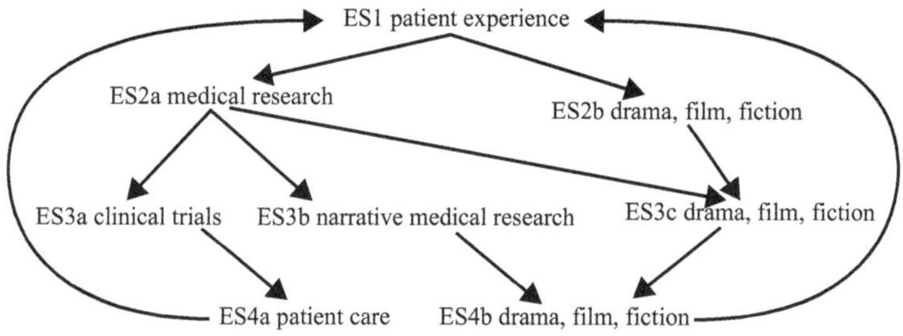

Figure. 4.1 Flowchart of translations from one Epistemic System (ES) to another in an expanded humanistic understanding of translational medicine

- *ES4a to ES1 to ES2b* would be something like the trajectory followed by Margaret Edson in writing *Wit:* before writing the play she worked in a research hospital as a unit clerk in the AIDS and cancer wing. She was not involved directly in (ES4a) patient care; but Gail Cameron (1999) reports her describing that job, and comments: "'I had such a low-level job that I saw a lot of things first hand and I was too insignificant for other people to notice.' Day to day, she observed how the nurses interacted with their patients and watched as patients relinquished much of the control they once had over their lives to hospital staff."
- *ES2a to ES3c to ES4b* would be the trajectory followed by the various interepistemic translations tracked in Essay 2: Rabelais and Burton translating medical research into literature, Sterne translating their literary TM into more literature, and so on.

What is not displayed on that line diagram, of course, is what Jakobson calls interlingual translation, or (in his gloss) "translation proper": Urquhart translating Rabelais in section 2.2.4; Portela translating Sterne in section 2.2.7; Robinson translating Kivi in 3.3.1 and Kruchyonykh in section 3.3.2, and so on. If one combinatory vector that I track through the book studies the Humanities of (Interepistemic) Medical Translation/Translational Medicine, that other one reports and speculates on the Medical Neuroscience of (Interlingual) Translational Humanities.

What both of those broad vectors share in common, of course, is translationality as transformationality: the constructivist/periperformativist realization (making-real) of our experience, which *always* changes things. I worry somewhat that readers will misread my invidious distinction (throughout section 2.3) between "objectivism" and "periperformativism" to be an attack on empirical science: if empirical science is mythologized as objectivism, as it often is in what Thomas Kuhn (1962/1970) calls "normal science," then my attacks on objectivism will be thematized as attacks on science. But I don't accept that particular myth of science. Science may be an ongoing *quest* for objective truth, but in experiential reality it is always only a series of periperformative constructions that, as Gerald

Weber discovers in *The Echo Maker*, stands far closer to the novel than it does to some pure prelapsarian "truth" in the Mind of God.

Indeed one might compare Gerald Weber's discoveries in *The Echo Maker* with, say, Michael Gazzaniga's discoveries in *Tales from Both Sides of the Brain: A Life in Neuroscience* (2015):

- arguably the discoveries about just how novelistic his scientific work has been are made not by Gerald Weber "himself" (whatever that might mean, in a novel character) but by Powers's narrator when focalized on Weber (i.e., seeing and presenting the world through Weber's consciousness);
- the discoveries Michael S. Gazzaniga makes about "a life in neuroscience" in his brilliant memoir, by contrast, are made by *him*, the author, who is also the model for *himself* as the genial, humanity-loving narrator, remembering the research done by *his earlier self*, Mike Gazzaniga, the character.

The mythic account of science would have it that the research findings reported by Gazzaniga over the half century of his career seek to "objectify" the results of the research as scientific fact. As I suggested earlier in the Conclusion, after all, in regard to Rokotnitz's depersonalizing rhetoric, that myth is built into the institutional requirements for the genre of scientific/scholarly publishing, so that we expect to find it when we read published scientific articles. The "reality" – an interactive, periperformative reality – is quite different. A sampling of Gazzaniga's scientific articles reveals the tentative communal rhetoric that is actually much more typical of science: "The general picture of callosal functions based on the animal studies tends to be supported in current early testing" (Gazzaniga et al. 1962, 1765), "these phenomena appear to be related to our left hemisphere's interpreter" (Gazzaniga 2000, 1293), and so on. This is science as what I have been calling periperformativism: the ongoing attempt to collaborate with colleagues in the creation of a plausible model of reality that is always provisional, always vulnerable to disagreement and debate, always at best subject to revision as new data are factored into the emerging model. And in the memoir (2015), as Gazzaniga-the-narrator tells the story of those discoveries by Gazzaniga-the-character and his friends and grad students, everything is even more fluid, even more tentative, even more collaborative, even more grounded in the periperformative interepistemic translations of *ES1 to ES2a to ES3b*. Gerald Weber seems to need Powers's narrator to help him discover just how periperformative/novelistic his interepistemic translations are; Michael Gazzaniga knows it "himself" (in his various "selves," which the memoir presents as networked rhizomatically through his many friends and colleagues).

My own faith in science is placed not in idealized myths of objectivity, but in the ongoing provisional/experimental networking of scientists like Gazzaniga, who know that they are working communally, dialogically, to develop and vet what they take to be plausible interpretations on complex sense-data. This to my mind is faith in science as translationality. It is faith in science as explanations that keep changing, because no explanation is ever the objective truth, and our attempts to reach through the conflicting evidence of our senses to "objective truth" invariably fail, to one degree or another, because the material world beyond our periperformative constructions keeps resisting us, keeps pushing back against our cultural grids and maps, thwarting our efforts to synthesize, consolidate, build elegant models of "reality" – but also providing us with our best clues as to what that world is actually like. (See Robinson 2010, reprinted as Robinson 2013b, 177–206, for an *elegant model* of this process.) At base science is a diligent collaborative attentiveness to those pushes, a willingness to let them transform our modeling, and indeed a constant search for more such pushes, just the right pushes to test our icotic assumptions.

To put that differently: science, like all scholarship, and like all storytelling, and indeed like all social interaction, is an unending collaborative attempt to create a coherent reality *out of* the astonishing resistance life puts up to our attempts to create a coherent reality.

Notes

1 See also my discussions (Robinson 1997a, 2016b) of Wendy Knox's production of my translation of Maaria Koskiluoma's expressionist stage adaptation of Maria Jotuni's *Huojuva talo* as *Tottering House*. The original 1983 Finnish production, directed by Eija-Elina Bergholm at the Oslo Theater Festival, for which Koskiluoma created the adaptation, staged domestic violence through epic-theatrical symbols: to show bleeding, for example, the actress playing the abused wife released a red ribbon. Wendy, an expressionistic director who was drawn to the play in the first place precisely because of its powerful expressionism, directed all the peripheral characters in that style but decided in the end that Lea, the abused wife, had to be played naturalistically. As I showed in my discussions, that decision resonated strongly with the abused women in the audience, but grated irritatingly on me, the translator, as a dramatistically incoherent (2) translation of my expressionistic translation of an expressionistic play – and Wendy ruefully agreed. It was a bad decision.

The takeaway from this story for our present purposes, it seems to me, is that the naturalistic pathos of *Wit* as Rokotnitz reports its staging is not an intrinsic textual feature – and not even an intrinsic aspect of "the play" as produced at the South Coast Repertory in 1995, the Long Wharf Theater in 1997, or, off-Broadway, the MCC Theater and Union Square Theater in 1998. It is, rather, a (2) *directorial translation*. It is a *decision*.

2 See LeDoux (2015, 121–33) for a thoroughgoing critique of the Darwinian "basic emotions theory" of Tomkins (1962/1992), Izard (1971, 1992, 2007), and Ekman (1977, 1984, 1999), and also of what he considers more sophisticated theories of innate "affect programs," especially as offered by Jaak Panksepp (1998, 2005, 2012). His comment:

> Most basic emotions theorists are psychologists, not brain researchers, and tend to view affect programs as placeholders for brain mechanisms. In general, they adhere to the idea that there are entities located in subcortical areas of the limbic system that constitute the affect program for each basic emotion, but are not strongly committed to hypotheses about which particular brain areas or circuits are responsible.
>
> (124)

He insists that the innate "affect programs" *not* be called emotions (20), and notes that "the recent notion that emotions are 'psychological constructions' is perhaps the cognitive-based theory of emotions that is closest to my own view" (20) – citing Barrett (2006a, 2006b, 2009a, 2009b, 2012, 2013), Barrett and Russell (2014), Russell (2003), Russell and Barrett (1999), Lindquist et al. (2006), Barrett et al. (2007a, 2007b), Lindquist and Barrett (2008), Clore and Ortony (2013).

LeDoux's (2015, 134–38) response to the Damasio model is more complex: while critiquing specific aspects of Damasio's adaptation of William James's theory of the emotions, he wholeheartedly supports Damasio's claim that feelings are becoming-cognitive mappings of emotions and other body states. See also Gazzaniga (1998, 118–20) for a resounding endorsement of the Damasio team's conclusions on the relations between emotions and feelings, and his early remark that "several adaptations in our brain modulate our emotional states: fear, anxiety, and sadness all help us in our decision making" (10).

Of course LeDoux published *Anxious* four years after Leys (2011): could LeDoux have changed his tune after Leys published her critique? No: in LeDoux (1984, 1996), the two works on which Leys's critique is based, he does pay considerable attention to automatic/unconscious emotional processing, as she charges, but also insists on the interplay between unconscious emotional response and conscious feelings – the neo-Jamesian model on which the Damasio team relies:

> In the *Emotional Brain,* continuing the fear theme, I argued that the conscious feeling of fear is due to the representation in consciousness, via attention and other neocortical cognitive processes, of unconscious ingredients that are consequences of activation of the amygdala threat-processing circuit. I proposed that we could study the nonconscious aspects of fear in animals and humans alike, but that the conscious feelings of fear are best studied in humans.
>
> (2015, 35)

I find no evidence at all of an "essential separation" between affective and cognitive processing in any of these affect theorists.

References

Aaltonen, Sirkku. 2013. "Theatre Translation as Performance." *Translation in the Theatre*, Special issue of *Target* 25.3, 385–406.

Abdallah, Kristiina. 2010. "Translators' Agency in Production Networks." In Tuija Kinnunen and Kaisa Koskinen, eds., *Translator's Agency*, 11–46. Tampere: Tampere University Press.

Abdallah, Kristiina. 2012. *Translators in Production Networks: Reflections on Agency, Quality and Ethics.* Joensuu: University of Eastern Finland.

Abdallah, Kristiina, and Kaisa Koskinen. 2007. "Managing Trust: Translating and the Network Economy." *Meta* 52.4: 673–87.

Abutalebi, Jubin, Pasquale Anthony Della Rosa, David W. Green, Mireia Hernandez, Paola Scifo, Roland Keim, Stefano F. Cappa, and Albert Costa. 2012. "Bilingualism Tunes the Anterior Cingulate Cortex for Conflict Monitoring." *Cerebral Cortex* 22.9: 2076–86.

Abutalebi, Jubin, Pasquale Anthony Della Rosa, Anna Kaarina Gonzaga, Roland Keim, Albert Costa, and Daniela Perani. 2013. "The Role of the Left Putamen in Multilingual Language Production." *Brain and Language* 125.3: 307–15.

Adolphs, Ralph. 2002. "Neural Mechanisms for Recognizing Emotion." *Current Opinion in Neurobiology* 12: 169–78.

Adolphs, Ralph, Hannah Damasio, Daniel Tranel, Gregory Cooper, and Antonio Damasio. 2000. "A Role for Somatosensory Cortices in the Visual Recognition of Emotion as Revealed by 3-D Lesion Mapping." *The Journal of Neuroscience* 20: 2683–90.

Adolphs, Ralph, Daniel Tranel, and Antonio R. Damasio. 1994. "Impaired Recognition of Emotion in Facial Expressions Following Bilateral Damage to the Human Amygdala." *Nature* 372: 669–72.

Adolphs, Ralph, Daniel Tranel, and Antonio R. Damasio. 1998. "The Human in Social Judgment." *Nature* 393: 470–4.

Ahsen, Akhter. 1984. *Trojan Horse: Imagery in Psychology, Art, Literature, and Politics.* New York: Brandon House.

Ahn, Jong-Su. 1990. *Leibniz's Philosophie und die chinesishe Philosophie.* Konstanz: Hartung-Gorre.

Ames, Roger T., and David L. Hall, eds. and trans. 2003. *Daodejing: "Making Life Significant": A Philosophical Translation.* New York: Ballantine.

Anderson, Benedict. 1983/2006. *Imagined Communities: Reflections on the Origin and Spread of Nationalism.* Revised edition. London: Verso.

Apter, Emily. 2005. *The Translation Zone: A New Comparative Literature.* Princeton: Princeton University Press.

Apter, Emily. 2013. *Against World Literature: On the Politics of Untranslatability*. London: Verso.

Apter, Emily, trans. 2014. *Dictionary of Untranslatables: A Philosophical Lexicon*. Translation of Cassin 2004. Princeton: Princeton University Press.

Atwood, Margaret. 2006. "In the Heart of the Heartland." *New York Review of Books* (December 21). Online at www.nybooks.com/articles/archives/2006/dec/21/in-the-heart-of-the-heartland/. Accessed April 23, 2016.

Austin, J. L. 1961. *Philosophical Papers*. Edited by J. O. Urmson and Geoffrey J. Warnock. Oxford: Oxford University Press.

Austin, J. L. 1962/1976. *How to Do Things With Words*. Edited by J. O. Urmson and Marina Sbisa. Cambridge, MA: Harvard University Press.

Badiou, Alain. 2012. *La République de Platon*. Paris: Fayard.

Baker, Mona. 2000. "Towards a Methodology for Investigating the Style of a Literary Translator." *Target* 12.2: 241–66.

Bakhtin, Mikhail. 1940/1984. *Rabelais and His World*. Translated by Hélène Iswolsky. Bloomington, IN: Indiana University Press.

Banissy, Michael J., and Jamie Ward. 2007. "Mirror-Touch Synesthesia Is Linked With Empathy." *Nature Neuroscience* 10.7 (July): 815–6.

Barrett, Lisa Feldman. 2006a. "Are Emotions Natural Kinds?" *Perspectives on Psychological Science* 1: 28–58.

Barrett, Lisa Feldman. 2006b. "Solving the Emotion Paradox: Categorization and the Experience of Emotion." *Personality and Social Psychology Review* 10: 20–46.

Barrett, Lisa Feldman. 2009a. "The Future of Psychology: Connecting Mind to Brain." *Perspectives on Psychological Science* 4: 326–39.

Barrett, Lisa Feldman. 2009b. "Variety Is the Spice of Life: A Psychological Construction Approach to Understanding Variability in Emotion." *Cognition and Emotion* 23: 1284–1306.

Barrett, Lisa Feldman. 2012. "Emotions Are Real." *Emotion* 12: 413–29.

Barrett, Lisa Feldman. 2013. "Psychological Construction: The Darwinian Approach to the Science of Emotion." *Emotion Review* 5: 379–89.

Barrett, Lisa Feldman, Kristen A. Lindquist, Eliza Bliss-Moreau, Seth Duncan, Maria Gendron, Jennifer Mize, and Lauren Brennan. 2007b. "Of Mice and Men: Natural Kinds of Emotions in the Mammalian Brain? A Response to Panksepp and Izard." *Perspectives on Psychological Science* 2: 297–311.

Barrett, Lisa Feldman, Kristen A. Lindquist, and Maria Gendron. 2007a. "Language as Context for the Perception of Emotion." *Trends in Cognitive Sciences* 11: 327–32.

Barrett, Lisa Feldman, and James A. Russell, eds. 2014. *The Psychological Construction of Emotion*. New York: Guilford.

Barth, John. 1967/1984. "The Literature of Exhaustion." In Barth, ed., *The Friday Book: Essays and Other Non-Fiction*, 62–76. Baltimore: John Hopkins University Press.

Bassnett-McGuire, Susan. 1980. *Translation Studies*. London: Routledge.

Baudrillard, Jean. 1981/1994. *Simulacra and Simulation*. Translated by Sheila Faria Glaser. Ann Arbor: University of Michigan Press.

Baudrillard, Jean. 2007/2011. *Why Hasn't Everything Disappeared?* Translated by Chris Turner. London: Seagull.

Bellos, David. 2011. *Is That a Fish in Your Ear? Translation and the Meaning of Everything*. Harmondsworth: Penguin.

Bergman, Mats. 2009. *Peirce's Philosophy of Communication: The Rhetorical Underpinnings of the Theory of Signs.* New York: Continuum.

Berman, Antoine. 1984. *L'Épreuve de l'étranger: Culture et traduction dans l'Allemagne romantique.* Paris: Gallimard.

Bermann, Sandra. 2014. "Performing Translation." In Sandra Berman and Catherine Porter, eds., *A Companion to Translation Studies,* 285–97. Chichester, UK: Wiley-Blackwell.

Blair, Rhonda. 2013. "Introduction: The Multimodal Practitioner." In Shaughnessy 2013: 135–46.

Blair, Rhonda, and Amy Cook. 2016a. "Introduction." In Blair and Cook 2016b: 1–15.

Blair, Rhonda, and Amy Cook, eds. 2016b. *Theatre, Performance and Cognition: Languages, Bodies and Ecologies.* London: Bloomsbury/Methuen Drama.

Bloom, Harold. 1980. *The Flight to Lucifer: A Gnostic Fantasy.* New York: Vintage.

Bloom, Irene, trans. 2009. *Mencius.* New York: Columbia University Press.

Blumczynski, Piotr. 2016a. "Translation as an Evaluative Concept." in Piotr Blumczynski and John Gillespie, eds., *Translating Values: Evaluative Concepts in Translation,* 327–49. London: Palgrave Macmillan.

Blumczynski, Piotr. 2016b. *Ubiquitous Translation.* London and New York: Routledge.

Bolgar, R. R. 1940. "Rabelais's Edition of the 'Aphorisms' of Hippocrates." *Modern Language Review* 35.1 (January): 62–6.

Bolgar, R. R. 1954/1964. *The Classical Heritage and Its Beneficiaries: From the Carolingian Age to the End of the Renaissance.* New York: Harper & Row.

Breen, Nora, et al. 2000. "Towards an Understanding of Delusions of Misidentification: Four Case Studies." *Mind and Language* 15.1: 74–110.

Brennan, Teresa. 2004. *The Transmission of Affect.* Ithaca, NY: Cornell University Press.

Brindley, Nicola. 2012. " 'The Truth of Our Scattering': (Post)Human Complexity in Richard Powers' *The Echo Maker.*" *49th Parallel* 28 (Spring). Online at fortyninthparalleljournal.files.wordpress.com/2014/07/5-brindley-truth-of-our-scattering.pdf. Accessed April 23, 2016.

Brook, Peter. 1968/2008. *The Empty Space: A Book About the Theatre: Deadly, Holy, Rough, Immediate.* New York: Simon & Schuster/Touchstone.

Brown, Huntington. 1933. *Rabelais in English Literature.* Cambridge, MA: Harvard University Press.

Brown, Malcolm Hamrick, ed. 2004. *A Shostakovich Casebook.* Bloomington, IN: Indiana University Press.

Burke, Kenneth. 1961/1970. *The Rhetoric of Religion: Studies in Logology.* Berkeley, CA: University of California Press.

Burn, Stephen J. 2008. "An Interview With Richard Powers." *Contemporary Literature* 49.2: 163–79.

Burn, Stephen J., and Peter Dempsey, eds. 2008. *Intersections: Essays on Richard Powers.* Champaign, IL: Dalkey Archive.

Burton, Robert. 1621/1871. *The Anatomy of Melancholy, What It Is, With All the Kinds, Causes, Symptoms, Prognostics, and Several Cures of It. In Three Partitions. With Their Several Sections, Members, and Subsections, Philosophically, Medically, Historically Opened and Cut Up. By Democritus Junior. With a Satirical Preface, Conducing to the Following Discourses.* New York: Widdleton.

Butler, Judith. 1990/1999. *Gender Trouble: Feminism and the Subversion of Identity.* Reprint. London: Routledge.

Butler, Judith. 1991. "Imitation and Gender Insubordination." In Diana Fuss, ed., *Inside/Out: Lesbian Theories, Gay Theories*, 13–31. London: Routledge.

Butler, Rex. 1999. *Jean Baudrillard: The Defence of the Real.* London: Sage.

Cameron, Gail. 1999. "Off Broadway." *Smith Alumnae Quarterly* (Fall). Reprinted online at www.mywhatever.com/cifwriter/content/56/wit3262.html. Accessed August 16, 2016.

Casper, Kevin. 2015. "'I'm so glad you're fake!': Simulacra Slapstick and the Limits of the Real." *Ephemera: Theory and Politics in Organization* 15.3: 581–600.

Cassin, Barbara. 2004. *Vocabulaire européen des philosophies: Dictionnaire des intraduisibles.* Paris: Seuil.

Cavell, Stanley. 1995. "What Did Derrida Want of Austin?" In Cavell, ed., *Philosophical Passages: Wittgenstein, Emerson, Austin, Derrida*, 42–65. Oxford: Blackwell.

Chan Wing-tsit. 1963. *A Sourcebook in Chinese Philosophy.* Princeton: Princeton University Press.

Charon, Rita. 2015. "Narrative Medicine: A Model for Empathy, Reflection, Profession, and Trust." In Brian Dolan, ed., *Humanitas: Readings in the Development of the Medical Humanities*, 207–23. San Francisco: University of California Medical Humanities Press.

Cheng Aimin. 2000. "Humanity as 'A Part and Parcel of Nature: A Comparative Study of Thoreau's and Taoist Concepts of Nature." In Richard J. Schneider and Lawrence Buell, eds., *Thoreau's Sense of Place: Essays in American Environmental Writing*, 207–220. Iowa City: University of Iowa Press.

Chesterman, Andrew. 2014. "Translation Studies Forum: Universalism in Translation Studies." *Translation Studies* 7.1: 82–90.

Ching, Julia, and Willard Oxtoby, eds. and trans. 1992. *Moral Enlightenment: Leibniz and Wolff on China.* Nettetal: Steyler.

Christiansen, Broder. 1909. *Die Philosophie der Kunst* ("The Philosophy of Art). Hanau: Clauss and Fedderson.

Christoffels, Ingrid K., Annette M. B. de Groot, and Judith F. Kroll. 2006. "Memory and Language Skills in Simultaneous Interpreters: The Role of Expertise and Language Proficiency." *Journal of Memory and Language* 54.3: 324–45.

Christy, Arthur. 1963. *The Orient in American Transcendentalism: A Study of Emerson, Thoreau, and Alcott.* London: Octagon.

Chukovsky, Korney Ivanovich. 1941/2014. *Vysokoe iskusstvo: Printsipy khudozhestvennogo perevoda* ("The High Art: Principles of Artistic Translation"). Edited by Konstantin Vasil'ev. St. Petersburg: Azbuka.

Chukovsky, Korney Ivanovich, and Andrey Venediktovich Fyodorov. 1930. *Iskusstvo perevoda* ("The Art of Translation"). Leningrad: Academia.

Clark, Andy. 1997. *Being There: Putting Brain, Body, and World Together Again.* Cambridge, MA: MIT Press.

Clark, Andy. 2004. *Natural-Born Cyborgs: Minds, Technologies, and the Future of Human Intelligence.* Oxford: Oxford University Press.

Clark, Andy. 2008. *Supersizing the Mind: Embodiment, Action, and Cognitive Extension.* Oxford: Oxford University Press.

Clark, Andy, and David J. Chalmers. 1998. "The Extended Mind." *Analysis* 58: 7–19.

Clore, Gerald L., and Andrew Ortony. 2013. "Psychological Construction in the OCC Model of Emotion." *Emotion Review* 5: 335–43.

Cohen, J. M., trans. 1955. François Rabelais, *Gargantua and Pantagruel.* Harmondsworth, UK: Penguin.

Coleman, Paul. 2003. "'The Taylor's Stitch': Sir Thomas Urquhart's Translation of Rabelais." *Cambridge Quarterly* 32.4: 299–309.

Connor, Peter, trans. 1991. Jean-Luc Nancy, "The Inoperative Community." Translation of Nancy 1986/2004. In Peter Connor, ed., *The Inoperative Community*, 1–42. Minneapolis, MN: University of Minneapolis Press.

Coover, Robert. 1967. *The Origin of the Brunists*. New York: Putnam.

Coover, Robert. 2014. *The Brunist Day of Wrath*. New York: Dzanc.

Costa, Albert, and Núria Sebastián-Gallés. 2014. "How Does the Bilingual Experience Sculpt the Brain?" *Nature Reviews Neuroscience* 15.5: 336–45.

Cousin, Victor. 1854. *The Philosophy of Kant*. London: John Chapman.

Craik, Roger. 1999. "Sir Thomas Urquhart's Translation of Rabelais." *Studies in Scottish Literature* 31.1: 151–68.

Crinion, Jenny, Robert Turner, Alice Grogan, Takashi Hanakawa, Uta Noppeney, Joseph T. Devlin, Toshihiko Aso, Shinichi Urayama, Hidenao Fukuyama, Kath Stockton, Keiko Usui, David W. Green, and Cathy J. Price. 2006. "Language Control in the Bilingual Brain." *Science* 312.5779: 1537–40.

Damasio, Antonio R. 1989. "Time-Locked Multiregional Retroactivation: A Systems Level Proposal for the Neural Substrates of Recall and Recognition." *Cognition* 33.1–2: 25–62.

Damasio, Antonio R. 1994. *Descartes' Error: Emotion, Reason, and the Human Brain*. New York: Putnam.

Damasio, Antonio R. 1999. *The Feeling of What Happens: Body and Emotion in the Making of Consciousness*. New York: Harcourt.

Damasio, Antonio R. 2003. *Looking for Spinoza: Joy, Sorrow, and the Feeling Brain*. New York: Harcourt.

Damasio, Antonio R. 2010. *Self Comes to Mind: Constructing the Conscious Brain*. New York: Vintage.

Damasio, Antonio, and Norman Geschwind. 1984. "The Neural Basis of Language." *Annual Review of Neuroscience* 7: 127–47.

Damasio, Antonio R., Daniel Tranel, and Hanna Damasio. 1990a. "Individuals With Sociopathic Behavior Caused by Frontal Damage Fail to Respond Autonomically to Social Stimuli." *Behavioural Brain Research* 41: 81–94.

Damasio, Antonio R., Daniel Tranel, and Hanna Damasio. 1990b. "Face Agnosia and the Neural Substrates of Memory." *Annual Review of Neuroscience* 13: 89–109.

Damasio, Antonio R., Daniel Tranel, and Hanna Damasio. 1991. "Somatic Markers and the Guidance of Behavior: Theory and Preliminary Testing." In Harvey S. Levin, Howard M. Eisenberg, and Arthur L. Benton, eds., *Frontal Lobe Function and Dysfunction*, 217–29. New York: Oxford University Press.

Damasio, Antonio R., Daniel Tranel, and Hanna Damasio. 1993. "Similarity of Structure and the Profile of Visual Recognition Defects: A Comment on Gaffan and Heywood." *Journal of Cognitive Neuroscience* 5: 371–72.

Davis, Kathleen. 2001/2014. *Deconstruction and Translation*. London: Routledge.

Darò, Valeria, and Franco Fabbro. 1994. "Verbal Memory During Simultaneous Interpretation: Effects of Phonological Interference." *Applied Linguistics* 15.4: 365–81.

Delabastita, Dirk, and Rainer Gutman, eds. 2005. "Fictionalising Translation and Multilingualism." Special issue of *Linguistica Antverpiensia* 4.

Deleuze, Gilles, and Félix Guattari. 1972. *Capitalisme et schizophrénie: L'anti-Œdipe*. Paris: Minuit.

Deleuze, Gilles, and Félix Guattari. 1975. *Kafka: Pour une littérature mineure*. Paris: Minuit.

Dennett, Daniel. 1991. *Consciousness Explained.* Boston: Little, Brown.

Dennett, Daniel. 2008. "Astride the Two Cultures: A Letter to Richard Powers, Updated." In Burn and Dempsey 2008, 151–61.

Derrida, Jacques. 1977/1988. "Limited Inc a b c . . ." In Gerald Graff, ed., Derrida, *Limited Inc,* 29–110. Translated by Samuel Weber. Evanston, IL: Northwestern University Press.

Di Pellegrino, Giuseppe, Luciano Fadiga, Leonardo Fogassi, Vittorio Gallese, and Giacomo Rizzolatti. 1992. "Understanding Motor Events: A Neurophysiological Study." *Experimental Brain Research* 91: 176–80.

Dobson, W. A. C. H., trans. 1963. *Mencius: A New Translation Arranged and Annotated for the General Reader.* Toronto: University of Toronto Press.

Dolan, Brian. 2015. "One Hundred Years of Medical Humanities: A Thematic Overview." In Brian Dolan, ed., *Humanitas: Readings in the Development of the Medical Humanities,* 1–30. San Francisco: University of California Medical Humanities Press.

Doyle, Charles Clay. 2008. " 'Ex Desuetudine Amittuntur Privilegia': Rabelais, Urquhart, and *Les Clercs.*" *Romance Notes* 48.2 (Winter): 151–5.

Dror, Itiel E., and Stevan Harnad, eds. 2008. *Cognition Distributed: How Cognitive Technology Extends Our Minds.* Amsterdam: John Benjamins.

Duke, James, and Jack Forstman, trans. 1977. Friedrich Schleiermacher, *Hermeneutics: The Handwritten Manuscripts.* Translation of Schleiermacher 1959. Atlanta: Scholars.

Edson, Margaret. 1993/2012. *Wit: A Play.* London: Nick Hern.

Ekman, Paul. 1977. "Biological and Cultural Contributions to Body and Facial Movement." In John Blacking, ed., *The Anthropology of the Body,* 39–84. London: Academic.

Ekman, Paul. 1984. "Expression and Nature of Emotion." In Klaus Scherer and Paul Ekman, eds., *Approaches to Emotion,* 319–43. Hillsdale, NJ: Erlbaum.

Ekman, Paul. 1985. *Telling Lies: Clues to Deceit in the Marketplace, Politics, and Marriage.* New York: Norton.

Ekman, Paul. 1999. "Basic Emotions." In Tim Dalgleish and Micheal Power, eds., *Handbook of Cognition and Emotion,* 45–60. Chichester, UK: Wiley.

Ellis, Hadyn D., and Michael B. Lewis. 2001. "Capgras Delusion: A Window on Face Recognition." *Trends in Cognitive Science* 5.4: 149–56.

Elman, Jeffrey L. 1994. "Learning and Development in Neural Networks: The Importance of Starting Small." *Cognition* 48: 71–99.

Ericsson, K. Anders, Neil Charness, Paul J. Feltovich, and Robert R. Hoffman, eds. 2006. *The Cambridge Handbook of Expertise and Expert Performance.* Cambridge: Cambridge University Press.

Ericsson, K. Anders. 2010. "Expertise in Interpreting: An Expert-Performance Perspective." In Gregory M. Shreve and Erik Angelone, eds., *Translation and Cognition,* 231–62. Amsterdam: John Benjamins.

Esselborn, Karl. 2007. "Übersetzungen aus der Sprache, die es nicht gibt: Interculturalität, Globalisierung und Postmoderne in den Texten Yoko Tawadas." *Arcadia* 42.2: 240–62.

Even-Zohar, Itamar. 1979. "Polysystem Theory." *Poetics Today* 1.1–2: 283–305.

Even-Zohar, Itamar. 1981. "Translation Theory Today: A Call for Transfer Theory." *Poetics Today* 2.4: 1–7.

Fabbro, Franco, and Valeria Darò. 1995. "Delayed Auditory Feedback in Polyglot Simultaneous Interpreters." *Brain and Language* 48.3: 309–19.

Falletti, Clelia, Gabrielle Sofia, and Victor Jacono, eds. 2016. *Theatre and Cognitive Neuroscience*. London: Bloomsbury/Methuen Drama.

Fay, Laurel. 1980. "Shostakovich Versus Volkov: Whose Testimony?" *The Russian Review* 39.4 (October): 484–93.

Ferrarin, Alfredo. 2004. *Hegel and Aristotle*. Cambridge: Cambridge University Press.

Festinger, Leon, Henry Riecken, and Stanley Schachter. 1956. *When Prophecy Fails: A Social and Psychological Study of a Modern Group That Predicted the Destruction of the World*. New York: Harper/Torchbooks.

Finger, Stanley. 1994/2001. *Origins of Neuroscience: A History of Explorations Into Brain Function*. Oxford: Oxford University Press.

Forster, Michael N., ed. and trans. 2002. Johann Gottfried Herder, "This Too a Philosophy of History for the Formation of Humanity." Translation of Herder 1774/1967. In Forster, ed., *Herder: Philosophical Writings*, 272–358. Cambridge: Cambridge University Press.

Foucault, Michel. 1980. *Power/Knowledge: Selected Interviews and Other Writings, 1972–1977*. Edited by Colin Gordon. Translated by Colin Gordon, Leo Marshall, John Mepham, and Kate Soper. New York: Pantheon.

Fowles, John. 1974/1984. *The Ebony Tower*. Boston: Little, Brown.

Freud, Sigmund. 1911/1957. "Formulations Regarding the Two Principles in Mental Functioning." Translated by Joan Riviere. In Alfred Ernest Jones, ed., Sigmund Freud, *Papers on Metapsychology: Papers on Applied Psycho-Analysis*, 13–21. Vol. 4 of Collected Papers. 5 vols. London: Hogarth and Institute of Psycho-Analysis.

Friederici, Angela D. 2006. "What's in Control of Language?" *Nature Neuroscience* 9.8: 991–2.

Frye, Northrop. 1957/1990. *Anatomy of Criticism: Four Essays*. Princeton: Princeton University Press.

Fyodorov, Andrey Venediktovich. 1953. *Vvedenie v teoriyu perevoda* ("Introduction to a Theory of Translation"). Moscow: Literatures in Foreign Languages.

Gabrakova, Dennitza. 2010. "'Wound in the Alphabet': The Punct(um) of the Text or the F(r)iction of Translation." In Christine Ivanovic, ed., *Yoko Tawada: Poetik der Transformation; Beiträge sum Gesamtwerk*, 385–93. Tübingen: Stauffenburg.

Gadamer, Hans-Georg. 1960/1990. *Wahrheit und Methode: Grundzüge einer philosophischen Hermeneutik*. Tübingen: Mohr.

Gallese, Vittorio, Luciano Fadiga, Leonardo Fogassi, and Giacomo Rizzolatti. 1996. "Action Recognition in the Premotor Cortex." *Brain* 119: 593–609.

Gane, Mike, ed. 1993. *Baudrillard Live: Selected Interviews*. London: Routledge.

Gazzaniga, Michael S. 1989. "Organization of the Human Brain." *Science* 245.4921: 947–52.

Gazzaniga, Michael S. 1998. *The Mind's Past*. Berkeley, CA: University of California Press.

Gazzaniga, Michael S. 2000. "Cerebral Specialization and Interhemispheric Communication: Does the Corpus Callosum Enable the Human Condition?" *Brain* 123.7: 1293–1326.

Gazzaniga, Michael S. 2005/2006. *The Ethical Brain: The Science of Our Moral Dilemmas*. New York: Harper Perennial.

Gazzaniga, Michael S. 2008/2009. *Human: The Science Behind What Makes Your Brain Unique*. New York: Ecco.

Gazzaniga, Michael S. 2011. *Who's in Charge? Free Will and the Science of the Brain.* New York: Ecco.

Gazzaniga, Michael S. 2015. *Tales From Both Sides of the Brain: A Life in Neuroscience.* New York: Ecco.

Gazzaniga, Michael S., Joseph E. Bogan, and Roger W. Sperry. 1962. "Some Functional Effects of Sectioning the Cerebral Commissures in Man." *Proceedings of the National Academy of Sciences* 48.10: 1765–69.

Gazzaniga, Michael S., Joseph E. Bogan, and Roger W. Sperry. 1965. "Observations on Visual Perception After Disconnexion of the Cerebral Hemispheres in Man." *Brain* 88.2: 221–36.

Gazzola, Valeria, and Christian Keysers. 2009. "The Observation and Execution of Actions Share Motor and Somatosensory Voxels in All Tested Subjects: Single-Subject Analyses of Unsmoothed fMRI Data." *Cerebral Cortex* 19: 1239–1255.

Geisel, Sieglinde. 2001. "Fremdkörper Sprache: Ein Spaziergang mit Yoko Tawada." *Neue Zürchner Zeitung* (February 23). Online at www.nzz.ch/2001/02/23/fe/article71hps_1.468004.html.

Genette, Gérard. 1991. *Fiction et Diction.* Paris: Seuil.

Ginzburg, Carlo. 1996. "Making Things Strange: The Prehistory of a Literary Device." *Representations* 56: 8–28.

González, Antonio Ballesteros. 1996. "Digression and Intertextual Parody in Nashe, Sterne, and Joyce." In David Pierce and Peter de Voogd, eds., *Laurence Sterne in Modernism and Postmodernism,* 55–64. Amsterdam: Rodopi.

Gorlée, Dinda L. 1994. *Semiotics and the Problem of Translation: With Special Reference to the Semiotics of Charles S. Peirce.* Amsterdam: Rodopi.

Gregg, Melissa, and Gregory J. Siegworth, eds. 2002. *The Affect Theory Reader.* Durham, NC: Duke University Press.

Grice, H. Paul. 1975/1988. "Logic and Conversation." In Grice, *Studies in the Way of Words,* 22–40. Cambridge, MA: Harvard University Press.

Grogan, Alice, 'Ōiwi Parker-Jones, Nilufa Ali, Jenny Crinion, S. Orabona, M.L. Mechias, Sue Ramsden, David W. Green, and Cathy J. Price. 2012. "Structural Correlates for Lexical Efficiency and Number of Languages in Non-native Speakers of English." *Neuropsychologia* 50.7: 1347–52.

Harris, Charles B. 2008. "The Story of the Self: *The Echo Maker* and Neurological Realism." In Burn and Dempsey 2008, 230–59.

Hartama-Heinonen, Ritva. 2008. *Abductive Translation Studies: The Art of Marshalling Signs.* Ph.D. dissertation, University of Helsinki. Imatra, Finland: International Semiotics Institute.

Harte, Tim. 2009. *Fast Forward: The Aesthetics and Ideology of Speed in Russian Avant-Garde Culture, 1910–1930.* Madison, WI: University of Wisconsin Press.

Hawley, Judith. 1993. "The Anatomy of *Tristram Shandy.*" In Marie Mulvey Roberts and Roy Porter, eds., *Literature and Medicine During the Eighteenth Century,* 84–100. London: Routledge.

Herder, Johann Gottfried. 1774/1967. *Auch eine Philosophie der Geschichte zur Bildung der Menschheit.* Frankfurt a. M.: Suhrkamp.

Hermans, Theo, ed. 1985/2014. *The Manipulation of Literature: Studies in Literary Translation.* London: Routledge.

Hermans, Theo. 1996. "The Translator's Voice in Translated Narrative." *Target* 8.1: 23–48.

Hermans, Theo. 1999/2014. *Translation in Systems: Descriptive and System-Oriented Approaches Explained.* London: Routledge.

Hermans, Theo. 2000. "Self-Reference, Self-Reflection and Re-Entering Translation." In Dirk de Geest, Ortwin de Graef, Dirk Delabastita, Koenraad Geldof, Rita Ghesquière, and José Lambert, eds., *Under Construction: Links for the Site of Literary Theory*, 259–74. Leuven: Leuven University Press.

Hervais-Adelman, Alexis, Barbara Moser-Mercer, and Narly Golestani. 2011. "Executive Control of Language in the Bilingual Brain: Integrating the Evidence from Neuroimaging to Neuropsychology." *Frontiers in Psychology* 2: 234.

Hervais-Adelman, Alexis, Barbara Moser-Mercer, Michel, C. M., and Narly Golestani. 2014. "fMRI of Simultaneous Interpretation Reveals the Neural Basis of Extreme Language Control." *Cerebral Cortex* 25.12 (December): 4727–39.

Hervais-Adelman, Alexis, Barbara Moser-Mercer, and Narly Golestani. 2015. "Brain Functional Plasticity Associated With the Emergence of Expertise in Extreme Language Control." *NeuroImage* 114: 264–74.

Heyvaert S., trans. 1992. Antoine Berman, *The Experience of the Foreign: Culture and Translation in Romantic Germany.* Translation of Berman 1984. Albany, NY: SUNY Press.

Highet, Gilbert. 1949/1976. *The Classical Tradition: Greek and Roman Influences on Western Literature.* New York: Oxford University Press.

Hinton, David, trans. 1998. *Mencius.* Counterpoint.

Hirstein, William, and Vilayanur S. Ramachandran. 1997. "Capgras Syndrome: A Novel Probe for Understanding the Neural Representation of the Identity and Familiarity of Persons." *Proceedings of the Royal Society of London B* 264.1380: 437–44.

Hollan, James, Edwin Hutchins, and David Kirsh. 2001. "Distributed Cognition: Toward a New Foundation for Human-Computer Interaction Research." In John M. Carroll, ed., *Human-Computer Interaction in the New Millennium*, 75–94. New York: ACM.

Holmes, James S. 1975. *The Name and Nature of Translation Studies.* Amsterdam: Translation Studies Section, Department of General Literary Studies, University of Amsterdam.

Holz-Mänttäri, Justa. 1984. *Translatorisches Handeln: Theorie und Methode.* Helsinki: Finnish Academy of Sciences.

House, Juliane. 1977. *A Model for Translation Quality Assessment.* Tübingen: Narr.

House, Juliane. 1996. *Translation Quality Assessment: A Model Revisited.* Tübingen: Narr.

Hurley, Robert, Mark Seem, and Helen R. Lane, trans. 1983. Gilles Deleuze and Félix Guattari. *Anti-Oedipus.* Vol. 1 of *Capitalism and Schizophrenia.* London: Athlone Press.

Hyman, Badley T., Gary W. van Hoesen, Antonio R. Damasio, and Clifford L. Barnes. 1984. "Alzheimer's Disease: Cell-Specific Pathology Isolates the Hippocampal Formation." *Science* 225.4667: 1168–70.

Ickes, William. 1997. *Empathetic Accuracy.* New York: Guilford.

Ickes, William, and Elliot Aronson. 2003. *Everyday Mind Reading: Understanding What Other People Think and Feel.* Amherst, NY: Prometheus Books.

Impola, Richard, trans. 1991. Aleksis Kivi, *Seven Brothers.* Translation of Kivi 1870/1984. New Paltz, NY: FATA.

Insel, Thomas R. 2010. "The Challenge of Translation in Social Neuroscience: A Review of Oxytocin, Vasopressin, and Affiliative Behavior." *Neuron* 65.6 (March 25): 768–79.

Iverson, Jana M., and Esther Thelen. 1999. "Hand, Mouth and Brain: The Dynamic Emergence of Speech and Gesture." *The Journal of Consciousness Studies* 6.11–12: 19–40.

Izard, Carrol E. 1971. *The Face of Emotion*. New York: Appleton-Century-Crofts.

Izard, Carrol E. 1992. "Basic Emotions, Relations Among Emotions, and Emotion-Cognition Relations." *Psychological Review* 99: 561–65.

Izard, Carrol E. 2007. "Basic Emotions, Natural Kinds, Emotion Schemas, and a New Paradigm." *Perspectives on Psychological Science* 2: 260–80.

Jakobson, Roman. 1959. "On Linguistic Aspects of Translation." In Reuben A. Brower, ed., *On Translation*, 232–9. Cambridge, MA: Harvard University Press.

James, William. 1890/1950. *Principles of Psychology*. 2 vols. New York: Holt.

Jameson, Fredric. 1992. *Postmodernism: The Cultural Logic of Late Capitalism*. Durham, NC: Duke University Press.

Johnson, Kent. 1997. *Double Flowering: From the Notebooks of Araki Yasusada*. New York: Roof Books.

Kaindl, Klaus. 2014. "Of Dragons and Translators: Foreignness as a Principle of Life; Yoko Tawada's 'St. George and the Translator.'" In Klaus Kaindl and Karlheinz Spitzl, eds., *Transfiction: Research Into the Realities of Translation Fiction,* 87–101. Amsterdam: John Benjamins.

Kaufman, Moisés. 2008. *33 Variations*. Play produced by the Arena Theater, Washington, DC.

Kelly, A. M. Clare, and Hugh Garavan. 2005. "Human Functional Neuroimaging of Brain Changes Associated with Practice." *Cerebral Cortex* 15.8: 1089–1102.

Keysers, Christian, and Valeria Gazzola. 2009. "Expanding the Mirror: Vicarious Activity for Actions, Emotions, and Sensations." *Current Opinion in Neurobiology* 19: 666–71.

Kirk, Eugene P. 1980. *Menippean Satire: An Annotated Catalogue of Texts and Criticism*. Garland.

Kivi, Aleksis. 1870/1984. *Seitsemän veljestä* ("Seven Brothers"). Vol. 1 in Eino Kauppinen, Simo Konsala, and Kai Laitinen, eds., Aleksis Kivi, *Kootut teokset* ("Collected Works"). 4 vols. Helsinki: Finnish Literature Society.

Klein, Denise, Robert J. Zatorre, Brenda Milner, Ernst Meyer, and Alan C. Evans. 1994. "Left Putaminal Activation When Speaking a Second Language: Evidence from PET." *Neuroreport* 5.17: 2295–7.

Klein, Denise, Brenda Milner, Robert J. Zatorre, Ernst Meyer, and Alan C. Evans. 1995. "The Neural Substrates Underlying Word Generation — A Bilingual Functional Imaging Study." *Proceedings of the National Academy of Sciences of the United States of America* 7: 2899–903.

Klein, Denise, Kelvin Mok, Jen-Kai Chen, and Kate E. Watkins. 2014. "Age of Language Learning Shapes Brain Structure: A Cortical Thickness Study of Bilingual and Monolingual Individuals." *Brain and Language* 131: 20–4.

Klein, Denise, Kate E. Watkins, Robert J. Zatorre, and Brenda Milner. 2006. "Word and Nonword Repetition in Bilingual Subjects: A PET Study." *Human Brain Mapping* 27.2: 153–61.

Kohler, Evelyne, Christian Keysers, M. Alessandra Umiltà, Leonardo Fogassi, Vittorio Gallese, and Giacomo Rizzolatti. 2002. "Hearing Sounds, Understanding Actions: Action Representation in Mirror Neurons." *Science* 297: 846–48.

Köpke, Barbara, and Jean-Luc Nespoulous. 2006. "Working Memory Performance in Expert and Novice Interpreters." *Interpreting* 8.1: 1–23.

Krings, Hans P. 1986. *Was in den Köpfen von Übersetzern vorgeht: Eine empirische Untersuchung zur Struktur des Übersetzungsprozesses an fortgeschrittenen Französischlernern*. Tübingen: Narr.

Kuhn, Thomas. 1962/1970. *The Structure of Scientific Revolutions.* 2nd ed. Chicago: University of Chicago Press.

Lach, Donald. 1957. *The Preface to Leibniz' Novissima Sinica.* Honolulu: University of Hawai'i Press.

Lai Yuen-Ting. 1998. "Leibniz and Chinese Thought." In Allison P. Coudert, Richard H. Popkin, and Gordon M. Weiner, eds., *Leibniz, Mysticism, and Religion,* 136–68. Dordrecht: Kluwer Academic.

Lamb, Jonathan. 1989. *Sterne's Fiction and the Double Principle.* Cambridge: Cambridge University Press.

LeDoux, Joseph E. 1984. "Cognition and Emotion: Processing Functions and Brain Systems." In Michael S. Gazzaniga, ed., *Handbook of Cognitive Neuroscience,* 357–68. New York: Plenum.

LeDoux, Joseph E. 1996. *The Emotional Brain.* New York: Simon and Schuster.

LeDoux, Joseph E. 2010. "From the Integrated Mind to the Emotional Brain." In Patricia A. Reuter-Lorenz, Kathleen Baynes, George R. Mangun, and Elizabeth A Phelps, eds., *The Cognitive Neuroscience of Mind: A Tribute to Michael S. Gazzaniga,* 89–98. Cambridge, MA and London: MIT Press/Bradford.

LeDoux, Joseph E. 2015. *Anxious: Using the Brain to Understand and Treat Fear and Anxiety.* New York: Viking.

Lefevere, André. 1992a. *Translation/History/Culture: A Sourcebook.* London: Routledge.

Lefevere, André. 1992b. *Translation, Rewriting and the Manipulation of Literary Fame.* London: Routledge.

Leighton, Lauren, trans. 1984. Kornei Chukovskii, *The Art of Translation: Kornei Chukovskii's the High Art.* Translation of Chukovsky 1941/2014. Knoxville: University of Tennessee Press.

Lemon, Lee T., and Marion J. Reis, eds. and trans. 1965. *Russian Formalist Criticism: Four Essays.* Lincoln: University of Nebraska Press.

Leslie, Kenneth R., Scott H. Johnson-Frey, and Scott T. Grafton. 2004. "Functional Imagining of Face and Hand Imitation: Towards a Motor Theory of Empathy." *Neuroimage* 21: 601–7.

Levin, Charles. 1996. *Jean Baudrillard: A Study in Cultural Metaphysics.* Hemel Hempstead: Prentice Hall Europe.

Lewis, Philip E. 1985. "The Measure of Translation Effects." In Joseph F. Graham, ed., *Difference in Translation,* 31–62. Ithaca, NY: Cornell University Press.

Leys, Ruth. 2011. "The Turn to Affect: A Critique." *Critical Inquiry* 37.3: 434–72.

Lincoln, Yvonna S., Susan A. Lynham, and Egon G. Guba. 2011. "Paradigmatic Controversies, Contradictions, and Emerging Confluences, Revisited." In Norman K. Denzin and Yvonna S. Lincoln, eds., *The SAGE Handbook of Qualitative Research,* 97–128. Fourth edition. Thousand Oaks, CA: Sage.

Lindenberger, Herbert. 1979. *Saul's Fall: A Critical Fiction.* Baltimore: Johns Hopkins University Press.

Linder, Birgit. 2003. "China in German Translation: Literary Perceptions, Canonical Texts, and the History of German Sinology." In Leo Tak-hung Chan, ed., *One Into Many: Translation and Dissemination of Classical Chinese Literature,* 243–83. Amsterdam: Rodopi.

Lindquist, Kristen A., and Lisa Feldman Barrett. 2008. "Constructing Emotion: The Experience of Fear as a Conceptual Act." *Psychological Science* 19: 898–903.

Lindquist, Kristen A., Lisa Feldman Barrett, Eliza Bliss-Moreau, and James A. Russell. 2006. "Language and the Perception of Emotion." *Emotion* 6: 125–38.

Loggia, Marco L., Jeffrey S. Mogil, and M. Catherine Bushnell. 2008. "Empathy Hurts: Compassion for Another Increases Both Sensory and Affective Components of Pain Perception." *Pain* 236: 168–76.
Lombez, Christine. 2005. "La 'traduction supposée' ou: De la place des pseudotraductions poétiques en France." *Linguistica Antverpiensia* 4: 107–21.
Luk, Gigi, David W. Green, Jubin Abutalebi, and Cheryl Grady. 2012. "Cognitive Control for Language Switching in Bilinguals: A Quantitative Meta-Analysis of Functional Neuroimaging Studies." *Language and Cognitive Processes* 27.10: 1479–88.
Lund, Mary Ann. 2006. "Robert Burton the Spiritual Physician: Religion and Medicine in the *Anatomy of Melancholy*." *The Review of English Studies* 57.232: 665–83.
Lutterbie, John. 2013. "Wayfaring in Everyday Life: The Unravelling of Intricacy." In Shaughnessy 2013, 103–15.
Marcus, Gary. 2008. *Kluge: The Haphazard Evolution of the Human Mind*. Boston: Houghton Mifflin.
Martín de León, Celia. 2013. "Who Cares If the Cat Is on the Mat? Contributions of Cognitive Models of Meaning to Translation." In Ana María Rojo López and Iraide Ibarretxe-Antuñano, eds., *Cognitive Linguistics and Translation: Advances in Some Theoretical Models and Applications*, 99–122. Berlin: DeGruyter/Mouton.
Massumi, Brian. 1980. "Foreword." In Gilles Deleuze and Félix Guattari, *A Thousand Plateaus: Capitalism and Schizophrenia*, Vol. 2. Minneapolis, MN: University of Minnesota Press.
Massumi, Brian. 2002. *Parables for the Virtual: Movement, Affect, Sensation*. Durham, NC: Duke University Press.
Matson, Alex, trans. 1929/1962. Aleksis Kivi, *Seven Brothers*. Translation of Kivi 1870/1984. American-Scandinavian Society.
McCloud, Scott. 1993. *Understanding Comics*. New York: Harper Perennial.
McDowell, Nicholas. 2005. "Urquhart's Rabelais: Translation, Patronage, and Cultural Politics." *English Literary Renaissance* 35.2 (March): 273–303
McHale, Brian. 2003. "'A Poet May Not Exist': Mock-Hoaxes and the Construction of National Identity." In Robert J. Griffin, ed., *The Faces of Anonymity: Anonymous and Pseudonymous Publication from the Sixteenth to the Twentieth Century*, 233–52. New York: Palgrave Macmillan.
McNeill, David. 1992. *Hand and Mind: What Gestures Reveal About Thought*. Chicago: University of Chicago Press.
Mechelli, Andrea, Jenny T. Crinion, Uta Noppeney, John O'Doherty, John Ashburner, J., Richard S. Frackowiak, and Cathy J. Price. 2004. "Neurolinguistics: Structural Plasticity in the Bilingual Brain." *Nature* 431: 757.
Melnick, David. 1983. *Men in Aida*. Berkeley, CA: Tuumba.
Mermikides, Alex, and Gianna Bouchard, eds. 2016. *Performance and the Medical Body*. London: Bloomsbury/Methuen Drama.
Miller, Michael B., Alan Kingstone, Paul M. Corballis, Jennifer Groh, and Michael S. Gazzaniga. 1999. "Manipulating Encoding of Faces and Associated Brain Activations." *Society for Neuroscience Abstracts* 25.1: 646.
Morrissey, Mary Beth Quaranta. 2014. *Suffering Narratives of Older Adults: A Phenomenological Approach to Serious Illness, Chronic Pain, Recovery and Maternal Care*. London: Routledge.
Moser, Barbara. 1978. "Simultaneous Interpretation: A Hypothetical Model and its Practical Application." In D. Gerver and H. W. Sinaiko, eds., *Language, Interpretation and Communication*, 353–68. New York: Plenum.

Moser-Mercer, Barbara, Sylvie Lambert, Valeria Darò, and Sarah Williams. 1997. "Skill Components in Simultaneous Interpreting." Paper presented at "Conference Interpreting: Current Trends in Research," Turku, Finland.

Mungello, David. 1977. *Leibniz and Confucianism: The Search for Accord*. Honolulu: University of Hawai'i Press.

Mungello, David. 1982. "Die Quellen für das Chinabild Leibnizens" (The Sources for Leibniz's Image of China). *Studia Leibniziana* 14: 233–43.

Muñoz Martín, Ricardo. 2010. "Leave No Stone Unturned: On the Development of Cognitive Translatology." *TIS: Translation and Interpreting Studies* 5.2: 145–62.

Muñoz Martín, Ricardo. 2013. "More Than a Way With Words: The Interface Between Cognitive Linguistics and Cognitive Translatology." In Ana María Rojo López and Iraide Ibarretxe-Antuñano, eds., *Cognitive Linguistics and Translation: Advances in Some Theoretical Models and Applications*, 75–94. Berlin: DeGruyter/ Mouton.

Naess, Arne. 1995. "The Systematization of the Logically Ultimate Norms and Hypotheses of Ecosophy T." In Alan Drengson and Yuichi Inoue, eds., *The Deep Ecology Movement: An Introductory Anthology*, 31–48. Berkeley, CA: North Atlantic Books.

Nancy, Jean-Luc. 1986/2004. "La Communauté désœuvrée." In Nancy ed., *La Communauté désœuvrée*, 9–102. Paris: Detroits.

Nida, Eugene A. 1964. *Toward a Science of Translating: With Special Reference to Principles and Procedures Involved in Bible Translating*. Leiden: Brill.

Nord, Christiane. 1991. *Text Analysis in Translation: Theory, Method, and Didactic Application of a Model for Translation-Oriented Text Analysis*. Amsterdam: Rodopi.

Nord, Christiane. 1997. *Translating as a Purposeful Activity: Functionalist Approaches Explained*. Manchester, UK: St. Jerome.

Nord, Christiane, trans. 2013. Katharina Reiß and Hans Vermeer, *Towards a General Theory of Translational Action: Skopos Theory Explained*. Manchester, UK: St. Jerome.

Nuland, Sherwin B. 1988. *Doctors: The Biography of Medicine*. New York: Knopf.

Osman, Jena, and Juliana Spahr, eds. 2003. *Chain 10: translucinación*.

Palmquist, Stephen R. 2000. *Kant's Critical Religion: Volume Two of Kant's System of Perspectives*. Aldershot: Ashgate.

Panksepp, Jaak. 1998. *Affective Neuroscience: The Foundations of Human and Animal Emotions*. New York: Oxford University Press.

Panksepp, Jaak. 2005. "Affective Consciousness: Core Emotional Feelings in Animals and Humans." *Consciousness and Cognition* 14: 30–80.

Panksepp, Jaak. 2012. *The Archaeology of Mind: Neuroevolutionary Origins of Human Emotion*. New York: Norton.

Parnell, Tim. 1996. "Sterne and Kundera: The Novel of Variations and the 'Noisy Foolishness of Human Certainty.'" In David Pierce and Peter de Voogd, eds., *Laurence Sterne in Modernism and Postmodernism*, 147–55. Amsterdam: Rodopi.

Penelhum, Terence. 1983. "Skepticism and Fideism." In Myles Burnyeat, ed., *The Skeptical Tradition*, 287–318. Berkeley, CA: University of California Press.

Perkins, Franklin. 2004. *Leibniz and China: A Commerce of Light*. Cambridge: Cambridge University Press.

Perloff, Marjorie. 2012. "In Search of the Authentic Other: The Poetry of Araki Yasusada." In Bill Friend, ed., *Scubadivers and Chrysanthemums: Essays on the Poetry of Araki Yasusada*, 23–50. Bristol: Shearsman.

Polan, Dana, trans. 1986. *Kafka: Toward a Minor Literature*. Translation of Deleuze and Guattari 1975. Minneapolis, MN: University of Minnesota Press.

Popkin, Richard H. 1979. *The History of Skepticism From Erasmus to Spinoza*. Berkeley, CA: University of California Press.

Popović, Anton. 1975. *Dictionary for the Analysis of Literary Translation*. Edmonton, CA: Department of Comparative Literature, University of Alberta.

Portela, Manuel, trans. 1998. Laurence Sterne, *A Vida e Opiniões de Tristram Shandy, o romance dos romances*. Translation of Sterne 1659/1986. Lisboa: Edições Antígona.

Portela, Manuel. 2000. "Typographic Translation: The Portuguese Edition of *Tristram Shandy*." In Joe Bray, Miriam Handley, and Anne C. Henry, eds., *Ma(r)king the Text: The Presentation of Meaning on the Literary Page*, 291–308. Aldershot, UK: Ashgate.

Porter, Catherine, trans. 1993. Gérard Genette, *Fiction and Diction*. Ithaca, NY: Cornell University Press.

Powers, Richard. 2006. "Echo Maker Roundtable #5." Online at www.edrants.com/echo-maker-roundtable-5/. Accessed April 26, 2016.

Powers, Richard. 2006/2007. *The Echo Maker*. London: Vintage.

Powers, Richard. 2007. "The Brain Is the Ultimate Storytelling Machine, and Consciousness Is the Ultimate Story." Interview with Alex Michod. *Believer* (February 8). Online at www.believermag.com/issues/200702/?read=interview_powers. Accessed April 28, 2016.

Prescott, Anne Lake. 2015. "Urquhart's Inflationary Universe." In Tania Demetriou and Rowan Tomlinson, eds., *The Culture of Translation in Early Modern England and France, 1500–1660*, 175–90. Houndmills: Palgrave Macmillan.

Pym, Anthony. 1990. "An Economic Model of Translational Equivalence." *Parallèles: Cahiers de l'École de Traduction et d'Interprétation de Genève* 12: 121–9.

Pym, Anthony. 1991. "Translational Ethics and the Recognition of Stateless Nations." *Fremdsprachen* 4: 31–5.

Pym, Anthony. 1992. *Translation and Text Transfer: An Essay on the Principles of Intercultural Communication*. Frankfurt a. M.: Peter Lang.

Pym, Anthony. 1995. "Translation as Transaction Cost." Meta 40.4: 594–605.

Pym, Anthony. 2004. *The Moving Text: Localization, Translation, and Distribution*. Amsterdam: Benjamins.

Pym, Anthony. 2010. *Exploring Translation Theories*. London: Routledge.

Pym, Anthony. 2016. *Translation Solutions for Many Languages: Histories of a Flawed Dream*. London: Bloomsbury.

Pym, Anthony, Miriam Shlesinger, and Zuzana Jettmarová, eds. 2006. *Sociocultural Aspects of Translating and Interpreting*. Amsterdam: Benjamins.

Rabelais, François. 1533. *Pantagruel: Les Horribles et espoventables faictz et prouesses du très renommé Pantagruel, roy des Dipsodes, filz du grand géant Gargantua, composez nouvellement par Maistre Alcofrybas Nasier*. Paris: n.p. Online at www.theeuropeanlibrary.org/tel4/record/3000022739058. Accessed June 1, 2016.

Ramachandran V. S. 1998. *Phantoms in the Brain*. New York: Morrow.

Ramírez, Álvaro. 2005. "'Don Quijote' and the Age of Simulacra." *Hispania* 88.1 (March): 82–90.

Reason, Matthew, Dee Reynolds, Marie-Hélène Grosbras, and Frank E. Pollick. 2013. "Researching Dance Across Disciplinary Paradigms: A Reflective Discussion of the Watching Dance Project." In Shaughnessy 2013, 39–56.

Regan, Shaun. 2001. "Translating Rabelais: Sterne, Motteux, and the Culture of Politeness." *Translation and Literature* 10.2: 174–99.

Reiß, Katharina, and Hans J. Vermeer. 1984. *Grundlegung einer allgemeinen Translationstheorie* ("Foundations of a General Theory of Translation"). Tübingen: Niemeyer.

Risku, Hanna. 2009. *Translationsmanagement: Interkulturelle Fachkommunikation im Informationszeitalter*. Second edition. Tübingen: Gunter Narr.

Risku, Hanna. 2010. "A Cognitive Scientific View on Technical Communication and Translation: Do Embodiment and Situatedness Really Make a Difference?" *Target* 22.1: 94–111.

Risku, Hanna. 2014. "Translation Process Research as Interaction Research: From Mental to Socio-Cognitive Processes." *MonTI: Monographs in Translation and Interpreting* (Special issue: Minding Translation): 331–53.

Rizzolatti, Giacomo, Luciano Fadiga, Vittorio Gallese, and Leonardo Fogassi. 1996. "Premotor Cortex and the Recognition of Motor Actions." *Cognitive Brain Research* 3: 131–41.

Robinson, Douglas. 1991. *The Translator's Turn*. Baltimore: Johns Hopkins University Press.

Robinson, Douglas. 1996. *Translation and Taboo*. DeKalb, IL: Northern Illinois University Press.

Robinson, Douglas. 1997a. "(Dis)Abusing Translation: Philip E. Lewis, 'The Measure of Translation Effects.'" In Robinson 1997b, 132–77.

Robinson, Douglas. 1997b. *What Is Translation? Centrifugal Theories, Critical Interventions*. Kent, OH: Kent State University Press.

Robinson, Douglas, ed. 1997/2002. *Translation Theory From Herodotus to Nietzsche*. Manchester, UK: St. Jerome.

Robinson, Douglas. 1997/2003/2012. *Becoming a Translator: An Introduction to the Theory and Practice of Translation*. London and New York: Routledge.

Robinson, Douglas. 2001. *Who Translates? Translator Subjectivities Beyond Reason*. Albany, NY: State University of New York Press.

Robinson, Douglas. 2003. *Performative Linguistics: Speaking and Translating as Doing Things With Words*. London: Routledge.

Robinson, Douglas. 2008. *Estrangement and the Somatics of Literature: Tolstoy, Shklovsky, Brecht*. Baltimore: Johns Hopkins University Press.

Robinson, Douglas. 2010. "Liar Paradox Monism: A Wildean Solution to the Explanatory Gap Between Materialism and Qualia." *Minerva* 14: 66–106. Online at www.minerva.mic.ul.ie/Vol14/Monism.pdf.

Robinson, Douglas. 2011. *Translation and the Problem of Sway*. Amsterdam: John Benjamins.

Robinson, Douglas. 2012. *First-Year Writing and the Somatic Exchange*. New York: Hampton Press.

Robinson, Douglas. 2013a. *Displacement and the Somatics of Postcolonial Culture*. Columbus, OH: Ohio State University Press.

Robinson, Douglas. 2013b. *Feeling Extended: Sociality as Extended Body-Becoming-Mind*. Cambridge, MA: MIT Press.

Robinson, Douglas. 2013c. *Schleiermacher's Icoses: Social Ecologies of the Different Methods of Translating*. Bucharest: Zeta Books.

Robinson, Douglas. 2014. "Response." *Translation Studies* 7.3: 346–9.

Robinson, Douglas. 2015a. *The Dao of Translation: An East-West Dialogue*. London: Routledge.

Robinson, Douglas. 2015b. "Towards an Intercivilizational Turn: Naoki Sakai's Cofigurative Regimes of Translation and the Problem of Eurocentrism." *Translation Studies* 8.3: 1–16.

Robinson, Douglas. 2016a. *The Deep Ecology of Rhetoric in Mencius and Aristotle*. Albany, NY: State University of New York Press.

Robinson, Douglas. 2016b. "Pushing-Hands and Periperformativity." In Douglas Robinson, ed., *The Pushing Hands of Translation and Its Theory: In Memoriam Martha Cheung, 1953–2013,* 193–216. London: Routledge.

Robinson, Douglas. 2016c. *Semiotranslating Peirce*. Tartu Semiotics Library 17. Tartu, Estonia: University of Tartu Press.

Robinson, Douglas. 2017a. *Critical Translation Studies*. London: Routledge.

Robinson, Douglas. 2017b. *Exorcising Translation: Towards an Intercivilizational Turn*. New York: Bloomsbury.

Robinson, Douglas. 2017c. *Aleksis Kivi and/as World Literature*. Leiden: Brill.

Robinson, Douglas, trans. 2017d. Aleksis Kivi, *The Brothers Seven*. Bucharest: Zeta Books.

Rockmore, Tom. 2002. *Marx After Marxism: The Philosophy of Karl Marx*. New York: Wiley-Blackwell.

Rokotnitz, Naomi. 2013. "Between Faulty Intellects and Failing Bodies: An Economy of Reciprocity in *Wit* and *33 Variations*." In Shaughnessy 2013, 117–31.

Ross, Don, David Spurrett, Howard Kinkaid, and G. Lynn Stephens, eds. 2007. *Distributed Cognition and the Will: Individual Volition in Social Context*. Cambridge, MA: MIT Press.

Ruskin, John. 1856/1891. "Of the Pathetic Fallacy." In Ruskin ed., *Modern Painters,* 157–72. Vol. 3. Fourth edition. London: George Allen.

Russell, James A. 2003. "Core Affect and the Psychological Construction of Emotion." *Psychological Review* 110: 145–72.

Russell, James A., and Lisa Feldman Barrett. 1999. "Core Affect, Prototypical Emotional Episodes, and Other Things Called Emotion: Dissecting the Elephant." *Journal of Personality and Social Psychology* 76: 805–19.

Sacks, Oliver. 1998. *The Man Who Mistook His Wife for a Hat, and Other Clinical Tales*. New York: Simon and Schuster.

Sager, Juan C., and Marie-Josée Hamel, trans. and ed. 1995. Jean-Paul Vinay and Jean Darbelnet, *Comparative Stylistics of French and English: A Methodology for Translation*. Amsterdam: John Benjamins.

Sakai, Naoki. 1997. *Translation and Subjectivity: On "Japan" and Cultural Nationalism*. Minneapolis, MN: University of Minnesota Press.

Sawday, Jonathan. 1995. *The Body Emblazoned: Dissection and the Human Body in Renaissance Culture*. London: Routledge.

Schleiermacher, Friedrich. 1813/2002. "Ueber die verschiedenen Methoden des Übersetzens." In Martin Rößler, with the assistance of Lars Emersleben, eds., *Akademievorträge,* 67–93. Part I of *Schriften und Entwürfe*. Vol. 11 of *Kritische Gesamtausgabe*. Berlin: BBAW.

Schleiermacher, Friedrich. 1959. *Hermeneutik, nach den Handschriften neu herausgegeben und eingeleitet von Heinz Kimmerle*. Heidelberg: Carl Winter.

Schmitt, Charles B. 1966. "Perennial Philosophy: From Agostino Steuco to Leibniz." *Journal of the Philosophy of Ideas* 27: 505–32.

Scoggin G. C. 1919. "A Popular Commonplace." *Classical Philology* 14.4 (October): 386–89.

Searle, John R. 1969. *Speech Acts: An Essay in the Philosophy of Language*. Cambridge and London: Cambridge University Press.

Searle, John R. 1975/1979. *Expression and Meaning*. Cambridge: Cambridge University Press.

Searle, John R. 1977. "Reiterating the Differences: A Reply to Jacques Derrida." In *Glyph One*, 198–211. Baltimore: Johns Hopkins University Press.

Sedgwick, Eve Kosovsky. 2003. *Touching Feeling: Affect, Pedagogy, Performativity*. Durham, NC: Duke University Press.

Shaughnessy, Nicola, ed. 2013. *Affective Performance and Cognitive Science: Body, Brain and Being*. London: Bloomsbury/Methuen Drama.

Shiavi, Giuliana. 1996. "There Is Always a Teller in a Tale." *Target* 8.1: 1–21.

Shields, David. 2010. *Reality Hunger*. New York: Knopf.

Shklovsky, Viktor. 1925/1983. *O teorii prozy* ("On the Theory of Prose"). Moscow: Sovyetsky pisatel'.

Shun Kwong-Loi. 1997. *Mencius and Early Chinese Thought*. Stanford, CA: Stanford University Press.

Singer, Tania, Ben Seymour, John O'Doherty, Holger Kaube, Raymond J. Dolan, and Chris D. Frith. 2004. "Empathy for Pain Involves the Affective But Not Sensory Components of Pain." *Science* 303 (February 20): 1157–62.

Smith, M. W. 2001. *Reading Simulacra: Fatal Theories for Postmodernity*. Albany, NY: State University of New York Press.

Snell-Hornby, Mary. 1988. *Translation Studies: An Integrated Approach*. Amsterdam: John Benjamins.

Snow, C. P. 1959/2001. *The Two Cultures*. London: Cambridge University Press.

Sonnby-Borgström, Marianne. 2002. "Automatic Mimicry Reactions as Related to Differences in Emotional Empathy." *Scandinavian Journal of Psychology* 43.5 (December): 433–43.

Spicer, Jack. 1957/2008. "After Lorca." In Peter Gizzi and Kevin Killian, eds., *My Vocabulary Did This to Me: The Collected Poetry of Jack Spicer*, 105–54. Middletown, CT: Wesleyan University Press.

Spivak, Gayatri Chakravorty. 2007. "Translation as Culture." In Paul St. Pierre and Prafulla C. Kar, eds., *In Translation – Reflections, Refractions, Transformations*, 263–76. Amsterdam: John Benjamins.

Stavrakaki, Stavroula, Kalliopi Megari, Mary H. Kosmidis, Maria Apostolidou, and Eleni Takou. 2012. "Working Memory and Verbal Fluency in Simultaneous Interpreters." *Journal of Clinical Experimental Neuropsychology* 34.6: 624–33.

Stein, Maria, Andrea Federspiel, Thomas Koenig, Miranka Wirth, Werner Strik, Roland Wiest, Daniel Brandeis, and Thomas Dierks. 2012. "Structural Plasticity in the Language System Related to Increased Second Language Proficiency." *Cortex* 48.4: 458–65.

Steiner, George. 1999. *The Portage to San Cristobal of A.H.: A Novel*. Chicago: University of Chicago Press.

Sterne, Laurence. 1759/1986. *The Life and Opinions of Tristram Shandy, Gentleman*. Oxford: Oxford University Press.

Stone, Donald, Jr. 1969. *France in the Sixteenth Century: A Medieval Society Transformed*. Englewood Cliffs, NJ: Prentice-Hall.

Suchman, Lucy. 2007. *Human-Machine Reconfigurations: Plans and Situated Actions*. Cambridge: Cambridge University Press.

Tawada Yōko. 2007. "St. George and the Translator." In Yoko ed., *Facing the Bridge*, 109–75. Translated by Margret Mitsutani. New York: New Directions.

Thompson, Evan. 2007. *Mind in Life: Biology, Phenomenology, and the Sciences of Mind.* Cambridge, MA: Harvard University Press.

Tomasello, Michael. 2008. *Origins of Human Communication.* Cambridge, MA: MIT Press/Bradford Books.

Tomkins, Silvan S. 1962–1992. *Affect Imagery Consciousness.* 4 vols. New York: Springer.

Toury, Gideon. 1980. *In Search of a Theory of Translation.* Tel Aviv: The Porter Institute for Poetics and Semiotics, Tel Aviv University.

Toury, Gideon. 1995. *Descriptive Translation Studies and Beyond.* Amsterdam: John Benjamins.

Toury, Gideon. 2005. "Enhancing Cultural Changes by Means of Fictitious Translations." In Eva Hung, ed., *Translation and Cultural Change: Studies in History, Norms and Image-Projection,* 3–17. Amsterdam: John Benjamins.

Traill, H. D. 1882. *Sterne.* Online at www.authorama.com/book/sterne.html. Accessed July 23, 2016.

Tranel, Daniel, and Antonio R. Damasio. 1985. "Knowledge Without Awareness: An Autonomic Index of Facial Recognition by Prosopagnosics." *Science* 228.21: 1453–54.

Tranel, Daniel, Antonio R. Damasio, and Hanna Damasio. 1988. "Intact Recognition of Facial Expression, Gender, and Age in Patients with Impaired Recognition of Face Identity." *Neurology* 38: 690–96.

Tranel, Daniel, Hanna Damasio, and Antonio R. Damasio. 1995. "Double Dissociation Between Overt and Covert Face Recognition." *Journal of Cognitive Neuroscience* 7: 425–32.

Urquhart, Thomas, trans. 1653–93/1994. François Rabelais, *Gargantua and Pantagruel.* Translation of Rabelais 1533. Edited by Peter le Motteux and John Ozell. New York: Knopf.

Van Norden, Bryan W., trans. 2008. *Mengzi: With Selections from Traditional Commentaries.* Indianapolis and Cambridge: Hackett.

Van Rooten, Luis. 1967. *Mots D'Heures: Gousses, Rames.* New York: Viking Adult.

Venuti, Lawrence. 1995. *The Translator's Invisibility.* London: Routledge.

Venuti, Lawrence, ed. 1998. *Translation and Minority.* Manchester, UK: St. Jerome.

Vinay, Jean-Paul, and Jean Darbelnet. 1958. *Stylistique comparée du français et de l'anglais: Méthode de traduction.* Paris: Beau-chemin.

Volkov, Solomon. 1979. *Testimony: The Memoirs of Dmitri Shostakovich, as Related to and Edited by Solomon Volkov.* Translated by Antonina W. Bouis. New York: Harper & Row.

Walpole, Horace. 1764/1901. *The Castle of Otranto.* London, Paris, New York, and Melbourne: Cassell.

Wechsler, Robert. 1998. *Performing Without a Stage: The Art of Literary Translation.* New Haven, CT: Catbird.

Weinsheimer, Joel, and Donald G. Marshall, trans. 1975/1989. Hans-Georg Gadamer, *Truth and Method.* London and New York: Continuum.

Welton, Martin. 2013. "*Footage*: Surface Feelings." In Shaughnessy 2013, 159–69.

Whittaker, Ruth. 1988. *Tristram Shandy.* Milton Keynes: Open University Press.

Wicker, Bruno, Christian Keysers, Jane Plailly, Jean-Pierre Royet, Vittorio Gallese, and Giacomo Rizzolatti. 2003. "Both of Us Disgusted in *My* Insula: The Common Neural Basis of Seeing and Feeling Disgust." *Neuron* 40.3 (October): 655–64.

Willett, John, ed. and trans. 1964/1992. *Brecht on Theatre: The Development of an Aesthetic.* New York: Hill & Wang.

Wolf, Michaela, ed. 2006. *Übersetzen – Translating – Traduire: Toward a Social Turn?* Münster: LIT.

Wolf, Michaela. 2011. "Mapping the Field: Sociological Perspectives on Translation." *International Journal of the Sociology of Language* 207: 1–28.

Wolf, Michaela, and Alexandra Fukari, eds. 2007. *Constructing a Sociology of Translation.* Amsterdam: Benjamins.

Yan Zhongying. N.d. "歌德" ("Goethe"). Chinese Encyclopedia Online. http://ap6.pccu.edu.tw/Encyclopedia/data.asp?id=9297. Accessed March 21, 2014.

Yudes, Carolina, Pedro Macizo, and Teresa Bajo. 2011. "The Influence of Expertise in Simultaneous Interpreting on Non-Verbal Executive Processes." *Frontiers in Psychology* 2: 309.

Yudes, Carolina, Pedro Macizo, and Teresa Bajo. 2012. "Coordinating Comprehension and Production in Simultaneous Interpreters: Evidence from the Articulatory Suppression Effect." *Bilingualism: Language and Cognition* 15.2: 329–39.

Zou Lijuan, Ding Guosheng, Jubin Abutalebi, Shu Hua, and Peng Danling. 2012. "Structural Plasticity of the Left Caudate in Bimodal Bilinguals." *Cortex* 48.9: 1197–1206.

Zempliner, Artur. 1970. "Gedanken über die erste deutsche Übersetzung von Leibniz' Abhandlung über die chinesische Philosophie." *Studia Leibniziana* 2: 223–31.

Zempliner, Artur. 1971. "Leibniz und die chinesische Philosophie." *Studia Leibniziana Supplementa* 5: 15–30.

Zukofsky, Paul, Celia Thaew Zukofsky, and Louis Zukofsky. 1969. *Catullus Fragmenta.* London: Turret.

Index

FSC
www.fsc.org
MIX
Papier | Fördert gute Waldnutzung
FSC® C083411

Kolibri 360 GmbH
Ferdinand-Jühlke-Straße 7
99095 Erfurt, Deutschland
produktsicherheit@kolibri360.de